MEMOIRS OF MY NERVOUS ILLNESS

DANIEL PAUL SCHREBER

Translated and edited by
IDA MACALPINE
RICHARD A. HUNTER

With a new introduction by
SAMUEL M. WEBER

MEMOIRS OF MY NERVOUS ILLNESS

Memoirs of My Nervous Illness

DANIEL PAUL SCHREBER

Translated and edited by

IDA MACALPINE

and

RICHARD A. HUNTER

With a new introduction by

SAMUEL M. WEBER

Harvard University Press
Cambridge, Massachusetts
London, England
1988

Printed in the United States of America
10 9 8 7 6 5 4 3 2 1

The Introduction to the 1988 Edition was originally published in German as the introduction to Daniel Paul Schreber, *Denkwürdigkeiten eines Nervenkranken,* © 1973 by Verlag Ullstein, Berlin.

Library of Congress Cataloging-in-Publication Data

Schreber, Daniel Paul, 1842–1911.
Memoirs of my nervous illness.

Translation of: Denkwürdigkeiten eines Nervenkranken.
Reprint. Originally published: London : W. Dawson, 1955.
Bibliography: p.
1. Schreber, Daniel Paul, 1842–1911—Mental health.
2. Paranoia—Patients—Germany—Biography. 3. Paranoia
—Case studies. I. Title.
RC520.S33A313 1988 616.89'7'00924 [B] 87-25133
ISBN 0-674-56515-0 (cloth)
ISBN 0-674-56516-9 (paper)

CONTENTS

INTRODUCTION TO THE 1988 EDITION

Samuel M. Weber
Translated by Benjamin Gregg

"Who's Ever Heard of Dr. Schreber?"

On 28 October 1884 elections to the German Reichstag were held. In the Saxon city of Chemnitz the candidate of the National Liberal Party suffered a crushing defeat. A local newspaper carried an article on this unsuccessful candidacy, headlined: "Who's ever heard of Dr. Schreber?"

For the hapless Doctor of Jurisprudence Daniel Paul Schreber, at the time Landgerichtsdirektor (chairman of the state court) in Chemnitz, the election returns marked the end of a political career even before it had started. The unsuccessful candidate sought to recover from the strains of the election campaign by taking the waters. But, again, the desired success never materialized: on 8 December 1884 the unknown Dr. Schreber was admitted to the Psychiatric Clinic at the University of Leipzig. There he remained for half a year before being discharged, apparently cured, at the beginning of June 1885, whereupon he resumed his work as a judge. His first and only attempt to establish himself in German politics had failed ingloriously, yet a different kind of "politics" and a different kind of glory was still in store for him.

Who's ever heard of Dr. Schreber? For the second son of the famous physician, orthopedist, and pedagogue Daniel Gottlieb Moritz Schreber, this was scarcely a pleasant question. His father—to this day revered by many as the inventor of the *Schrebergarten* (a small, private allotment garden within an urban area)—was in his time a leading proponent of German orthopedic gymnastics and was anything but unknown. His books numbered among the bestsellers of the nineteenth century; the most successful of his publications—*Medical Indoor Gymnastics; or, A System of Hygienic Exercises for Home Use To Be Practiced Anywhere without Apparatus or Assistance by Young and Old of*

Either Sex, for the Preservation of Health and General Activity—had reached by 1909 its thirty-second edition and a total of 205,000 copies printed. The *Biographical Lexicon of Outstanding Physicians of All Times and Peoples* (edited by Dr. August Hirsch) remarks that Dr. Schreber's achievements in orthopedics and remedial gymnastics "contributed greatly to the development and popularization of active, so-called German remedial gymnastics, based on scientific physical training, in distinction to passive, so-called Swedish remedial gymnastics."[1] Because the titles of his works distinctly characterize the interests and endeavors of their author, several deserve to be mentioned, beginning with one which suggests that the family's political activism did not begin with Daniel Paul: *Physical Training from a Medical Standpoint, also a Matter of State*. Other books by the elder Schreber include: *Detrimental Carriage and Habits of the Child, Callipaedics or Rearing unto Beauty through the Natural and Uniform Promotion of Normal Bodily Development, Anthropos, the Structural Wonder of the Human Organism, The Pangymnastikon; or, the Complete System of Gymnastics Using Only One Piece of Equipment,* and—last but not least—*The Family Friend as Educator and Conductor to Domestic Happiness, to Popular Health and to the Refinement of Man, for the Fathers and Mothers of the German People*.

Thus Dr. Schreber senior was no simple orthopedist but rather a reformer filled with missionary zeal. The subtitle of one of his books expresses his goal most clearly: *A Doctrine of Happiness for the Physical Life of Man*. Not for a moment did he ever doubt that his efforts to raise the gymnastics movement to the level of a science would be of epoch-making significance for the German people. Accordingly, the *Pangymnastikon* begins with the proclamation: "We salute German gymnastics as a sign of the revivification of the robust German popular spirit in a perfected and ennobled form corresponding to the level of general cultural development."[2]

This development, according to D. G. M. Schreber, reaches its zenith in the gymnastics movement:

> For centuries the vital German popular spirit wrestled in silent, open battle with the dark powers of medieval popery and jesuitism, without ever permitting them to smother its vigor . . . Until 1618, and despite many earlier tests, this vigor managed to preserve itself in many essential aspects of spiritual and physical life . . . Of these beautiful blossoms of popular German national life, the monstrosity of the Thirty

Years' War destroyed nearly all traces . . . It took many, many years before the still glorious embers of the German popular spirit, mired deep in the ruins and ashes left behind, could again burst forth in individual flames. Yet even these various figures, the great spirits of a German nation now regenerating itself, were merely heralds of a better age which they, despite their valiant works, were never themselves to know. Two whole centuries were to pass before the era of rejuvenation could begin for the life of the German people and for its vital forces. Praise be to God! We, the generations now living, have entered this era, have crossed its threshold . . . Gymnastics is thus no passing fashion, but the young and ennobled instinct of the old but still healthy root of Germanic national life.[3]

"Silent, open battles" against "dark powers"; "beautiful blossoms" destroyed by a "monstrosity"; "ruins and ashes" following the devastation; and, above all, the inextinguishable flames "still shining forth," impatiently awaiting a better age: these set the stage for the scene that would be fully performed only by Daniel Paul Schreber. His father's contribution to this development can be summed up by the epigraph to his *Pangymnastikon:* "The prevailing institution of gymnastics suffers in general from a random plurality of different forms of exercise. What we need is a *system.*"[4]

Accordingly, Moritz Schreber saw his mission as that of bestowing scientific cultivation upon the "young and ennobled instinct of the . . . still healthy root of Germanic national life." Long before he invented the garden that was to immortalize his name, he was convinced that his historical mission could only be that of gardener to the German spirit and body. As an educator he strove to separate, even in children, the "noble" from the "base spores"; as a physician he was convinced that moral improvement is inseparable from the body's condition. For the epigraph to his first book—*The Book of Health*—he chose a quotation by Rückert: "Bear in mind that a god resides in your body and that the temple at all times must be spared desecration."[5] For his son, too, a god was to reside in the body, but the temple was not to escape desecration.

Indeed, not even Dr. Schreber senior was spared. In 1851, during his daily gymnastic exercises, a heavy iron ladder fell on his head, inducing a chronic headache that affected him until his death in 1861. During this period of declining health the elder

Dr. Schreber is supposed to have experienced "hallucinations with a pathological urge to murder" (according to the medical history written by his son).[6]

The family friend of the German people, a man who aspired to lead its fathers and mothers to domestic happiness, to contribute to popular health and to the ennoblement of man, left behind a wife, two sons, and three daughters. The oldest son, Daniel Gustav, became a lawyer, as his brother, Daniel Paul, did soon after him. Whether Daniel Gustav ever achieved his father's goals, we do not know; we know only that he was named Gerichtsrat (judge) in 1877 and that, several weeks later, he took his life with a gun. He was thirty-eight years old, his brother thirty-four.

What, then, do we know about Dr. Schreber? Up to his electoral defeat, not very much. We are, however, able to make several conjectures about his childhood and upbringing, since his father had very definite ideas about child rearing. The following passage from his *Book of Health* demonstrates his philosophy quite clearly:

> The tempers of the small child, making themselves known by the child's screaming and crying for no apparent reason, . . . expressing nothing more than whim, the first emergence of obstinacy, . . . must be confronted in a positive manner . . . by quickly diverting the child's attention, through stern admonitions or, if all else fails . . . by repeated, physically perceptible admonitions . . . In this way—and only in this way—the child becomes conscious of its dependence on the external world and learns . . . submission . . . This kind of procedure is necessary but once, or at most twice—and one will have become master of the child forever.[7]

That the author of these lines became "master" of his child—indeed, "forever"—is just as certain as the fact that one of these children, Daniel Paul, never, for the rest of his life, ceased to cry out against this authority.[8] Other than that, most of what we know about the life of Daniel Paul Schreber derives from what he wrote about himself and from the descriptions contained in the medical records of the various asylums where he spent twelve years of his life.[9] According to one such report Schreber "was quite gifted and had always been an excellent pupil. He is described as being of good-natured and sociable character. In his later life he demonstrated great talent and climbed the rungs of the career ladder relatively quickly. His last position was that of Senatspräsident [president of a panel of judges] at the Superior Country Court [court of appeal] at Dresden. He led, as far as we know, a thoroughly respectable life."[10]

The single event that might have cast a faint shadow on this thoroughly respectable life—prior to his illness—was his marriage to Sabine Behr, daughter of a senior director at the Municipal Theater in Leipzig, hence a match the Schreber family hardly considered suitable. Not only did Schreber have a famous father; for three hundred years the family itself had been prominent for its outstanding lawyers and scholars. Daniel Paul's great-grandfather, Daniel Godefredus Schreberus (as he called himself with his latinized name), was the first Schreber to attain literary renown, through works that reveal a clear affinity to the pursuits of descendents such as Daniel Gottlieb Moritz Schreber. We find for example that the grandfather of the man who invented the Schrebergarten was himself concerned with agricultural problems as impediments to human progress. One might mention his *Report on the Caterpillars Which in 1751 and in the Current Year Caused Great Devastation to the Harvest in Thuringia and Adjoining Areas of Saxony,* as well as his *Instructions on Stabilizing Quicksand and Making Arid Fields into Meadows,* published in Leipzig in 1764.[11] A family tradition like this can hardly have been without consequence for the little known Dr. Daniel Paul Schreber, especially following his unsuccessful candidacy for the Reichstag. Shortly thereafter, he was afflicted with hypochondria, in particular, with the notion that he was becoming emaciated. Finally, it became necessary to commit Dr. Schreber to the Psychiatric Clinic at the University of Leipzig, in a "very unstable state of mind" according to the hospital records, and concerned that he would "die any moment of a heart attack."[12] Again, we know very little about this first sojourn in the Leipzig clinic, which lasted six months. The extant medical records mention speech impediments, two suicide attempts, hypersensitivity to noise and a "weepy disposition." Schreber himself writes only about certain difficulties in using the scales, whose construction was unfamiliar to him, and whose accuracy he was therefore unable to verify. He nonetheless allows that these "are only minor points on which I place little importance," (*M,* p. 62). His weight remained a primary cause of concern for him, however: he was still claiming at the time of his discharge to have lost thirty to forty pounds ("gained 2 lbs.," a report states laconically).[13] In the Leipzig clinic Schreber met for the first time Dr. Paul Emil Flechsig, the clinic director who treated him and whose photograph stood for many years on the desk of Schreber's wife.

After being discharged in 1885, Schreber resumed his work as a judge and "spent eight happy years with my wife, on the whole quite happy ones, rich also in outward honors and marred only from time to time by the repeated disappointment of our hope of being blessed with children" (*M,* p. 63). The high point of these years was Schreber's appointment as Senatspräsident at the Dresden Superior State Court. In the period immediately preceding his official appointment, when he had already been informed of it, he dreamed that his "earlier neuroses had returned." Stranger still is the following incident: "One morning while still in bed (whether still half asleep or already awake I cannot remember), I had a feeling which, thinking about it later when fully awake, struck me as highly peculiar. It was the idea that it really must be rather pleasant to be a woman succumbing to intercourse. This idea was so foreign to my whole nature that I may say I would have rejected it with indignation if fully awake" (*M,* p. 63).

Following worsening insomnia and states of anxiety, he placed himself—shortly after assuming his new office—once again under the care of Dr. Flechsig. The initial session was encouraging: Flechsig displayed "a remarkable eloquence which affected me deeply" (*M,* p. 65), Schreber recalled; but his condition declined rapidly despite Flechsig's eloquence and that of his assistant, Dr. Täuscher—"I cannot deny him also my recognition [*Anerkennung*] of the excellent way he spoke to me on that occasion" (*M,* p. 67). Yet Schreber was soon to be occupied with voices and discourses of a much different nature—indeed, ceaselessly for the next eight years in which he was institutionalized, until his discharge in 1902 (and no doubt even after that). He recorded the history of these years in a book which brought the fame that had eluded him in politics. *Memoirs of My Nervous Illness,* published in 1903, made its author the "most frequently quoted patient in psychiatry," according to Macalpine and Hunter (*M,* p. 8), as he became "the Schreber case."

Although the *Memoirs* went through only one edition, a large part of which was bought up and destroyed by horrified family members, the book was quickly declared a textbook by the psychiatric community, and Schreber was celebrated as a perfect example of paranoia. Whether these developments were known to Schreber himself is not certain, but in any case they fulfilled a wish he formulates at the end of his book: "And so I believe I am not mistaken in expecting that a very special palm of victory will eventually be mine. I cannot say with any certainty what form it will take. As possibilities I would mention . . . that great fame will be attached to my name surpassing that of thousands of other people much better mentally endowed" (*M,* p. 214).

Eight years after the *Memoirs* appeared, Freud published his "Psycho-Analytic Notes on an Autobiographical Account of a Case of Paranoia (Dementia Paranoides)" and transformed the Schreber case from a psychiatric case into a psychoanalytic one whose renown, while limited, has been tenacious. In the same year that Freud's essay appeared (1911), when that "special palm of victory" was finally his, Daniel Paul Schreber died in the Leipzig asylum where since 1907—for the third time—he had been hospitalized. For the final portion of his life we are again dependent upon medical records. The important events in the period following his discharge in 1903 are the death of his mother, with whom he had then lived for a time, as well as his wife's stroke shortly before the third onset of his own illness. His years of institutionalization are marked both by increasing isolation and by repeated efforts to communicate nonetheless. The author of the *Memoirs* often tried to "express his wishes in undecipherable written characters." Again and again, he is said to have called out, in a tormented voice, "Ha—ha!"[14]

Who, then, has ever heard of Dr. Schreber? Other than the psychiatrists and the psychoanalysts, who knew him only as a "case," few people indeed. Walter Benjamin counted *Memoirs* among his collection of books authored by the mentally ill. Elias Canetti devotes two chapters of *Crowds and Power* to Schreber, again as a "case," though not as a purely psychological one; he treats Schreber as a paragon of the "ruler."[15] And today in France "Le Président Schreber" belongs to the canon of the often mentioned but rarely read.[16] Will we ever learn who he was?

The Schreber Case: Reason on Trial

Perhaps the question seems unnecessary: after all, we have Schreber right here, in our very hands, before our eyes; we need only read the book to become acquainted with it—and with him. But what do we mean by "know" and by "read"? It may not be entirely unwarranted, before turning to the text itself, to linger a moment on this question. For "knowing" can mean many things, as Hegel's well-known distinction, between the "well-known" and "knowing well" (between *bekannt* and *erkannt*) reminds us:

> The well-known, just because it is familiar, is not known well. The commonest way in which we deceive either ourselves or others about knowledge is by assuming it to be familiar, and accepting it on that account; with all its pros and cons, such knowing never gets anywhere, and it knows not why. Subject and Object, God, Nature, Understanding, sense experience and so on, are uncritically taken for granted as familiar, established as valid, and made into fixed points of departure and return. While these remain unmoved, the knowing activity goes back and forth between them, thus moving only on their surface.[17]

Even the most cursory look at how Schreber's *Memoirs* has been received to date reveals a discrepancy between the "fixed points" of the text and the interpretation by its readers, mainly psychiatrists and psychoanalysts, who generally seek in it the familiar and the long-known, and who—*mirabile dictu*—find it there. What Freud asserted critically, of the "interest felt by the practical psychiatrist in such delusional formations as these," namely that "marvelling is not the beginning of understanding,"[18] also holds for such readers. What is at issue here is whether this text is to be read solely as a case, and if so, then as what kind. Schreber himself was convinced that his was "a quite remarkable case, unique in the field of psychiatric experience" (*M,* p. 292): an exemplar, perhaps, but a unique and therefore notable one. His physician, Geheimrat (Privy Councillor) Dr. Weber, saw the matter quite differently:

> But however varied and differently coloured the individual cases of mental illness may be, however characteristic and singular an individual case may appear to careful observation, yet . . . one cannot deny that . . . certain groupings emerge, certain complexes of pathological manifestations, which in their development, course and outcome, in the involvement of single psychic functions are more or less demarcated from each other [and] . . . have led to the delineation of a certain number of different disease forms. As

> colourful and inexhaustible the individual variations of cases of mental illness may be, as constant are the main outlines, and apart from the arabesques of the individual case the basic characteristics of the forms of illness are repeated with almost surprising, monotonous regularity. (*M*, p. 317)

The case is—so to speak—clear as daylight. As "colourful and inexhaustible" the individual characteristics that depart from the norm may be, the "main outlines" are nonetheless "constant"—and repeat themselves with the same monotonous regularity as Dr. Weber's rolling sentences. The individual case may well be "varied and differently coloured," but this is the coloring of an arabesque, a variation that celebrates the individual detail without ever questioning its membership within a larger whole. One immediately knows of what the exemplar is an example; only a madman or the ignorant layperson would ever place it into question: "Considered from this scientifically established point of view [Dr. Schreber's] mental illness and its peculiarities, far from not being known to psychiatry, clearly belong to a well-known and well-characterized form of mental illness, paranoia, and shows all its important distinguishing features" (*M*, p. 317).

Dr. Weber's exposition demonstrates clearly what for traditional psychiatry (yet not for it alone) an exemplar or case is: subsumption under the well-known, "paranoia," by identifying "all its important distinguishing features." If psychiatrists celebrated the Schreber case, then, they did so because they saw it not as something unique, but rather as a particular example, replete with "all [the] important distinguishing features"—symptoms—of paranoia.

We find that psychiatrists essentially knew Schreber long before they ever met him either in person or through his writing. They valued his writing but only as a particular case in which they thought they found what they had already always known: that cluster of characteristics which they termed "paranoia." As an individual case Schreber mirrored their knowledge, and the persons thus reflected were delighted. In this individual instance of the pathology of paranoia, psychiatry discovered its own image and thought it had thereby recognized Dr. Schreber as well.

That the consequences of this attitude are not merely academic is shown by the following example: during the lawsuit, in which Schreber challenged his being placed under tutelage for reasons of mental illness, Dr. Weber in several court-ordered opinions expresses his view that the proposed publication of *Memoirs* was only further evidence of the author's mental derangement. That Schreber "felt the urge to describe the history of his latter years" might, Dr. Weber allows, still be "understandable":

> But the patient harbours the urgent desire to have his "Memoirs" . . . printed and made available to the widest circles and he is therefore negotiating with a publisher—until now of course without success. When one looks at the content of his writings, and takes into consideration the abundance of indiscretions relating to himself and others contained in them, the unembarrassed detailing of the most doubtful and aesthetically impossible situations and events, the use of the most offensive vulgar words, etc., one finds it quite incomprehensible that a man otherwise tactful and of fine feeling could propose an action which would compromise him so severely in the eyes of the public, were not his whole attitude to life pathological, and he unable to see things in their proper perspective, and if the tremendous overvaluation of his own person caused by lack of insight into his illness had not clouded his appreciation of the limitations imposed on man by society. (*M,* pp. 282–283)

Of Dr. Weber's argument—whose significance cannot be underestimated in a lawsuit concerning nothing less than the individual's right to determine the course of his own life—Freud remarks: "Surely we can hardly expect that a case history which sets out to give a picture of deranged humanity and of its struggles to rehabilitate itself should exhibit 'discretion' and 'aesthetic' charm."[19]

No doubt about it: the contrast apparent here between the traditional psychiatrist and the founder of psychoanalysis marks a change, from a concept of science characterized by a narcissistic self-satisfaction with the well-known, to an effort to bring these "fixed points" into motion and to pose questions which might lead to new knowledge. And yet—or perhaps, therefore—the question of the structure and goal of this knowledge becomes unavoidable. Even though Freud's reading is incomparably more differentiated and productive than a traditional psychiatrist's was or ever could be, for Freud, too—and even more so for his epigones—Schreber's text remained a description of a particular instance or case, a medical record. Not the least of Freud's interests in the Schreber case was to confirm psychoanalytic theory in an area where it was less at home: psychosis. In his interpretation of the case Freud attempts to demonstrate that the conceptual apparatus of psychoanalysis is legitimate. The goal, he writes, is to find with the aid of psychoanalysis "a translation of the paranoic mode of expression into the normal one," the "normal" mode being none other than the language of psychoanalysis. In a certain sense, then, and like traditional psychiatry, Freud's discourse preserves the "fixed points of departure and return" criticized by Hegel. With his own peculiar mixture of tact and purposiveness, Freud explores Schreber's proliferating phantasms, drawing them ever closer to a fixed point within his theory in order finally to be able to assert in an unmistakably triumphant tone: "Thus in the case of Schreber we find ourselves once again on the familiar ground of the father-complex."[20] Yet the translation from a paranoic mode of expression (Schreber's) to a normal one (the psychoanalytic) succeeds almost two well, and Freud feels compelled to refer to the independence of the theory: "These and many other details of Schreber's delusional structure sound almost like endopsychic perceptions of the processes whose existence I have assumed in these pages as the basis of our explanation of paranoia. I can nevertheless call a friend and fellow-specialist to witness that I had developed my theory of paranoia before I became acquainted with the contents of Schreber's book."[21]

Freud did not, he asserts, plagiarize Schreber, although the similarity of their views leads him to ask, "whether there is more delusion in my theory than I should like to admit, or whether there is more truth in Schreber's delusion than other people are as yet prepared to believe."

This remark is not mere coquetry on Freud's part; rather, it indicates what is essentially new in a theory that, unlike traditional psychiatry, no longer unquestioningly presupposes a boundary between madness and truth, between the pathological and the normal, between irrationality and reason. Hence the special structure of psychoanalytic "translation": it is no longer merely a *procedure of subsumption* but now also a *practice of reading and interpretation:*

> [Schreber] himself not infrequently presses the key into our hands, by adding a gloss, a quotation or an example to some delusional proposition in an apparently incidental manner, or even by expressly denying some parallel to it

> that has arisen in his own mind. For when this happens, we have only to follow our usual psycho-analytic technique—to strip his sentence of its negative form, to take his example as being the actual thing, or his quotation or gloss as being the original source—and we find ourselves in possession of what we are looking for, namely a translation of the paranoic mode of expression into the normal one.[22]

Freud's method of reading no longer consists merely in collecting, describing and uncritically evaluating characteristic traits (*Merkmale*); on the contrary, it focuses on what might be called the text's "stains" or "marks" (*Male*), on that which is incidental, which has been added, that which is considered unimportant and has been denied: not *Merkmale,* but *Male* are sought after and noted down, as the carriers of a meaning expressible only through disguise and distortion.

Psychoanalysis, then, at least in Freud's version, is not a theory of *Merkmale,* which takes the subject's statements merely as the neutral expression of a content; rather, it attempts to understand forms of articulation as if they themselves were the contents, as in dreams, jokes, and slips of various kinds. Freud's approach to dreams considers a dream not as the *formation of meanings* but as the *deformation of wishes,* not as *Darstellung* but as *Entstellung*. The distinction is crucial. Whereas an expressivist theory neglects the conditions under which the expressed arose in favor of its meaning, Freud tries to work out just these conditions. His concept of the unconscious works less with definite contents than with mechanisms of articulation like "condensation," "displacement," and a "concern with the ability of something to be expressed" (*Rücksicht auf Darstellbarkeit*), the goal of which is not the expression or communication of meaning, but its distortion in the service of censorship.

This theory of unconscious articulation as distortion allows Freud to question the uniqueness of the Schreber case from the very start of his study. The key question is whether "a printed case history can take the place of personal acquaintance with the patient."[23] Freud's answer derives from the peculiar nature of paranoia. Paranoics possess "the peculiarity of betraying . . . precisely those things which other neurotics keep hidden as a secret." Furthermore, as Freud explains, this betrayal always takes place "in a distorted form." But this interpretation only establishes the possibility of examining paranoic persons psychoanalytically; the problem of a text as a substitute for the bodily presence of the analysand requires additional grounding. This Freud finds in the peculiar mode of the paranoic form of expression: paranoics "say only what they choose to say." It is a question of paranoic speech as a pure *discourse of the will:* "Since paranoics cannot be compelled to overcome their internal resistances," they are not willing to enter into the dialogue of analysis and therefore can be examined using their written expressions just as if they were personally present. They say only what they want to say—and yet in so doing they say (or write) something else: for they betray themselves, indeed even more so than the neurotic, precisely because they say only what they want to say—"in a distorted form," to be sure. But what can "distortion" mean in this context?

In one of his last essays Freud treats this issue in the context of the biblical presentation and distortion of the story of Moses. Freud argues for a twofold understanding of the word "distortion": "We might well lend the word *Entstellung* [distortion] the double meaning to which it has a claim but of which today it makes no use. It should mean not only 'to change the appearance of something' but also 'to put something in another place, to displace.' "[24]

Freud's description of the biblical text as distortion is equally valid for the paranoic's text, and in particular for *Memoirs of My Nervous Illness:*

> Thus almost everywhere noticeable gaps, disturbing repetitions and obvious contradictions have come about—indications which reveal things to us which [the text] was not intended to communicate. In its implications the distortion of a text resembles a murder: the difficulty is not in perpetrating the deed, but in getting rid of its traces . . . Accordingly, in many instances of textual distortion, we may nevertheless count upon finding what has been suppressed and disavowed, hidden away somewhere else, though changed and torn from its context. Only it will not always be easy to recognize it.[25]

Distortion, according to Freud, is to be understood not only as the deformation of something originally undistorted, but as a change of location, or a displacement, as well. Yet this word "displacement" also denotes a mechanism of unconscious articulation: the displacement of psychic intensities—called "cathexis" or "occupation"—from one representation to another, along a chain of associations. The distortion of a text mirrors in this way the dislocation of the subject, which is a necessary effect of the unconscious. The subject of the unconscious—according to Freud, the subject itself—is no longer constituted by the identity and transparence of self-consciousness, no longer the Cartesian *cogito* or the Hegelian *Begriff,* no longer the subject of knowledge and the will alone, but also and above all, that of *unconscious desire:* that is, the subject of the unconscious is mediated by an irreducible heterogeneity, a foreignness—by a dislocation that no dialectic can overcome or transcend.

Hence, a different kind of reading is required to unravel the discourse of a will that says only what it wants to say and thus always, as distortion (and this is especially clear in the case of paranoia), is already displaced, relocated, moved somewhere else, recorded in a text of desire that, like desire itself, is articulated through gaps, repetitions, contradictions: in short, it is expression through the contours of a conflict. Consequently, what till now we have called "knowing," displaces and distorts itself. Insofar as the objects of unconscious knowledge are constituted by a conflict of desire, they resist being grasped conceptually; as with dreams, an untranslatable, idiosyncratic, singular residue always remains.[26] It persists, however, not as the arabesque of a unique occurence, but as the necessary, if idiosyncratic, materialization and localization of a process of articulation. Although such a process includes logical thought and makes reason possible, it itself is not governed by reason. The unconscious articulates a "case" (*der Fall*) of reason; it lures reason into a trap (*die Falle*) and fells it there. It is in this sense, perhaps, that the *case* of Schreber lives up to its title and becomes "worthy of thought": *denkwürdig,* and not merely "memorable."

The History of an Illness: Body, Soul, and Nerves

However one reads it, Schreber's text *Memoirs* is not an easy one. It operates alternately on three levels, all different yet closely connected: the first recounts the history of Schreber's illness, his life in asylums, his efforts to have the order placing him under tutelage rescinded; the second is devoted to his "personal experiences," as he calls them; the third deals with that all-encompassing context, the "cosmic order" (*Weltordnung*) and its crises—a context which provides the meaning of all that appears and all that is experienced. For the sake of simplicity, let us begin with the external history of Schreber's illness—that is, with his case—so that we can subsequently enter with him into his own trap.

The period of his second hospitalization lasted from November 1983, when he was admitted to the Leipzig clinic, until his discharge at his own request (following his successful lawsuit against his tutelage) from the State Asylum Sonnenstein in Pirna (near Dresden) on 20 December 1902. The extant medical bulletins describe his initial condition as follows:

> At first more hypochondrical complaints, that he suffers from a "softening of the brain, will soon die," etc., at the same time mixed with delusions of persecution, that "he has now been made happily insane." Also hallucinations now and then, which gave him quite a fright . . . He thinks he is dead and has begun to rot, that he is no longer in a condition "fit for burial"; that he is "plague-stricken," probably as a result of olfactory hallucinations; that his penis was twisted off by means of a "nerve probe"; he thinks he is a woman, but also often claims he must repulse energetically "the homosexual love of certain persons." All of these things tormented him greatly so that he wished for death; he tried to drown himself in the bathtub and for many weeks demanded daily "the glass of cyanide destined for him." The auditory and visual hallucinations sometimes became so strong that he spent hours at a time in a chair or in bed completely inaccessible, squinting his eyes. The delusions of his senses apparently were of ever-changing content, referring in the more recent period of his stay at the Leipzig clinic to his belief that he was being tortured to death in a ghastly manner. He then lost himself more and more in a mystic-religious dimension, maintaining that God spoke openly to him, that vampires and devils make game of him. He said he wanted to convert to the Roman Catholic Church in order to avoid being persecuted. He then saw apparitions, heard sacred music and, finally, apparently thought he was in another world. At least he considered everything around him to be spirits, taking his environment to be a world of illusions . . . At that time Flechsig considered him dangerous to himself and to others.[27]

This description, which coincides in part with what I quoted from the *Memoirs* above, has the advantage of bringing into bold relief two aspects that will prove decisive in Schreber's case: first, his *body* as the favored object of his imaginings (at first in a mostly negative sense: he claims to suffer from a softening of the brain, to feel himself to be dead, to have begun to decay, to be plague-stricken, to have had his penis twisted off, and so on); and second, the aspect of *language,* in the form of verbal hallucinations ("God spoke openly to him"). The homosexual aspect also appears ("he thinks he is a woman"), and this in connection both with fantasies of castration and with illusions of persecution (that he had to repulse the "homosexual love of certain persons")—a complex that Freud places at the very center of his interpretation.

Above all, a reading of the medical bulletin, as well as the memoirs themselves, reveals the increasing significance of linguistic phenomena for Schreber. Even his initial inaccessibility seems to have actually been a form of *listening:* "He was in a state of great psychic excitation, at the outset inaccessible, sullen, almost gloomy. He was uncomfortable with any and all conversation. He hallucinated intensely, showed little interest in his surroundings, but stood around in the same position with a frightened look on his face, staring out into the distance. It was observed in the garden how he placed his hands on his ears, listening intensely."

If at first he refused all communication with physicians and nurses, one of his "reasons," it appears, was his concern with other "communications": "At times obviously harassed by voices, never spoke to anyone about this." Later, in his memoirs, Schreber argues that he did not articulate his visions and experiences because their complexity exceeded the capacity of oral communication—as anyone who reads the memoirs will agree.

On the surface Schreber remains, for a period, passive ("is never occupied with anything, does not read anything," the medical record remarks). Yet already in November 1894 there are signs of a turn toward activity, toward behavior that will be of the greatest significance for his later development. "On the whole somewhat more lively, writes shorthand and draws figures on paper": Schreber begins to write.

From this point on writing assumes an increasingly important role in his life, in addition to the hallucinatory transformations of his body. A description of his condition in June 1895 reads: "Completely under the influence of delusions. Maintains that his body is completely changed, that one of his lungs has almost completely disappeared, that everything that he sees around him is merely appearance. That the world has perished . . . Calm again for periods. Writes many letters, also in Italian, signed himself once 'Paul Höllenfürst' [literally, "Prince of Hell"]. He addressed one letter to 'Mr. Ormuzd *in coelo*.' "

Thus, Schreber not only listens, he writes. Shortly thereafter he adds a new component: he not only writes, he screams. The "bellowing miracle" appears on the scene. *What* he screams about is not without interest: "Often screams out the window at night, always the same terms of abuse, or 'I am Senatspräsident Schreber.' " These terms of abuse may well have been intended for that other Schreber, who recommended that one make oneself master of his child forever. The abuse, and the bellowing of his name and high official title, all point to Schreber's struggle for his own identity, a battle to be waged within language and by means of language.

In 1896, as his interest in his immediate environment slowly begins to reawaken, Schreber's body is subjected to a new form of alteration. Whereas previously it has been mainly an object of decomposition and destruction, it is now increasingly affected by a more positive change: "Has let himself go in his appearance, inadequately dressed, shows the physician his naked upper body, claiming that 'he now has almost female breasts.' The only real changes are greater fat deposits, given that the patient has gained greatly in weight." With the onset of what in the *Memoirs* is called "unmanning" or "transformation into a woman," his body assumes a new function: it becomes an object to be looked at, gazed upon, thus Schreber's willingness to show the doctor his exposed upper body.

"Seems quite preoccupied with sexual notions, likes very much to look up nudes in illustrated magazines, evidently draws them as well. In a letter to his wife—in Italian—writes that the nights are very pleasant because he always has 'un pou die volupte feminae' [*sic*]." This mingling of the sexes not only takes place in Schreber's body, but applies as well to a divine interlocutor: "Continues to bellow, often quite offensive terms of abuse: 'The sun is a whore' or 'God is a whore.' " Already at an earlier time Schreber had been greatly preoccupied with the sun, and he had been observed standing "for a long time in one place, emotionless, looking into the sun and all the while making the most bizarre faces." At the conclusion of his book he maintains that the sun pales before his very gaze. In any case, seeing and being seen gain in significance.

He now becomes ever more "talkative and accessible, reads more." In 1897 he conducts a "lively correspondence with wife and relatives, written in a polite and proper manner, the letters betraying not the slightest sign of illness. Talks about his sickness apparently with complete insight." Only the old "bellowing sessions and face-making" continue, joined by several new forms of coquetry: "Adorns himself with colorful ribbons, now and then engages in quite trivial dalliances." "Often naked in his room, laughing and yelling in front of a mirror, adorned with colorful ribbons."

At the beginning of 1899 he speaks for the first time about the content of his experiences, in a "detailed letter to his wife . . . The lucidity and logical acuity with which he develops his system is striking." From this period onward he is increasingly occupied with the question of his tutelage, which as early as 1895—and without his knowledge—had been declared temporarily, and later in March 1900 was upheld as permanent. Schreber contested this ruling at about the time he was writing his *Memoirs*. The major portion was written between February and September of 1900, too early to play a role in the initial appeal proceedings, which ended in 1901 in Schreber's favor. The text, enlarged by several "postscripts" as well as by an appendix ("In What Circumstances Can a Person Considered Insane Be Detained in an Asylum against His Declared Will?"), was submitted as testimony in the appeal proceedings, which on 14 July 1902 lead to the recision of Schreber's tutelage by the Royal State Superior Court.

The court's argumentation is of interest even today. Its verdict found that the plantiff was unquestionably mentally ill; whereas Schreber himself maintained that, although he was *nervously ill,* he was not *mentally ill,* in otherwords, that his experience was of an objective nature. Despite this disagreement, the court did accept Schreber's view that the decisive issue was not his mental state but, rather, whether he was capable of taking care of his own affairs and defending his own interests. The court agreed with the plaintiff that he was indeed entirely capable of doing this. Remarkable however is the court's assessment of the *Memoirs*. Recall that for Geheimrat Dr. Weber, director of the asylum, well-known court psychiatrist, and Schreber's physician, the intention to publish the text was in itself proof of

Schreber's mental illness. The court firmly rejected this opinion, arguing first that such intent does not violate the author's objective interests (that is, it did him no financial harm); and second that:

> One also cannot maintain that the contents of the "Memoirs" are such as to compromise [the] plaintiff himself. The manuscript is the product of a morbid imagination and nobody reading it would for a moment lose the feeling that its author is mentally deranged. But this could not possibly lower the patient in the respect of his fellow men, particularly as no one can miss the seriousness of purpose and striving after truth which fill every chapter. As Dr. Schreber remarks correctly, the worst that could happen to him would be that one consider him mad, and this one does in any case. (*M*, p. 354)

This opinion manifests a liberality that surprisingly—although perhaps not entirely uninfluenced by its authors' collegial relation to the plaintiff, as well as by his high position—belongs to an Enlightenment tradition whose influence on German jurisprudence was surely not overwhelming at the time. Yet we should not overlook the precondition for such tolerance: fools, like poets, enjoy greater freedom than average citizens, precisely because they are fools. There is a further component to be noted here, one to which we will return: the court's recognition of Schreber's "seriousness of purpose and striving after truth, which fill each chapter." However much it may otherwise have erred, the court nonetheless acknowledged that Schreber was only trying to be *more rational than reason itself.* Hence all the more surprising is the court's argument in making allowances for Schreber's style of discourse, which Dr. Weber had strongly censured: "One cannot be offended by the strong language in the book. It is not [the] plaintiff's; he only repeats what the voices of spirits spoke into him in earlier years when he was most severely hallucinated" (*M*, p. 355).

To appreciate adequately the significance of this concession, one need only juxtapose it to the opinion of Dr. Weber, concerning the relationship of Schreber's madness to his other views: "It is true that every delusional system," Dr. Weber writes, "must somehow influence all the patient's ideas because its bearer is an 'individual,' that is, indivisible . . ." (*M*, p. 318). By contrast, the court seems prepared to place this principle of the indivisible individual into doubt: it considers Schreber's text (whether dictated to him or composed by him) as a different language, one foreign to him ("merely a reproduction of phantom voices"). The Royal State Superior Court at Dresden thus accepts that an author is not necessarily—at least *de jure*—responsible for "his" text.

The Cosmic Order; or, The Gap in the Vosges

Having familiarized ourselves with the case history of Daniel Paul Schreber, we should now turn to the remarkable history of his *nervous illness*—however distorted or abridged this account may be. Schreber himself starts with an explication of the "Cosmic Order,"[28] that is, with a world that has not yet fallen into disorder. This world—like its divine creator—consists mainly of nerves: God is "from the very beginning . . . only nerve," and he creates the world when his nerves transform themselves into "rays," which can then become anything at all. Humans are likewise nerve, in the sense that their souls are contained in nerve.

Let us dwell on these nerves for a moment, since they form the fundamental elements of Schreber's universe. In terms of their composition they are very strange things indeed. They evidently unite the highest interiority and immanence, on the one hand, with the greatest externality and heteronomy, on the other. The nerves—"nerves of understanding,"[29] as they are called—are like monads, inasmuch as every single mental nerve "represents the entire mental individuality of a human being": the number of nerves a person has influences the *duration* of his identity, but not his *identity* itself. To this extent the nerves represent that which is internal and identical in a person. Yet as parts of the body—they are essentially corporeal in that they occupy space and are material—the nerves are necessarily dependent on external impressions and impulses in order to be "jarred into vibration."

The nerve, as the inner essence of humans, requires the external and the foreign in order to function. The relationship between internal and external, between the identical and the heterogeneous, is governed by identity, insofar as the original and lawful conditions which constitute the Cosmic Order obtain. God externalizes Himself as rays which transform themselves into the Creation; this Creation stands in a relation of otherness to God, it is His Other, until death, when the nerves of the human—or, more precisely, of the human *corpse*—slowly, in a process of purification, re-ascend into the heavenly fields, there to be taken into God and to dissolve within Him. As long as the Cosmic Order prevails, it is governed by what Georges Bataille has called a "restricted economy": an economy of identity where nothing is lost, where every externalization is dialectically reappropriated, where every expenditure yields a return.[30] The Cosmic Order, the World-as-yet-*still*-in-Order, follows reason and its laws, which are concentrated in one of the messages Schreber "receives," and which might very well have served as a motto for his entire work: "All nonsense cancels itself out" (*Aller Unsinn hebt sich auf; M,* pp. 151, 226).

But there is a hitch in this system or structure: the reason and cause, the beginning and end of this Cosmic Order, God, is likewise "to begin with . . . only nerve." Hence the aspect of the heteronomical and the nonidentical, which characterizes every nerve, characterizes God as well. Accordingly, Schreber's God is different from His more orthodox predecessors: He is corporeal—material and localized—subject (at least in part) to the laws of time and space. Moreover, heavenly existence consists in a "state of blessedness" which Schreber describes as "uninterrupted enjoyment" (*M,* p. 51). And this propensity for hedonism, rooted in the neural nature of God and of the souls that return to Him, is not without certain risks for God Himself. As a nerve, God depends upon others, on the nerves of humans, for instance. This is not a problem as long as He approaches their corpses to suck out the nerves (for which death is merely a form of sleep) and to draw them heavenward. Difficulties arise only in those exceptional cases where God, perhaps out of ignorance (for He knows the human only externally, as a cadaver), approaches the living human and—as Schreber describes it—"attaches" Himself to the human, forming a "nerve attachment."[31] As long as it is the exception, for example, in the case of "highly gifted people (poets, etc.)," the nerve attachment does not cause any problems. However, "such 'nerve attachment' was not allowed to become the rule, as already mentioned, because for reasons which cannot be further elucidated, the nerves of *living* human beings, particularly when in a state of *high-grade excitation,* have such power of attraction for the nerves of God that He would not be able to free Himself from them again, and would thus endanger His own existence" (*M,* p. 48).

In this case the normal course of things in the Cosmic Order would be completely reversed, with fatal consequences. Before these consequences, which form the *Memoirs*' real point of departure, can be discussed, several other characteristics of the Cosmic Order should be mentioned, if briefly; first, that it consists of beings who are not only corporeal, only nerve to start with, but who are equally determined by their language. As Schreber writes, "it seems to lie in the nature of rays that they must *speak* as soon as they are in motion; the relevant law was expressed in the phrase 'do not forget that rays must speak,' and this was spoken into my nerves innumerable times, particularly early on" (*M,* p. 121).

Here we confront a further peculiarity of Schreber's text: the objects he discusses are no less language than he himself is—a slightly disjointed, slightly twisted language, "the so-called 'basic-language,' a somewhat antiquated but nevertheless powerful German, characterized particularly by a wealth of euphemisms" (*M,* pp. 49–50). Everything that Schreber says about the Cosmic Order is based on communications he receives that utilize the "basic-language," characterized not only by shifts of meaning (though not always euphemistic ones), but also by a tendency not to finish sentences: "The souls were in the habit—even before the conditions contrary to the Cosmic Order had started—of giving their thoughts (when communicating with one another) grammatically incomplete expression; that is to say they omitted certain words which were not essential for the sense" (*M,* p. 70). It is as if the tendency of souls (or rays) not to complete their sentences was bound up with their character as transitional beings: they are aspects of an externalizing movement that emanates from a divine being and leads back to it. Blessedness, understood as the final goal of nerves returning to God, corresponds to meaning, understood as the final goal of a basic-language expression: both are intended and approximated, yet never quite attained.

It becomes increasingly clear that in this kind of Cosmic Order, crises and disruptions are, as it were, programmed, prior to all intervention from without. A God who is Himself all nerve and therefore dependent on external stimulation, who knows the human being only externally (as a cadaver), who now and then engages in a nerve attachment despite the risks involved; a language whose words have inverted meaning, whose sentences are begun but never finished, trusting in a meaning that is never more than approximate; above all, the entire, apparently stable, restricted economy, including God, subject to the "unfathomable law" of the "power of attraction," "according to which rays and nerves mutually attract one another," in a reciprocity that "harbors a kernel of danger for the realms of God" (*M,* p. 59): all of this points to catastrophe as an immanent possibility of this order itself.

When it does take place, the catastrophe assumes the remarkable form of a *rip* or *tear:* "This 'miraculous structure'[32] [the Cosmic Order] has recently suffered a rent, intimately connected with my personal fate" (*M,* p. 54)—thus begins Schreber's description of the misfortune which has befallen the Cosmic Order like a pestilence, wrenching it out of joint. The extra-ordinary nature of this tear in the wondrous structure has already been alluded to: it originates externally, as it were out of nothing, and it not only *sunders,* it *joins,* or is joined to Schreber's personal fate. A peculiarity of this special tear is that it sunders *in that it joins*. As Schreber writes:

> It is impossible even for me to present the deeper connections in a way which human understanding can fully grasp. My personal experiences enable me to lift the veil only partially; the rest is intuition and conjecture. I want to say by way of introduction that the leading roles in the genesis of this development, the first beginnings of which go back perhaps as far as the eighteenth century, were played on the one hand by the names of Flechsig and Schreber (probably not specifying any individual member of these families), and on the other by the concept of *soul murder.* (*M,* p. 54)

At the beginning stands the joining of two names—Flechsig and Schreber, at first independent of their individual carriers—as well as the dark concept of "soul murder." According to Schreber, the latter seems to consist in one person's somehow taking "possession of another person's soul" (*M,* p. 55). This, he asserts, actually took place in the course of a feud between the Schreber and Flechsig families, both of which "belonged, it was said, to 'the highest nobility of heaven' " (*M,* p. 55),[33] families that had had a falling out when the Flechsig family "had been outstripped in some way or other by members of the Schreber family" (*M,* p. 57). A certain "Daniel Fürchtegott Flechsig" (who, like the other Flechsigs named by Schreber, bears the names of his own ancestors)[34] actually managed to lure God into a nerve attachment, never to release him: "He resisted[35] breaking off the attachment into which divine rays had directly or indirectly entered with him, or made it dependent on conditions which could not be denied him, considering the souls' natural weakness of character compared with that of living men, and in any case it was not thought possible to keep up permanent nerve attachment with a single human being" (*M*, p. 57). The Flechsig family thus attained an incredible power, which it used against the Schrebers: "One can imagine that in this way something like a conspiracy may have arisen between such a person and the elements of the anterior realms of God [the purified souls returning to God] to the detriment of the Schreber race [*Geschlecht*], perhaps in the direction of denying them offspring or possibly only of denying them choice of those professions which would lead to closer relations with God such as that of a nerve specialist" (*M*, p. 57).

The obscurity of these events is rendered still more obscure by the censor, to whom the *Memoirs*' third chapter—dealing with "some events concerning *other members of my family*, which may possibly in some way be related to the presumed soul murder" (*M*, p. 61)—fell victim. Yet it becomes increasingly apparent to Schreber that his encounter with Paul Emil Flechsig in the Leipzig University Psychiatric Clinic was no mere coincidence, but rather the result of considerable planning. Even though the plot was initiated by the Flechsig family, God's complicity seems ever more certain to Schreber: "It occurred to me only much later, in fact only while writing this essay did it become quite clear to me, that God Himself must have known of the plan, if indeed He was not the instigator, to commit soul murder on me, and to hand over my body in the manner of a female harlot (*M*, p. 77).

On the one hand this description clearly shows that soul murder concerns not only the "surrender of a *soul* to another person" or the appropriation of "his *mental* powers" (*M*, p. 58; my emphasis); it also concerns the body, and this could hardly be otherwise since, in Schreber's Cosmic Order, soul and mind are bound to the body's nerves. On the other hand, it becomes clear that the composition of the *Memoirs* is not simply a report; rather, it is part of, and participant in, the experience it recounts.

This explanation also sheds light on the peculiar goal of the conspiracy against Schreber, which was initiated by soul murder: his body is to be surrendered to Professor Paul Emil Flechsig, as a "female prostitute" for purposes of sexual pleasure.

This implies the "unmanning" of Daniel Paul Schreber, his "transformation into a woman" for purposes that contravene the Cosmic Order. Subsequently all sorts of "miracles" are directed at his body with the intention both of transforming him into a woman and also of destroying his physical "integrity" (see especially chapter 12). His limbs are wounded and lamed; his internal organs destroyed, removed from his body and replaced with new ones. Not only is his body attacked, but his mind is as well, at first through the body. One description of these attacks may serve for many:

> These concerned firstly my *head;* secondly . . . also the *spinal cord,* which next to the head was considered as the seat of reason. One therefore attempted to pump the spinal cord out, which was done by so-called "little men" placed in my feet . . . The effect of the pumping out was that the spinal cord left my mouth in considerable quantity in the form of little clouds, particularly when I was walking in the garden . . . The miracles directed against my *head and the nerves of my head* happened in manifold ways. One attempted to pull the nerves out of my head, for a time even (during the nights) to transplant them into the head of M. who slept in the next room . . . Serious devastation was caused in my head by the so-called "flights of rays," . . . the effect of which was that my skull was repeatedly sawn asunder in various directions. (*M,* pp. 135–136)

These attacks on the integrity of his body and mind produce just the opposite of what was intended: the more he is assaulted, the more attractive his sorely tested nerves become, the greater the number of souls entering into and dissolving within him, the greater the danger to, and temptation of, God Himself (in His two forms of the lower God, Ariman, and the higher, Ormuzd). For the conspirators had overlooked and misconstrued the laws of the Cosmic Order: all the damage done by the "impure rays" (unpurified souls, called "tested souls" in the "basic language") can be reversed by "pure rays." The conspirators misunderstand above all the nature of emasculation. As Schreber slowly learns, emasculation is "connected with the basic plan on which the Cosmic Order seems to rest" (*M,* p. 72), a plan that, in the case of catastrophes, makes possible the survival of the human race through divine insemination. After initial resistance, Schreber thus consents to the plan for his unmanning so as to ensure this survival against all eventualities. It would seem that the Cosmic Order's restricted economy, despite all the violations of it, will once again be able to defend and maintain itself, at least in the opinion of Daniel Paul Schreber, who places himself—his body, his mind, and his work—at the service of truth and science. Schreber's emasculation, the heightening of his nerves' attraction and the saturation of his body with "female nerves of lust" (*weibliche Wollustnerven*), influencing in turn souls, rays, and ultimately the lower God Himself, implies not so much the possibility of impregnation as the certainty of demise: in the seductive power of the nerves, lust and death are mixed. But since souls "were used to uninterrupted enjoyment, and were therefore not or only little capable of temporary sacrifice or temporary denial of pleasure in order to procure permanent advantages in the future, a quality which is peculiar to human beings" (*M*, p. 75), they are all the more vulnerable to this danger. For the

> dissolution in my body of the rays (which are separated from the totality of God's nerves) due to my power of attraction amounts to the end of their independent existence, like death is to man. It was therefore a matter of course that God should make all attempts to avoid the fate of having to perish in my body with more and more parts of His totality, and indeed one was not very particular in choosing the means of prevention. *But the attraction lost all its terror for these nerves, if and to the extent they met a feeling of soul-voluptuousness in my body* in which they also participated. They then regained in my body a more or less adequate substitute for the lost heavenly Blessedness which itself consisted in enjoyment similar to voluptuousness. (*M*, pp. 149–150)

The whole plot of his *Memoirs* is played out as repetitions and variations of this scenario: the divine assault, at first with Flechsig and then without him, on the integrity of Schreber's body and mind; Schreber's counterattack, together with World-Order elements (pure rays), which leads to an increase in his power of attraction; and, consequently, the danger to God, in turn calling forth the next heavenly assault, and so on.

These assaults are directed not only at the body, but also—once it became obvious that this body is inviolable, even for God—increasingly at his mind, with the goal of driving Schreber "mad," or at least making him appear so, thereby diminishing his power of attraction. Schreber, however, leaves no doubt as to which of two adversaries is closer to insanity: for the divine plan overlooks the simple fact "that the nerves, even of a demented human being, would, in a state of highly pathological excitement retain their power of attraction" (*M*, pp. 120–121).

Mainly *linguistic* means are employed in these assaults on Schreber. I shall examine two of them more closely: the "system of notation" (*Aufschreibsystem*) and "compulsive thinking" (*Denkzwang*). Schreber describes a system of notation in which "*books or other notes* are kept in which . . . have been *written-down* all my thoughts, all my phrases, all my necessaries, all the articles in my possession or around me"—in short, anything at all having to do with Schreber. The writing is done by random, thoughtless souls, "bound" to some distant celestial bodies (an invention of Flechsig's to protect the souls from Schreber's power of attraction): "Their hands are led automatically, as it were, by passing rays for the purpose of making them write down" (*M*, p. 119).

The purpose of the notes made in this way is, on the one hand, to exhaust Schreber's store of thoughts—"this of course is quite absurd, because human thinking is inexhaustible," Schreber remarks—and, on the other hand, to provide material for the rays, which must talk continuously, "to fill in these pauses." Moreover, by means of this system of notation the rays, "in a manner hard to describe," are supposed to be "made unreceptive to the power of attraction of such a thought" (*M*, p. 122).

The system of notation reveals the entwinement of language and body, of desire and defense, that characterizes Schreber's text. The system is supposed to exhaust Schreber by establishing a complete inventory of his discourse; any and all of his linguistic expressions are to be fixed, that is, they are to be written down and removed from his control so as to neutralize, if not eliminate, his nerves' power of attraction. But, despite the "mental torture" caused him by the rays' know-it-all attitude—any thought or expression of Schreber's is met with: "We have this already" (already "written down" or "recorded")—he overcomes the system of notation, indeed not least of all by himself becoming a note taker: he writes his *Memoirs*. Only when writing is Schreber free from the power of his persecutors: "For all miracles are powerless to prevent the expression of ideas in writing" (*M*, p. 298).

I will return to the significance of Schreber's writing. But first let us examine the second attempt to destroy his mind by linguistic means: compulsive thinking. As the term suggests, this consists in "a human being having to think incessantly" (*M,* p. 70), as a result either of direct questioning ("What are you thinking about now?") or of those unfinished phrases that characterize the basic language as such, and that practically force the listener to complete them. The compulsion to introduce what has been omitted has to do with the "nature of nerves": "that if unconnected words or started phrases are thrown into them, they automatically attempt to complete them to finished thoughts satisfactory to the human mind." (*M,* p. 172).

The nerves are thus driven by a kind of *horror vacui* to complete the meaning still outstanding, regardless of the intentions of their subject (Schreber). The completion usually consists in nothing more than the repetition of often-heard phrases, hence it requires no special mental effort. If, for instance, Schreber hears the words, "It will be," then his nerves complete the phrase in a nonarbitrary way: " . . . done now, the joint of pork," whereby Schreber knows full well that "joint of pork" here signifies—in keeping with the basic language's twisted logic—nothing other than himself. "It was meant to express that I was done, i.e. that my power of resistance against the attacks on my reason by the rays must by now be exhausted" (*M,* p. 173). That Schreber should be called, of all things, a joint of pork becomes somewhat more understandable when we read why the voices resist finishing their sentences. Their goal is not only to force Schreber to expend his powers, thereby reducing his power of attraction, but also to prevent a development more dangerous still. As Schreber writes, "whenever expressed in a grammatically complete sentence, the rays would be led straight to me, and entering my body . . . temporarily increase its soul-voluptuousness. Not-finishing-a-sentence has apparently the effect that the rays are, as it were, held up half way, and could therefore withdraw before having added to the soul-voluptuousness in my body" (*M,* p. 173).

Earlier it was not Schreber who, as a joint of pork, had to fear the mouths of others; rather, the situation was reversed: "While conditions prevailed which were at least somehow in consonance with the Cosmic Order, that is before tying-to-rays and tying-to-celestial-bodies was started . . . , a momentary uniform *feeling* was enough to make the freely suspended souls jump down from the sky into my mouth, thus ending their independent existence" (*M,* p. 173).

As the Cosmic Order was to some extent still intact, hence before the *tear* in its texture occurred or widened, *saying* a sentence to the point of its meaningful completion meant destroying the speaking rays *in Schreber's mouth.* This again confirms the entwinement of speech and lust, of meaning and death. Thus it comes as no surprise that God and the rays (the voices) attempt everything to prevent this fatal completion: writing things down, tying (distant planets) to Earth, using sentences left incomplete, and using speech that has been slowed and distended in the extreme. No wonder they attempt—through "wonders"—to make incompetent (*ent-mündigen*) Schreber's mouth (*Mund*), to expropriate his linguistic expressions and communicative competence by means of compulsive thinking (which, as we have seen, implies *compulsive speech* as well); or more directly through a system of "misrepresentations," compelling Schreber's nerves to give answers he had not intended, which are foreign to him; or, more directly still, by means of the "bellowing miracle," forcing Schreber to bellow whether he wants to or not.

To Schreber, all this seems an abominable disregard for the Cosmic Order, resulting from its critical fissure. Still, he gives us good reason to mistrust such an easy explanation. The simple model of an undamaged, unwounded earlier state, torn or ripped by the intrusion of some calamity—or "apparition" (*Gesicht*), in the antiquating basic language—is difficult to reconcile with the peculiar structure of the nerves. Their "inherent" dependence on the external and the foreign, on stimulation and on unmitigated pleasure—this, their exogenic, exotic *lust principle,* destroys all order, all identity, and every restricted economy of expenditure-without-loss. At least for the nerves of Schreber's Cosmic Order[36] before and after the crisis, lust means *loss.* As long as God Himself, although participating in this process, could nonetheless be deemed to stand above it, as the beginning and the end, it seemed possible to amortize the loss of lust expended through a gain in identity. But when God Himself is drawn into the vortex of attraction—through a nerve attachment—this illusion can no longer be sustained. "Voluptuousness has become 'God-fearing' " (*M,* p. 210), say the voices, yet they express themselves here, as so often, euphemistically: it is not lust that has become God-fearing (beginning with Daniel Fürchtegott [literally, "God-fearing"], Flechsig and Schreber's nerve contact), but God who has learned to fear lust. And not without reason. For He is no longer involved with mere cadavers—like the physician who views a body mainly as a muscular mechanism; now He is engaged with fresh, living, excited *nerves,* nerves that have as their target nothing less than His existence and identity. And since God's identity, together with His economy of expenditure and reappropriation, represent here nothing other than a *fantasy of reason* (or, better, reason's nightmare), this struggle of identity with lust, this crisis of identity, acquires a more than merely "pathological" interest.

As much as one may attempt to distinguish the Before and After of the Cosmic Order, Schreber's text shows how they in fact overlap, how the After and the Exterior have always been present in the Interior of the Order of the World, as nerve. I have already mentioned a peculiarity of the voices, which was characteristic of them even before the crisis set in: their tendency not to finish sentences. Nonetheless one could still imagine that the act of speaking would guarantee the purity of identity and of the internal against everything foreign and external. It is spoken language in which Schreber (precisely in his struggles) places so much trust as that form of articulation which can most powerfully protect the subject's identity and property—"the human language (spoken aloud) . . . is the *ultima ratio* for preserving the sanctity of my house."[37] It is spoken language that can protect identity and property above all in Schreber's tormented head, the walls of which offer no protection against the ray-voices. Again and again he describes how the voices' "original" language, which continued to give "expression to genuine feeling," increasingly degenerates into rote phrases, "drummed" into "speaking birds," created by miracle (*M,* p. 85) to torment Schreber with their nonsense. How does Schreber describe this original language in his own text?

The language of souls and rays, God's basic language, is, we recall, a "language of nerves." According to Schreber, this can best be imagined "when one thinks of the processes by which a person tries to imprint certain words in his memory in a definite order, as for instance a child learning a poem by heart which he is going to recite at school, or a priest a sermon he is going to deliver in church. The words are *repeated silently* . . . that is to say a human being causes his nerves to vibrate in the way which corresponds to the use of the words concerned, but the real organs of speech . . . are either not set in motion at all or only coincidentally" (*M,* p. 69).

Because of its very structure, this nerve language is anything but an expression of "genuine feeling": it is much less an expression than an impression, something remembered, not the expression of something inward but the emergence in the interior of something outward (*Auswendiges*), something "learned by rote" (*auswendig gelernt*), a system of assertions not much different from the much derided system of notation that is employed just as thoughtlessly. Schreber's language (or bellowing), expropriated in part by the rays, differs from the nerve language in one respect: that of control or disposition over speech. In "normal" circumstances (those which correspond to the Cosmic Order), the use of a particular nerve "depends only on the will of the person whose nerves are concerned," in keeping with "man's natural right to be master of his own nerves" (*M,* pp. 69–70). We should not, however, lose sight of the fact that the language of the nerves is, in and of itself, foreign to the subject, owing to the constitution of his own nerves (as mentioned above). Whether it wants to or not, as nerve the subject does not speak, it is spoken. Although Schreber does not *say* this in so many words, he *writes* it; or, perhaps more precisely, it writes him.

There would be much more to say about this silent contradiction between what Schreber wants to say out loud, and what, in a sense, writes itself between the lines, about this other showplace of unconscious distortion, where the entwinement of meaning, lust and death, the inversion of internal and external, of that which is one's own and that which is foreign appears in a new and fateful manner: much could be said about the place where the subject is no longer master of "his" language, but rather is subjected to it. But instead of discussing these matters, we will have to content ourselves with this brief mention in order to continue the retelling of Schreber's story.

From the time he begins writing there is for this author no question as to how his story is to end. All human and divine assaults on him are frustrated by the Cosmic Order's laws and by the power of his nerves: their power of attraction steadily increases, his body swells up, stuffed full of souls and rays, filled with nerves of female lust; and in his mind—steeled by compulsive thinking, which has taught him to seek the cause and the purpose, the reason and the essence of things and not to dwell on their simple appearance—there can be no doubt as to the outcome. The book closes with Schreber's brilliant and unquestionable victory on all fronts. With the cultivation of femininity "inscribed . . . on my banner" (*M,* p. 149), Schreber marches ever closer to his goal, that of being unmanned and impregnated by God; he proceeds less in a military goose-step than in a seductive goosed-step, the meandering step of lust, in order thus to complete his seduction of God, thereby destroying his final resistance: "The experience of years has confirmed me in this view; indeed I believe that God would never attempt to withdraw (which always impairs my bodily well-being considerably) but would follow my attraction without resistance permanently and uninterruptedly, if only I could *always* be playing the woman's part in sexual embrace with myself, *always* rest my gaze on female beings, *always* look at female pictures, etc." (*M,* p. 210).

Schreber's main goal is to be God's own spectacle, continuously looking at women but more important, as the perfect woman in coitus with herself, *being looked at.* For God, however—that is, for the higher God, Ormuzd, who in distinction to His lower part, Ariman, has not yet succumbed entirely to Schreber's charms—matters appear somewhat differently. "Definitively tied" (*M,* p. 209) to Schreber's nerves, to his body, with a desire for continual pleasure and for unceasing passion, this God sees nothing in the world except Schreber. The diagnosis of a delusional relationship, Schreber remarks (*M,* pp. 251–252), applies less to him than to God, for whom he has become "the sole human being," and "the center of His interest." God has eyes for Schreber only: he stares, fixated, at him—and here a remarkable comparison occurs to Schreber—as "one used to say for many years after the 1870 war about the foreign policy of the French, that they stared at the gap in the Vosges as if hypnotized" (*M,* p. 232).

God stares at Schreber like . . . *Gott in Frankreich.* Yet surely God can hope for no more from this welcome sight than the French could from the gap in the Vosges. Is God perhaps pleased *because* he can observe the woman "in sexual embrace with [herself]"? Can it be that the spectacle helps him to forget, at least momentarily, that wretched and grevious hole?

Returning to Freud: Lacan

To answer these and other questions raised by a reading of the *Memoirs,* it is useful, if not indispensable, to return to the interpretation given by orthodox, mainstream Freudian psychoanalysis. It has generally limited itself to confirming Freud's reading, while at the same time reducing that reading to its most problematic and schematic aspect: the thesis of denied or rejected homosexuality as the core of paranoia and *a fortiori* of Schreber's case. The psychoanalytic studies that have followed Freud have indeed discovered information about the Schreber case, some of it significant—the works of Baumeyer, and Niederland, are particularly noteworthy.[38] Yet, with few exceptions, they have neglected to question either Freud's premises or their influence on his reading of the case. In what follows I shall briefly discuss two exceptions. But first to Freud himself.

Freud's central intention is expressed in the very title of his treatise: that of developing, by means of the Schreber case, a psychoanalytic theory of paranoia in general. At the heart of Freud's interpretation is the subject's defense against his own homosexual desires, which have been repressed, and which, owing to some external cause, reimpose themselves upon consciousness with renewed force. Insofar as the subject cannot or will not accept these wishes consciously (at the time of the Schreber treatise Freud had not yet conceptualized the superego), he must take recourse in various forms of defense, so as to make his own wishes unrecognizable as wishes. Freud describes these forms of defense as transformations of the sentence, "I (a man) love him": the various possible transpositions of subject, verb, and object generate the various forms of paranoia: delusions of persecution, erotomania, delusions of jealousy, and megalomania.[39]

Applied to Schreber, the theory implies a fixation on the father and older brother, which is later transferred to Flechsig and to God. Of Schreber's two main fantasies, the first, transformation into a woman, is primarily (whereas the second, saving mankind through divine impregnation, is only secondarily) a rationalization or a compromise, designed to justify the (desired) sacrifice of masculinity.

"We find ourselves," says Freud, "on the familiar ground of the father-complex," or more precisely on that of the so-called negative Oedipus. The reasons for this negation are decisive, yet Freud mentions them only incidentally, as if in passing. Homosexual fixation, in his view, is not so much the cause of a psychic process as its result: an effect of an Oedipal conflict. Under threat of castration by the father, the child abandons the mother as an object of love, but only in order to identify with her and assume her role. This, however, leaves the problem of castration largely unresolved, and indeed urgent, insofar as such identification with the mother—the archetype of being transformed into a woman—is, without castration, utterly unthinkable. Hence, whereas the threat of castration is repulsed by homosexuality—although not, of course, by homosexuality alone—at the same time it is also recognized, confirmed, and continually repeated. This process is what Freud elsewhere, in his essay on fetishism, calls "disavowal" (*Verleugnung*).[40]

Various objections have been made to this reading of Freud, which reduces his essay on Schreber to a schematic statement and, as we shall see, in no way exhausts it. Ferenczi very cautiously raised the first objections; although he agreed with Freud that a relationship obtains between paranoia and homosexuality, he did not find this an adequate explanation. Ferenczi then remarked that this aspect failed to account sufficiently for the *specificity* of paranoia vis-à-vis homosexuality. The question remained: "What conditions have to be fulfilled for infantile bi- or ambisexuality to develop into either homosexual neurosis, or paranoia?"[41]

This question has been addressed by two of the few authors who have sought to adhere to psychoanalytic theory while still attempting to examine critically Freud's Schreber interpretation: Ida Macalpine and Richard Hunter, who appended to their translation of the *Memoirs* into English their own thoughtful analysis. They turn the Freudian thesis around, asserting that what is primary is the fantasy not of emasculation but of the redeemer, a mythological-archaic (so-called heliolithic) fantasy of begetting that derives not from the Oedipus complex or from pre-Oedipal fixations, nor indeed from any sexual-genital source at all, but rather from an inborn, deeply felt wish to bring forth life and thereby overcome the limits of mortality. The weakness of such an interpretation—which owes more to Jung than to Freud—are, for Schreber's text at least, self-evident and require no further discussion. Yet the "somatic hallucinations," to which Macalpine and Hunter rightly call attention, are no better explained by being referred to a procreation fantasy than to a castration complex (in the strict sense). Even more serious is the fact that Macalpine and Hunter, no less than Schreber's other psychoanalytic commentators, completely ignore the aspect of paranoic discourse emphasized by Freud: its tendency to dissemble and distort. Thus, they base their arguments against the causality of castration, homosexuality, and so on, and in favor of the begetting fantasies, on a most unreliable witness: on Schreber himself or, rather, on his explicit statements, on what he *wants to say* (in distinction to what he actually *describes*). In their discussion we often read: "Schreber himself considered . . . ," and "Schreber makes this point clear . . ." (*M,* p. 398); such appeals to authority only make clear how little Freud's successors, whether orthodox or not, understand about the distorting intention of unconscious articulation, which, as in dreams, does not want to be understood and which *betrays itself* only as distortion.

Despite the shortcomings of an interpretation that would replace Freud's thesis with one even less adequate—one which can explain psychic conflict only in terms of the frustration of childlessness—Macalpine and Hunter are able to point out weaknesses in the Freudian and above all post-Freudian readings insofar as they invoke the Oedipal relation too schematically. Macalpine and Hunter emphasize that in clinical practice with paranoics, as well as in Schreber's case, the decisive point is not homosexuality as such but rather insecurity or confusion about one's sexual identity. The sun, God's main organ or instrument, is not simply a father, as Freud would have us believe, but equally "a whore" ("the sun is a whore," Schreber bellows),[42] and also "God": "O damn, it is extremely hard to say that God allows himself to be f. . . . ." (*M,* p. 159), the voices say. Macalpine and Hunter point to Schreber's multiple interest in questions of origin, genealogy, and creation. Finally, they focus attention on his body fantasies (largely neglected by Freud) as a decisive element in Schreber's delusional system.

There can be no doubt that such aspects must be included in any satisfactory interpretation of the *Memoirs*. It is equally clear that neither the thesis of repulsed homosexuality nor that of "heliolithic" fantasies of begetting is sufficient to do justice to the dynamics of Schreber's text. The fact that Schreber's most significant fantasies concern the *body* on the one hand, and *language* on the other; that body and language stand in the closest possible relation to each other; and, not least of all, that Schreber *writes,* that we are dealing here with a text which does not stand apart from what it describes, but which itself is included in it: none of this is taken into account, either by Freud or by Macalpine and Hunter. Only the French psychoanalyst Jacques Lacan has made such questions the center of his interpretation. He was the first to redefine boldly Freud's conceptual apparatus as being of an inherently linguistic nature. Inasmuch as Lacan's reading of Schreber's *Memoirs* presupposes a certain familiarity with the linguistic Freud interpretation, we need to consider a basic outline of the latter before going any further.

In his "return to Freud" Lacan starts with the notion that the structure of Freud's concept of the unconscious—its radical heterogeneity—is determined by the structure of language. Lacan understands language in terms of the semiotics of the Genevan linguist and founder of "structuralist" linguistics, Ferdinand de Saussure. Saussure's fundamental insight is that language, like any system of symbols, can function only on the basis of *differences*. Thus in order to denote something, it is essential first of all that the carriers of meaning, called "signifiers," differ from each other: only insofar as they are disparate can they refer to a positive content, what Saussure calls the "signified."

Lacan uses this differential or "diacritical" theory of linguistic articulation to conceptualize the symbolization process of unconscious desire. Hence desire—which for Lacan as for Freud is essentially unconscious, whether as wish, drive, or "libido"—is characterized by the fact that its objects are not real objects, not "signifieds" (to use Saussure's terminology) identical with themselves, but rather "signifiers," that is, elements which refer to something else, not through their internal constitution but through their differential relations to other elements, which are equally "signifiers." On this view reality in the ordinary sense of the word is accessible to the subject *only as an aftereffect of a symbolization process:* disturbances in the process affect its relationship to reality. And this is precisely the case with Schreber. But how should this disturbance be thought of, and what are its consequences?

Certainly it should not be thought of in terms of the simple concept of *projection:* even Freud, who often uses the concept in his Schreber essay, corrects himself in the end: "It was incorrect to say that the perception which was suppressed internally is projected outwards; the truth is rather, as we now see, that what was abolished internally [*das innerliche Aufgehobene*] returns from without."[43] But *what* is it that is abolished, only to return from without, as reality? Freud's answer is unambiguous: "His father's most dreaded threat, castration, actually provided the material for his wishful phantasy (at first resisted but later accepted) of being transformed into a woman."[44]

According to Freud, *castration*—at least initially—forms the core of what has been "abolished internally" and "returns from without." Important is how one understands this castration: whether as a real fact of a real development, or as an aspect of a structure that manifests itself within the development, yet whose function transcends the development and organizes it. These two styles of thought—the genetic and the structural—are both found in Freud and are related to each other in somewhat the same manner as are the manifest and latent content of a dream. Against the tendency of many psychoanalysts to read Freud only genetically, and thereby to assimilate his thought to egopsychology (for the temporality and conceptual apparatus of the genetic perspective are inseparably linked to the primacy of the ego), Lacan tries to elaborate the primacy of the structural aspects in Freud.

One can particularize this issue in terms of Macalpine and Hunter's criticism of Freud's interpretation of Schreber's case. Freud, they claim, grasps the case exclusively in terms of the Oedipus complex, as a *sexual* problematic. Yet Macalpine and Hunter tacitly follow the psychoanalytic establishment they so severely criticize, insofar as they construe the Oedipal aspect to be a *genetic* category, from which the "Oedipal = genital = sexual" equation derives. Castration, they agree, is tied to a specific Oedipal = genital phase of development, whereas in Schreber's case much earlier and more archaic phases are decisive, phases in which castration and Oedipus have no place. Freud's procedure, however, militates in and of itself against any such schematization; he always approaches linear phenomena from a structural standpoint. Thus, in Schreber's case he considers the "fixation" on the phase of early (pregenital) narcissism to be motivated by the rejection of castration. Lacan argues that for Freud the Oedipal relation is never limited to a purely genetic phase, but rather determines the subject's entire development by providing the minimal symbolic structure that constitutes unconscious desire from the start.[45] How does this structure then come to prevail in the subject?

Lacan's answer is: by means of the "phallus," and of the "castration" that mediates it. Castration names the confrontation of the subject with the symbolic structure of its desire. As Freud shows, the discovery that the mother lacks a penis marks the decisive moment when castration begins to affect the child: this discovery brings with it the certainty that something like not having a penis is possible as a permanent condition. More important, since the child assumes that everyone has a penis, he interprets the absence of the organ as implying the reality of castration. Castration is thereby regarded as a real possibility. Castration thereby transforms the object of desire into that which it has always already tended to be, although the subject only gradually develops an organ for it: into a *signifier*. For the phallus is neither something (the penis of the mother), nor is it simply *nothing* (the castration of the mother); rather, it marks the differential relationship making possible, and structuring, the articulation of gender identity. The phallus—for Lacan, the *signifier of desire as such*—signifies something that neither is, nor is not: it signifies a difference. Hence, what until now has appeared to be either real or purely psychic—castration, the phallus, and the Oedipal structure—reveals itself to be eminently *linguistic* within the individual subject's economy and history. Castration marks the subject's access to the differential-symbolic structure of articulated desire.

Yet the extent of this access depends, says Lacan, on another linguistic relationship: that of the subject to the "Name-of-the-Father" (*Nom-du-Père*). That castration and the father are connected is, of course, nothing new to psychoanalysis; new and significant is the attempt to understand this connection as an essentially symbolic one, that is, in the differential-diacritical sense (in sharp contrast to the traditional notion of symbol). The Name-of-the-Father can be no normal name: it was Saussure who emphasized that the function of language as a system of signification is to be distinguished from the operation of naming.[46] To the extent that the name emphasizes the identity with the named, Lacan's concept of the symbolic as a movement of differences generating identity (the signified) as its aftereffect has little to do with it. According to Lacan, what the Name-of-the-Father signifies is nothing other than the dead father, for only insofar as he is dead, can the father have an effect as a symbol. Lacan refers in this context to Freud's *Totem and Taboo,* which he considers to be a mythical reconstruction not of actual primal history but of symbolic necessity, a reconstruction that cannot be understood in terms of traditional logic: for the function of the father has a psychic effect precisely because a name can distinguish itself from the named and can therefore develop its symbolic power independently of the person who bears it.

According to Lacan, Schreber rejects or "forecloses" the Name-of-the-Father. In contrast to the normal process of repression—which on the one hand implies a kind of recognition or acknowledgment of the repressed as its precondition, and on the other hand entails the continual presence of the repressed as an unconscious cathexis—Lacan's concept of "foreclosure" (a translation of Freud's *Verwerfung*) seems to entail the "Aufhebung" Freud speaks of, the exclusion of something that returns from without, as reality. This *Aufhebung* as *Verwerfung* differs from repression in that it leaves no traces from which future symbolization could be structured, but simply a hole, a gap in the symbolical or, more precisely, a rent in the Symbolical.

Here I break off the discussion of Lacan without any excessive apologies for its distortions, which result both from the fragmentary, highly elliptical character of Lacan's discourse, as well as from the fact that a comprehensive description of Lacan's thought in this context is simply not possible.[47] Presupposing Lacanian theory as a working hypothesis, I shall in closing bring together certain aspects of the *Memoirs* having to do with the decisive relation between language and body. In this way I would like to indicate a direction for interpreting—in other words, a *manner of reading*—Schreber's text.

The Wondrous Wound; or, A Man Called Schneider

Schreber employs a simple "example" both to characterize compulsive thinking and to show how it not only misses its goal of destroying his mind, but brings about the exact opposite: "I meet a person I know by the name of Schneider. Seeing him the thought automatically arises 'This man's name is Schneider' or 'This is Mr. Schneider.' With it 'But why' or 'Why because' also resounds in my nerves" (*M*, pp. 179–180).

Normally, Schreber continues, one would consider such questions to be absurd and reject them with justified indignation: "What a silly question, the man's name is simply Schneider." Yet, "my nerves were unable or almost unable to behave like this . . . This very peculiar question 'why' occupies my nerves automatically—particularly if the question is repeated several times—until their thinking is diverted in another direction" (*M*, p. 180).

It is important to observe very carefully the nature of this "diversion" of thought: "My nerves perhaps answer first: Well, the man's name is Schneider because the father was also called Schneider." But this answer, which traces the name's origin back to the father, is unsatisfactory: "This trivial answer does not really pacify my nerves. Another chain of thought starts about why giving of names was introduced at all among people, its various forms among different peoples at different times . . . Thus an extremely simple observation under the pressure of compulsive thinking becomes the starting point of a very considerable mental task, usually not without bearing fruit" (*M,* p. 180).

One must not underestimate the significance of this "considerable mental task," generated as a by-product of compulsive thinking: it ultimately made possible Schreber's reconstruction of the Cosmic Order and of its crisis, as well as his composition of the *Memoirs*. The example alluded to is important not least of all for this reason. That it is not merely an arbitrary example—if such a thing is even possible—can be shown on a number of grounds. First, Schreber's concern with names is a very old one: his interest in "etymological questions" is, he says, stimulated particularly by compulsive thinking, which "has interested me in earlier days of health" (*M,* p. 179). Second, the names of his ancestors as well as those of Flechsig play a decisive role in his fantasy of soul murder: one notes formulations like "I presume that at one time a bearer of the name Flechsig—a human being carrying that name—succeeded in . . . " (*M,* p. 56); or that "the names of Flechsig and Schreber (probably not specifying any individual member of these families)" played "leading roles" (*M,* p. 54) in the soul murder. Even the theological implications of the Name-of-the-Father are present in Schreber's delirious genealogy (Paul *Theodor* Flechsig, Abraham *Fürchtegott* Flechsig, and so on).[48] Finally, the entire Cosmic Order is constructed by means of (and is constituted as) a series of names that, to Schreber, prove the objectivity of his own experience, since he did not earlier know these names "themselves."

All this would suggest that Schreber's example of naming was no mere fortuitous idea. Let us therefore examine it somewhat more closely. Unfortunately Schreber does not elaborate on the "considerable mental task" involved in his thoughts on naming. We are provided with only two details: first, the man Schreber meets is already known to him; second, his name is "Schneider." Yet there is a third detail as well, if only a negative one, one that has been disavowed: identifying the father as the origin of the name is, Schreber thinks, "trivial" and it does not "calm" his nerves, which search for the true "reason" that surely lies elsewhere. These are the elements of the example.

The fact that in our culture family names generally come from the father is something that Schreber considers trivial, something that hardly puts him at ease. The name itself suggests why this should be the case: the man named Schneider is so named not only because it was his father's name, or his grandfather's, or his great-grandfather's, but perhaps because an ancestor actually *was* a *Schneider* (a tailor). Or are *we* perhaps falling prey to the kind of compulsive thinking Schreber described?

Perhaps—except that a reading of the *Memoirs* reveals that tailors are at work everywhere: this is suggested first of all by the tear or rip in the Cosmic Order, but also by sentences that are only begun (*angeschnitten,* literally, cut into); by souls that are cut off (*abgeschnitten,* literally, cut up or away) from the total mass of divine nerves; by organs that are cut out (*herausgeschnitten*) and limbs that are dissected (*zerschnitten*). But above all, we are interested here in a different kind of cut, one discussed in the first postscript to the *Memoirs,* which concerns "miracles." Again, this is "a minor example" chosen by Schreber to "serve as proof" for the divine miracles being directed against him: "On 5th October 1900 while being shaved I received a small cut, which had quite frequently happened before. Walking through the garden afterwards I met the Government Assessor M.; he noted at once the inconspicuous little piece of sponge covering my cut (of about this size O) and asked me about it; I told him truthfully, that the barber had cut me" (*M,* p. 219).

This is but a minor incident, certainly, yet for Schreber (and hence for us as well) "extremely interesting and instructive." What actually took place? Schreber is nicked by the barber, whom he takes to be merely a tool of God, who "acted on the muscles of the barber's hand to give it a rapid movement," causing the cut. Schreber attempts to protect and hide the wound with a small piece of sponge, which he also illustrates, life-size, in the text. But this attempt at concealment is in turn thwarted, again by God, and this immediately draws the attention of the Government Assessor M. to the small mark; the hidden wound is discovered and becomes the object of a conversation initiated by the question, "What is that on your mouth?" The conversation, Schreber continues, satisfies the vanity of the rays, which—not unlike humans—are especially flattered when "recognition of their achievement or industry . . . is remarked on" (*M*, p. 219). Not much happens in this minor example, yet it may well be that the essential elements of Schreber's phantasm are collected here. What are these elements, and what is their phantasmic structure?

First, there is God, the "cutter" (*Schneider*), who wounds Schreber. Second, Schreber attempts not only to protect the wound but, more important, to hide it with a small piece of sponge, which *is then seen* in place of the wound. This insignificant piece of sponge is seen by God and becomes the object of a conversation that pleases the rays, since they (or their works) are thus observed and respected. On the one hand the wound is protected and hidden, on the other it is seen and talked about as something that is hidden. It is seen and talked about, however, not only by the Government Assessor M., but also—and this is the crucial point—by Schreber himself, who makes this minor incident into the subject of his first postscript. He describes the scene and reveals its true meaning: he gives the wound its true name—which comprehends its apparent name, "wound" (*Wunde*)—and at the same time sublates it. For, as the voices proclaim in recognition of Schreber's victory over God, "all nonsense cancels itself out." Yet here nonsense signifies "wound," and its sublation (*Wunder*) signifies "wonder" or "miracle." Like the small circle that Schreber draws in his text—not entirely trusting in the power of words, of verbal description—by means of his explanation the wound is supposed *to close* and at the same time to *heal itself,* as a wonder.

In this (phantasmic) light, the question of the Government Assessor M. implies a kind of Having that in fact entails a violation of the very thing to be possessed, namely, the body ("What is that on your mouth?"), but that, as a *miracle,* indicates a real possession. For Schreber *has* those rays—that is, God himself—in his body, as female nerves of lust radiating an irresistible attraction.

If it is thus the nature of miracles to destroy the body's integrity—be it Schreber's body or an inorganic one—then this integrity can be reestablished through a text that renames all *Wunden* to *Wunder* and reduces the latter to their cause, a text that ultimately consists in their absorption in Schreber's body.

For this reason, the body constitutes the ultimate goal of the *Memoirs*' composition and publication. This "essay, which seems to be growing to the size of a scientific work" (*M*, p. 123), will be published solely in the belief that it "would be of value both for science and the knowledge of religious truths" (*M*, p. 31); this *scientific* work has no other goal than to proffer its author's body—in its altered form, saturated with female nerves of lust—as an object of viewing: "I can do no more than *offer my person as object of scientific observation for the judgment of experts*. My *main motive in publishing this book* is to invite this" (*M*, p. 251).

Should this observation and judgment not be possible within his lifetime, Schreber hopes "that at some future time such peculiarities of my nervous system will be discovered by *dissection of my body*, which will provide stringent proof" (*M*, p. 251).

What Schreber would like to see established is the fact that *he holds God within his body*, that the *Wunde* of castration—which *is* not, and yet which is *not* nothing, insofar as it allows gender difference to articulate itself—has corporeal existence as a *Wunder*. Schreber's text attempts to control this difference, which structures both language and the subject (as a sexual being), by making the difference *visible*, so as to repeat and reverse the moment—the "apparition," as the voices say—when castration was discovered. Whereas as a woman Schreber is unmanned, he nonetheless *has it in him:* and like a woman, he can hope to *be* what he (no longer) *has*.

This is not only represented, it is linguistically distorted. The canceling out of nonsense—of that difference which, according to Saussure, makes possible language as well as the meaning it signifies—is followed by the return of the names, from without, announced by voices which still carry within them that rejected or foreclosed difference. Thus the cut leaves its traces in the "overlapping" (*Überschneidung*, literally, "over-cutting") of wound and wonder; and in Schreber's firm belief (*Überzeugung*, literally, "over-begetting") in a divine "spontaneous generation,"[49] one without difference and prior to all distinction (prior to all castration); and in many other examples whose play can only be considered exemplary.

But since his language seeks to dissolve into something seen, into an "apparition," I will close with an *image* that perhaps describes most clearly the movement and aspiration of the *Memoirs*. In the postscript concerning "hallucinations," Schreber renders the rays as he "can see them *only* with my mind's eye" (*M*, p. 227): "The filaments aiming at my head and apparently originating from the sun or other distant stars do *not* come towards me in a straight line but in a kind of circle or parabola, similar perhaps to the way the chariots in the games of the old Romans drove round the *Meta,* or a special variety of skittles where the ball fastened to a string is first thrown around a post before it strikes the ninepins" (*M,* p. 228).

The rays, instead of coming at him directly, take a detour, just as, during the tournament, the Roman chariots of war drove around the *meta*. The *meta* were columns at the upper and lower end of the Roman circus around which the racers had to drive seven times. Schreber's *Memoirs* are the parable of this parabola whose course runs seven times around a divided middle before disappearing into it.

NOTES

1. Quoted in Franz Baumeyer, "Der Fall Schreber," *Psyche* 9 (1955–56): 536.
2. D. G. M. Schreber, *Das Pangymnastikon* (Leipzig, 1860), p. 2.
3. Ibid., p. 4.
4. Ibid., p. vi.
5. Alfons Ritter, *Schreber, das Bildungssystem eines Arztes* (Ph.D. diss., University of Erlangen, 1936), p. 19.
6. Baumeyer, "Der Fall Schreber," p. 515.
7. Quoted in William G. Niederland, "Schrebers 'angewunderte' Kindheitswelt," *Psyche* 22, no. 3 (1969): 200; trans. Benjamin Gregg. Niederland's analyses of D. G. M. Schreber's writings reveal the extent to which the father's text furnished the material for the son's delusional ideas. The voices' language is derived often literally from that of the father, while the orthopedic apparatus invented by the father recur in the son's book as a "head-compression machine" or as the "compression-of-the-chest miracle."
8. See references to the "bellowing miracle," in Daniel Paul Schreber, *Memoirs of My Nervous Illness,* trans. Ida Macalpine and Richard A. Hunter (Cambridge, Mass.: Harvard University Press, 1988), pp. 165 and passim. *Memoirs* hereafter cited as *M*.
9. See, however, Han Israels, *Schreber, Father and Son* (Amsterdam: Han Israels, 1981), for the most complete biographical study to date of the two Schrebers.

10. Quoted in Baumeyer, "Der Fall Schreber," p. 515.
11. See also his translation from the French: *Abhandlung von dem wahren Sitze des Rotzes [Treatise on the True Seat of Nasal Mucus]* (Liepzig, n.d.). Perhaps the following reference will suffice to indicate Daniel Paul Schreber's heartfelt if strained relationship to his ancestors: to demonstrate the senselessness of the devine "miracle," Schreber mentions "miracles . . . used to create anew lower animals" and insects, but adds: "all to no purpose whatsoever, as . . . the newly created insects belong to a species which in any case already exists in vast numbers, so that there is no need to call them into life afresh" (*M,* p. 196). *Novae Species Insectorum* by Johann Christian Daniel Schreber (a great uncle) appeared in 1759.
12. Quoted in Baumeyer, "Der Fall Schreber," p. 514.
13. Ibid.
14. Ibid., pp. 519–520.
15. Walter Benjamin, *Gesammelte Schriften,* vol. 4, pt. 2 Frankfurt am Main: Suhrkamp Verlag, 1972), pp. 615ff. Elias Canetti, *Crowds and Power,* trans. Carol Stewart (New York: Farrar, Straus and Giroux, 1984).
16. Exemplary for this type of nonreading is the book by Gilles Deleuze and Felix Guattari, *L'Anti-Oedipe* (Paris: Editions de Minuit, 1972), pp. 18–26, 66–67, and passim (*Anti-Oedipus: Capitalism and Schizophrenia,* trans. Robert Hurley, Mark Seem, and Helen R. Lane; Minneapolis: University of Minnesota Press, 1983; pp. 12–19, 56–57).
17. G. W. F. Hegel, *Phenomenology of Spirit,* trans. A. V. Miller and J. N. Findlay (Oxford: Oxford University Press, 1977), p. 18. Translation emended by Benjamin Gregg: *Sinnlichkeit* ("sense experience") is translated by Miller as "sensibility," and *sowohl des Ausgangs als der Rückkehr* ("departure and return") as "starting and stopping."
18. Sigmund Freud, "Psycho-Analytic Notes on an Autobiographical Account of a Case of Paranoia (Dementia Paranoides)," in *Standard Edition of the Complete Psychological Works of Sigmund Freud,* 24 vols., ed. James Strachey, trans. Strachey in collaboration with Anna Freud and assisted by Alix Strachey and Alan Tyson (London: Hogarth Press and the Institute of Psycho-Analysis, 1953–1974), vol. 12, pp. 17–18.
19. Ibid., p. 37, n. 1.

20. Ibid., p. 35.
21. Ibid., p. 79.
22. Ibid., p. 35.
23. Ibid., p. 9.
24. Sigmund Freud, "Moses and Monotheism," in *Standard Edition,* vol. 23, p. 43.
25. Ibid., p. 43.
26. "Indeed, dreams are so closely related to linguistic expression that Ferenczi has truly remarked that every tongue has its own dream-language. It is impossible as a rule to translate a dream into a foreign langauge . . ." (Freud, *The Interpretation of Dreams,* in *Standard Edition,* vol. 4, p. 99, n. 1). Cf. Jacques Derrida, "Freud and the Scene of Writing," in Derrida, *Writing and Difference,* trans. Alan Bass (Chicago: University or Chicago Press, 1978), pp. 196–231.
27. This and all subsequent quotations in this section are from Baumeyer, "Der Fall Schreber," pp. 515–518.
28. *Weltordnung,* translated by Macalpine and Hunter as "Order of the World"—*Gregg's note.*
29. *Verstandesnerven,* translated by Macalpine and Hunter as "nerves of intellect" (*M,* p. 45)—*Gregg's note.*
30. See Georges Bataille, *La part maudite* (Paris: Editions de Minuit, 1967). On the concept of "restricted economy," see also Jacques Derrida, "From Restricted to General Economy," in Derrida, *Writing and Difference,* pp. 251–277. Here an interpretation remains to be made which would reveal the social mediation of Schreber's delusional system not only in the sense of shared notions, but as a structuring factor. One would have to investigate especially the heightened problematic of identity of a (double) God who appears on the one hand as a transcendent Creator, and on the other as a limited subject, the phantasmal presentation of the bourgeois individual.
31. *Nervenanhang,* translated by Macalpine and Hunter as "nerve-contact."
32. Compare this formulation with the subtitle of a book by Schreber's father: *Anthropos: The Structural Wonder of the Human Organism.* No wonder, then, that Schreber remarks in a footnote that, once again, this is "an expression which I did not invent. I would have ["*hätte,*" translated by Macalpine and Hunter as "had"—Gregg's note] spoken," he continues, "of [a] *miraculous organization* . . ." (*M,* p. 54).

33. Regarding the Schreber Family's title—the "Margraves of Tuscany and Tasmania"—see Niederland, "Schrebers 'angewunderte' Kindheitswelt," pp. 216ff.
34. See William G. Niederland, "Three Notes on the Schreber Case," *Psychoanalytic Quarterly,* 20 (1951): 579–591.
35. *Widersetzte,* translated by Macalpine and Hunter as "may have resisted"—*Gregg's note.*
36. And, according to Freud and Bataille, not for Schreber's nerves!
37. *M,* p. 175, n. 96. The function of spoken language in the constitution and preservation of identity becomes quite clear here: it is no accident that in Schreber's book, that which is heterogeneous and foreign to the ego makes use of written language—the system of notation—as an instrument (which is dead, automatic, and mindless) against the desire and power of Schreber's nerves. On the general problematic of the priority of phonetic language in Western thought, see Jacques Derrida, *Of Grammatology,* trans. Gayatri Chakravorty Spivak (Baltimore: Johns Hopkins University Press, 1976).
38. In addition to Baumeyer, "Der Fall Schreber," see also Franz Baumeyer, "Noch ein Nachtrag zu Freuds Arbeit über Schreber," *Zeitschrift für Psychosomatische Medizin 16* (1970): 243–245; William G. Niederland, *The Schreber Case: Psychoanalytic Profile of a Paranoid Personality* (New York: Quadrangle Books, 1974). The non-psychoanalytic investigations of Han Israels, *Schreber, Father and Son,* should also be mentioned here.
39. See Freud, "Case of Paranoia, pp. 63ff.
40. Freud, "Fetishism," in, *Standard Edition,* vol. 21.
41. Sandor Ferenczi, "On the Part Played by Homosexuality in the Pathogenesis of Paranoia," in, Ferenczi and Otto Rank, *Sex in Psycho-Analysis,* trans. Ernest Jones (New York: Dover, 1956), p. 156; translation emended by Benjamin Gregg.
42. *M,* p. 270. It should be noted that Schreber does not himself record these (his own) expressions; they are mentioned solely in Dr. Weber's court-ordered medical opinion.
43. Freud, "Case of Paranoia," p. 71.
44. Ibid., p. 56.
45. In this context one should refer to Melanie Klein, who thought she had traced the beginnings of the triadic,

Oedipal relation to earliest childhood. See the essays collected in Klein, *The Psychoanalysis of Children* (Atlantic Highlands, N.J.: Humanities Press, 1969).

46. Ferdinand de Saussure, *Course in General Linguistics,* trans. Wade Baskin (New York: McGraw-Hill, 1964).
47. See Jacques Lacan, "On a Question Preliminary to Any Possible Treatment of Psychosis," in, Lacan, *Ecrits: A Selection,* trans. Alan Sheridan (New York: Norton, 1977). See also Samuel Weber, *Rückkehr zu Freud: Jacques Lacans Ent-Stellung der Psychoanalyse* (Berlin: Ullstein, 1978). An English translation, *Return to Freud,* trans. Michael Levine, is forthcoming from Cambridge University Press.
48. Cf. Lacan, *Ecrits,* p. 580.
49. See *M,* p. 191: "In the previous chapter I expressed my opinion that *spontaneous generation* (parentless generation) does actually occur"; that Schreber would very much have liked to have stood *above all begetting* on the strength of his *convictions* can at least be surmised.

MEMOIRS OF MY NERVOUS ILLNESS

TRANSLATORS' INTRODUCTION

Family History

Daniel Paul Schreber came of a distinguished family. His father, Daniel Gottlob Moritz Schreber, of Leipzig (15th October 1808–11th November 1861), the son of an advocate, was a physician and lecturer at Leipzig University where he founded an Institute of Orthopaedics. He was also an educationalist and social reformer with an apostle-like mission to bring health, happiness and bliss to the masses through physical culture. He advocated gymnastics in the treatment of disease, and organized outdoor games and playing fields for the young. In German-speaking countries small allotment gardens are called *Schrebergärten* after him. He published a number of books of which the titles alone, quite apart from their text, show that he was eccentric, not to say a crank.

Chapter III of Schreber's Memoirs originally dealt with " other members of my family ". Unfortunately it was considered unfit for publication in the German edition. However, in other places Schreber mentions his mother who was still alive, an older and a younger sister, a brother-in-law and sister-in-law, and " the memory of my brother ".

Schreber says he knew his family tree, of which he was very proud, " extremely well ". He refers several times to events affecting members of the Schreber family in the eighteenth century. The voices said that the Schrebers " belonged to the highest heavenly nobility ", to which he explains only persons of outstanding achievement were raised. The following famous Schrebers were ancestors; all shared the Christian name Daniel.

* For instance, one of his books is called GLÜCKSELIGKEITSLEHRE FUR DAS PHYSICHE LEBEN DES MENSCHEN (perhaps best translated as HOW TO ACHIEVE HAPPINESS AND BLISS BY PHYSICAL CULTURE.) His most widely known work is MEDICAL INDOOR GYMNASTICS which reached eight editions in the first six years and between thirty and forty in all, was translated into seven languages, into English from the 3rd edition in 1856 and from the 26th in 1912. It starts as follows " Man is so to speak a *double being* consisting of a miraculous intimate union of a mental with a bodily nature ". This is an example of the philosophical speculations about the origin of man and the nature of the human soul, coupled with high-flung zeal to improve mankind, which pervades all his publications. Certain passages in the Memoirs bring home how much our author was a chip off the old block.

Daniel Gottfried Schreber (?–1777), Professor of Agriculture and Economics, was a prolific writer on many subjects, including mineralogy, economics, history, etc. Of his many books, seventeen are preserved in the British Museum, London. His son, Schreber's great uncle, Johann Christian Daniel (von) Schreber (1739–1810) was the most famous. He was active in many fields of science, Professor of Medicine and Superintendent of the Botanical Garden at the University of Erlangen, ennobled in 1791, and among many other honours elected Fellow of the Royal Society of London. He participated in a work on public administration and finance (*Cameral–Statistik*) with his father. Thirty-two of his works are preserved in the British Museum, London, including NOVAE SPECIES INSECTORUM*, a "work of prime importance as it contains the first description of twelve insects, with illustrations, and the author makes use of the Linnean nomenclature, now universally adopted" (Griffin, 1939). Many of his books are on botany, and he published an Atlas of the Mammalia.

Personal History

Little is known of the author of the Memoirs†, probably because the family did not wish to publicize any details about him. It is even said that they bought up and destroyed most copies of the Memoirs. Freud (1911), from private information supplied by a physician in Dresden, gave Schreber's age as 51 at the beginning of his second illness in 1893, making the year of his birth 1842. From the Memoirs we know that he was happily married, except that the couple were "repeatedly disappointed in our hope of being blessed with children". Baumeyer (1951) claimed to have found mental hospital records showing that Schreber was admitted to an Asylum for the third time in 1907 following the death of his wife, and died there in 1911. It has, however, not been possible to confirm this.

Schreber followed the legal profession and in 1893 was promoted to the high office of *Senatspräsident*, i.e. President of a panel of Judges at the Court of Appeal (the Superior Country Court) at Dresden, at a comparatively early age. This was the Supreme Court of the Kingdom of Saxony, which at that time had a population of between

* Curiously, newly created insects played a large part in Schreber's delusions! (Cf. Memoirs, Chapter VIII).

† During our search for more information about Schreber, particularly the period following publication of the Memoirs, we came into possession of information relating to his parents and collaterals. None of it unfortunately has a direct bearing on the understanding of his psychosis, and we have therefore not included it.

4 and 5 millions. Only the Imperial German High Court in Leipzig was superior to it.

Some light is thrown on Schreber's personality by the subjects which interested him and by some of the books he says he "read repeatedly in the ten years preceding my illness". Apart from his profession these included natural history, particularly the doctrine of evolution, the natural sciences, astronomy and philosophy. From other parts of the book it appears he was widely read in the history of religion and literature, interested in etymology, and fond of music. His Greek was fluent: the voices talked in Greek "when I read a Greek book". His candidature for the *Reichstag* in 1884 bespeaks his interest in public affairs and politics. Dr. Weber, Superintendent of Sonnenstein Asylum, testified in Court that Schreber had wide and varied cultural interests, and was well informed on all matters of art, history, public welfare, administration—in fact on all general topics. He also stressed Schreber's unimpeachable honesty and outstanding intelligence, with which the Judges agreed.

History of Illness

Schreber suffered twice from a "nervous illness". The first illness started in the autumn of 1884 and was described as "severe hypochondriasis without any incidents bordering on the supernatural". At the beginning of December 1884 he was admitted to the Psychiatric Clinic of the University of Leipzig as a patient of its Director, Professor Paul Emil Flechsig.* He was discharged early in June the following year, and had fully recovered by the end of 1885 when he resumed his position as Judge at the Country Court in Leipzig, one of five Governmental Districts into which Saxony was divided.

The second illness, the subject proper of the Memoirs, started in October 1893 and "still persists". In the middle of November 1893, that is six weeks after taking up office as *Senatspräsident* to which he had been raised, he was admitted to the same Clinic, again under Flechsig. In June 1894 he was sent from Flechsig's Clinic to Lindenhof, Dr. Pierson's Private Asylum in Coswig near Dresden.† After a fortnight there he was transferred to Sonnenstein Asylum in Pirna, near Dresden, the first German Public Mental Hospital, situated in the Kingdom of Saxony.‡ Schreber

* See legend to Flechsig's portrait (Plate 1).

† A Private Asylum for about 95 patients of both sexes.

‡ See plates 2, 3 and 4.

was puzzled why his transfer to Sonnenstein was interrupted by a short stay at Lindenhof. He wondered whether it was designed to break the journey, whether his rooms at Sonnenstein were not ready; possibly it was a question of expense. Schreber himself mentions that he was more severely hallucinated and out of contact at Dr. Pierson's Asylum, the "Devil's Kitchen", as he called it, than he had been before: he may therefore have become too dangerous to keep in a small private asylum.

He remained at Sonnenstein Asylum for almost nine years, and there wrote his Memoirs. In the Preface to the book dated December 1902, he stated his intention to leave the Asylum early in 1903. He had succeeded in having his tutelage* rescinded in the Court of Appeal in September 1902 and from then on was free to discharge himself. The "Open Letter" to Professor Flechsig which also prefaces the Memoirs was written from Dresden in March 1903, which means he must have left the Asylum by then. There are no subsequent reliable data about him.

The "Memoirs"

The Memoirs were not originally planned as a book. During the years of his illness Schreber kept notes in shorthand, at first on little scraps of paper; later he made entries in diaries and notebooks, which he called his "Little Studies". When in 1900, after seven years in asylums, he had recovered sufficiently to strive for independence and restoration of his legal capacity, he started to write the Memoirs from these notes and jottings in anticipation of his release, in order to give his wife and others who would then be around him "at least an approximate idea of my religious conceptions so that they may have some understanding of the necessity which forces me to various oddities of behaviour". The oddities refer to his habit of wearing cheap jewellery, ribbons, or other feminine ornaments for severals hours a day, and to attacks of compulsive bellowing which set in when the process of transformation into a woman was impeded. Only in the process of writing did the work grow "into a scientific treatise", and with it Schreber intended to make available to a wider public a full account of his experiences, observations and reflections while "suffering from a nervous illness". The book's purpose was now to invite qualified men of science to investigate and examine his body, and

* German legal procedure for dealing with cases of insanity: by order of the Court the patient was placed under the care of a guardian or Committee of the person, deprived of the management of his affairs and disposal of his person.

observe future developments on him to verify " what other people think are delusions and hallucinations ", namely that his body was gradually being transformed into a female body, a process he called " unmanning ". Schreber believed that he was unique in such a transformation and that it had never previously been observed on a human being: if confirmed and established as a fact by men of science, new evidence would be provided about divine creative power and the nature of God, and proof furnished of the continuance of life after death and of the existence of a living God, which would lead to a new conception of religious truths. Believing himself the sole object of these divine miracles, Schreber felt it was his duty to spread this knowledge which would " in the highest degree act fruitfully and as a blessing to mankind ".

Schreber's Memoirs, then, were not prompted by litigious intent, nor by a desire to place blame on doctors, institutions and other public authorities, nor published for the sake of sensationalism or personal gain; this in itself sets the Memoirs far above other self-descriptions of mental patients.

Appendix to the Memoirs

The Appendix to the Memoirs is made up of documents from the files of the Court about Schreber's tutelage, that is the Court orders depriving him of the management of his affairs and legally detaining him in the Asylum, and their later suspension. He had entered the Psychiatric Clinic in Leipzig voluntarily in November 1893; when he " learned some years later ", apparently in 1899, that he had been placed under temporary tutelage as early as 1895, " I approached the authorities demanding a decision as to whether the temporary tutelage was to be made permanent or whether it could be rescinded ". Contrary to his expectation, a formal order for his tutelage was made by the District Court, Dresden, in March 1900. Because Schreber considered " the grounds for the decision unsubstantiated " he contested this order in the Country Court of Dresden. To his surprise it was confirmed by the Court in April 1901. He then took the matter to the Superior Country Court in Dresden, the highest Appeal Court of Saxony, playing an active part himself in conducting his case and in the pleadings in Court; especially in formulating the legally excellent grounds for his appeal. He succeeded in having his tutelage rescinded by this Court in September 1902, although obviously still mentally ill. He was thus free again to manage himself and his affairs, and at liberty to leave the Asylum.

Appended to the Memoirs are: Schreber's grounds for his appeal, three extensive expert reports on his mental state and the development of his illness by Dr. G. Weber, a well-known medico-legal expert and Superintendent of Sonnenstein, under whose care Schreber had been since 1894; also the Superior Court's Judgment in full. In them the involved psychiatric and legal questions raised by insanity are fully discussed, the case being very carefully tried because of Schreber's social position. They give to Schreber's own story a framework of objectivity which still allows full clinical evaluation of 'the Schreber case' today. Even by themselves they are of great interest: the relation of insanity to legal responsibility, the question of partial or total disturbance, whether insight precludes insanity in law, and the fundamental issue whether insanity is a disturbance of emotions or intellect or both, are discussed in exactly the same way in Courts today as they were over fifty years ago.

Reviews of the Memoirs

The book was favourably reviewed when it appeared. "Dr. Schreber's Memoirs stand sky-high above publications of other mental patients ... Written without malicious intent, they contain the story of his mental illness from his point of view and are of the greatest interest ... The great clinical value of this book is further enhanced by the inclusion of Court documents and medical reports ... The Memoirs deserve the closest study" (Pelman, 1903). Another reviewer said "Never before have the symptoms of paranoia been offered in such detail and so completely ... because of his high intelligence and logical training, Schreber's presentation must be called perfect by the well-informed physician. The book is therefore recommended to all psychiatrists" (Windscheid, 1904). Pfeiffer (1904) stressed the book's value from the legal point of view as well as its clinical descriptions. Dr. Weber considered "the Memoirs ... not only valuable from the scientific medical point of view ..., but they also afford ample support of practical value for understanding the patient's behaviour" because they "deal in the most detailed manner with the history of his illness of many years' duration, both in its external relations and in its inner development".

What makes the Memoirs an "invaluable book" (Freud, 1923) for the understanding of mental illness in general? In short, it is that despite the severity of his psychosis, Schreber's superior intelligence and legal training ennabled him "to make sense of it", that is to systematize it, as it abated. In other words, Schreber was able to speak and formulate feelings and ideas in words, where other psychotics are overwhelmed and therefore mute. Further, had he not kept notes during his illness, it is extremely doubtful, as Schreber himself says, whether he could have remembered so much of it, nor told it in so faithful and consecutive a fashion.

Such a complicated narrative would have been impossible to present in speech: the situation of an interview itself colours a patient's utterances and determines their choice, as he is bound to be influenced by the listener. Dr. Weber stated in Court that " These writings are to be given all the more weight because in general the patient is little inclined to reveal his pathological ideas to other people, and further because these ideas are elaborated in so complicated and subtle a manner, that he himself admits that rendering them by word of mouth is difficult ". This is true of all seriously ill patients: even did they wish to reveal the trends and inner connections of their fantasies and thoughts, the content of their hallucinations and delusions—in fact what their illness is about—they could not do so, least of all in coherent form in conversation. To write such a frank autobiographical account required Judge Schreber's intellect, his determination to grapple with his madness, his training in logical thinking, his inborn quest for truth, his integrity, absolute frankness, and finally admirable courage in laying his innermost thoughts and feelings bare before other people, knowing that they thought him mad.

Symptomatology

Schreber describes what happened to him and in him from the beginning of his illness, including two years during which he was so violent and noisy that—to his great indignation—he had to be confined in a padded cell at night, be accompanied by three attendants in the Asylum's garden, and forcibly fed; when he was negativistic, withdrawn, mute and immobile for long periods, impulsive, repeatedly attempted suicide, massively hallucinated and deluded about his own body and his surroundings, suffered from unbearable insomnia, tortured by compulsive acting and obsessive thinking. We follow the intense struggle with his delusions, his first glimpses of insight and how he slowly resumed contact with " the outside world ". Finally we see a transvestite emerge from this state of " acute hallucinatory insanity ", with a complicated system of delusions side by side with unimpaired capacity for clear and logical reasoning, which allowed him to play a decisive part in having his tutelage rescinded. With great acuity and keen logic he "argued right from wrong premises" (Locke, 1690), so that as Dr. Weber said in Court, "little would be noticeable" of his insanity "to an observer not informed of his total state".

So manifold were the symptoms he displayed at one time or another that almost the whole symptomatology of the entire field of psychiatric abnormality is described. Comparison with the items listed in a current textbook on psychiatry (Henderson and Gillespie, 1951) in the chapter on 'Symptomatology', allowed us to tick off nearly all as touched on in the Memoirs.

Schreber enters Psychiatry and Psychoanalysis

Schreber is now the most frequently quoted patient in psychiatry; how did he enter it? Extensive self-descriptions have occasionally been published, a not dissimilar case for instance by Haslam (1810). But they are forgotten. Their value being merely narrative and descriptive, they added little to knowledge of the psychotic mind; in part this was because they were read without gain by psychiatrists as one could not discern meaning or sense in them. Thus they had more literary and anecdotal than psychiatric value. Although it was widely recognized in the second half of last century that psychotic products were indicative of a "second personality" or "second mind", and stemmed from "unconscious mentation" or "unconscious cerebration"*, this could not be utilized in clinical psychiatry for lack of a technique of investigating the "unconscious" and its mechanisms; and therefore nothing was known of its connections with conscious mind. In brief, reading the story of one psychotic did not help to understand another.

It was left to Freud to discover the technique of investigating and tracing out the unconscious, of discovering its mechanisms and its relation to conscious mind. Thus Freud for the first time made the content of mental symptoms understandable, his historic contribution to mental science. When he discovered the phenomena of transference, free association, dreams as "the royal road to the unconscious", the importance of sexuality, the mechanisms of

* There was even controversy about priority in the use of this term: referring to Carpenter's (1837) "Voluntary and Instinctive Actions of Living Beings", Tuke (1891) says "With his name has been associated the phrase 'unconscious cerebration'. and although, I think, it must be admitted that in the regrettable contention for priority which occurred between Dr. Carpenter and Professor Laycock, the latter's claims are well founded, Dr. Carpenter's exposition of mental automatism was able, and on the whole formed a valuable contribution to psychology".

repression, condensation, projection, sublimation, of symbolism, slips, etc., he demonstrated that mental symptoms are not haphazard products of the mind, but are determined, have a meaning, and can be traced to their unconscious origin and connections and hence sense made of them.* Only since Freud replaced philosophical and psychological speculation by providing a new technique for investigating the unconscious mind, has it been possible to speak of a pathology of the mind, *psychopathology*, to assess the significance of symptoms and search for the mental mechanisms of psychiatric symptom formation.

The impact of Freud's discoveries on psychiatry is put succinctly by Bleuler, one of his earliest supporters, in the introduction to his classic DEMENTIA PRAECOX OR THE GROUP OF SCHRIZOPHRENIAS (written 1908, published 1911, but not translated till 1950): "*The whole conception of dementia praecox originates with Kraepelin; we owe to him alone the grouping and descriptions of individual symptoms . . . A major part of attempting to enlarge the pathology further is nothing but the application to dementia praecox of Freud's ideas*" (Bleuler's italics). In this book Bleuler moved away from the sterile classificatory excercises based on a descriptive nosology of the previous century, to an attempted psychopathology of mental disease made possible by Freud's work. In this way he cut across the rigid Kraepelinian diagnostic entities, particularly the division of psychoses into two supposedly fundamentally different types: dementia praecox and manic-depressive insanity.† At one time there was also a third, paranoia. Bleuler quotes repeatedly from Schreber's Memoirs, utilizing the insight to be gained from them. It may therefore be said that it was Bleuler who, stimulated by Freud's work, introduced Schreber into psychiatry, as he did the mind into dementia praecox. Meyer also attempted to understand the psychoses in their mental develop-

* Progress in science is dependent on and follows the discovery of new techniques. Although this is more evident in the physical branches of medical science it is equally true of psychology, the science of the mind. The only discovery in technique of investigating the mind is the one made by Freud. Hence the great impetus it gave to mental science. But the demonstration of a dynamic unconscious and its relation to conscious mind and how it can be investigated, is not the same as the merits or demerits of the classical psychoanalytic technique as a form of psychiatric treatment, which in itself raises quite different problems. Nor should his fundamental discovery of the laws of the unconscious be confused or even equated with the theoretical superstructure of psychoanalytic interpretations and hypotheses built on them; these remain debatable and open to discussion, as in Schreber's case.

† In the history of psychiatry classificatory zeal has always varied inversely with psychological understanding.

ment and stood out for the psychogenesis of dementia praecox.* He also frequently referred to Schreber, at first in connection with Bleuler's remarks, later to Freud's study as well.

Yet Schreber really came into his own only when Freud seized the opportunity provided by the Memoirs to apply his method for the first time to the case material of a mental hospital patient. In 1911 he published "Psychoanalytic Notes upon an Autobiographical Account of a Case of Paranoia (Dementia Paranoides)", now known as the Schreber case.† Freud interpreted Schreber's illness as the outcome of conflict over unconscious homosexuality:‡ an upsurge of unconscious homosexuality was unacceptable to Schreber's personality because of its implied castration threat, and the ensuing struggle led to his mental illness and withdrawal from reality. Bleuler (1912), reviewing Freud's analysis of the Schreber case as a clinical psychiatrist friendly to psychoanalysis, was guarded about Freud's interpretation and the construction he put upon the illness. He doubted whether unconscious homosexuality, though obviously playing a part in the symptomatology of the case, could account aetiologically or phenomenologically for Schreber's illness, paranoid schizophrenia.

Psychoanalysis and the Psychoses

But by psychoanalysts, Freud's thesis was immediately and generally accepted as forming the basis of 'paranoia'. Thenceforth paranoid symptom formation was considered as explained by conflict over unconscious homosexuality and established as identical with the old entity paranoia. Despite Freud's statement that in his study he had not attempted to cover the "much wider concept of dementia praecox", his theoretical formulations arising

* Like Bleuler he also opposed the concept of separate disease entities among the psychoses, particularly the sharp division between dementia praecox and manic-depressive insanity. Despite these efforts developments of the last two decades have again increased the cleavage; the symptom of depression, itself of infinite variety and significance, has been raised to the status of a disease *sui generis* under the impact of physical procedures, and has reached a popularity as a diagnosis hardly envisaged even by Kraepelin. This shows the close interaction of classification and therapy; the latter depending on *ad hoc* assessment, forces a symptomatological diagnosis; as Nasse (1818) says "the more remedies, the more names for diseases and the less understanding".

† It is possible that Freud's attention had been drawn to Schreber's Memoirs by Bleuler as they were at the time co-editors with Jung of JAHRBUCH FUR PSYCHOANALYTISCHE UND PSYCHOPATHOLOGISCHE FORSCHUNGEN, a biannual publication started in 1909 and discontinued in 1912, in which this study first appeared.

‡ Having its origin in the boy's inverted Oedipus situations, i.e. his homosexual attachment to a father figure.

from it were nevertheless imperceptibly extended in psychoanalysis to schizophrenia and the psychoses in general; as such they entered psychiatric literature as "the psychoanalytic theory of psychosis" Psychoanalytic studies of the psychoses are based on what came to be regarded as fundamental tenets, despite terminological confusion and "obvious logical fallacies" (Menninger, 1942). "Perhaps no psychoanalytic theory of a psychosis rests on firmer foundations or has been less frequently attacked" than "Freud's brilliant analysis of the Schreber case" (Knight, 1940).

According to Redlich (1952) "Most of the . . . psychological propositions about schizophrenia . . . may be traced back to . . . Freud's ingenious discussion of the Schreber case". Zilboorg (1941) says that "Freud's views on schizophrenia . . . were based . . . on . . . the Schreber case . . . later clinical studies corroborated Freud's views that certain aspects of unconscious homosexuality are the determining factor in the development of schizophrenia". Fenichel (1945) gives a long list of confirmatory publications.

More than half a century has passed since the publication of the Memoirs: today Schreber is mentioned in almost all textbooks of psychiatry, usually under the heading of paranoia or schizophrenia, and almost invariably in connection with Freud's name, whether in confirmation or rejection of his thesis. But the Memoirs themselves seem not to have been consulted again: psychiatric and psychoanalytic texts quote only those passages extracted by Freud in support of his interpretation. Schreber's Memoirs are quoted as interpreted by Freud, but they are not read: "Freud's study of Dr. Schreber" is accepted as one of "the best real-life descriptions of schizophrenics" (Gillies, 1950). Clearly a kind of myth has developed around this almost legendary name: it seems as if to be quoted but not read is the hallmark of the literary and scientific classic. As a result Freud's analysis had never been re-evaluated by investigation of the original Memoirs until recently (Macalpine and Hunter, 1953). Perhaps this was partly due to the book having long been very scarce and never before translated.

Historically seen, an interesting development has taken place: Freud selected from the vast symptomatology of Schreber's psychosis the elements of persecution, and concentrated his attention on material which seemed to lend weight to his thesis that unconscious homosexuality was the aetiological factor in the illness. This had important and far reaching consequences. First, tracing Schreber's illness back—like the psychoneuroses—to the Oedipus-complex, Freud treated it as if it were a neurosis, while at the same time maintaining a distinction between neurosis and psychosis (Freud, 1924).* In this way a confusion of terminology arose which continues to beset much of psychoanalytic theory, practice and writing. Second, 'paranoid' symptoms became synonymous with persecutory fears or delusions and in this sense were elevated to the signal symptom, and indeed hallmark of psychosis†. This led to neglect of other, often much earlier, disturbances of emotion, feeling, association, bodily sensations, etc., not in relation to other people but primarily in the patient's relation to himself, his mind and his body, which almost invariably precede the development of a psychosis.

Classification

The third consequence of the general acceptance of Freud's analysis of the Schreber case concerns psychiatric classification. Freud who himself did not profess to be a psychiatrist, used psychiatric terminology freely and without regard. He accepted Kraepelin's dementia praecox concept, and also Bleuler's group of schizophrenias, assuming them to be identical though objecting to their names. At the same time he thought it "essential . . . that paranoia should be maintained as an independent clinical type however frequently the picture it presents may be complicated by the presence of schizophrenic features" (F. 463).‡ Yet he tried vaguely to combine dementia praecox, paranoia, and schizophrenia, by reintroducing Kahlbaum's old term paraphrenia for Schreber's illness: "It would seem to me the most convenient plan to give dementia praecox the name of *paraphrenia*. This term has no special connotation, and it would serve to indicate a relationship with paranoia (a term which may be regarded as fixed) and would further recall hebephrenia, an entity which is now merged in

* In "A Neurosis of Demoniacal Possession in the Seventeenth Century" Freud (1923) speaks of Schreber's psychosis and equates it with the painter's illness, which both in title and text is called a neurosis.

† The central importance given to this term could not be better illustrated than by the British school of psychoanalysis postulating a 'paranoid' (persecutory) position in the first year of life.

‡ Quotations from Freud's (1911) "Psychoanalytic Notes upon an Autobiographical Account of Paranoia (Dementia Paranoides)" are given as (F . . .); the page number refers to the translation in *Collected Papers*, 1949, **3**, 390–470.

dementia praecox. It is true that the name has already been proposed for other purposes; but this need not concern us, since the alternative applications have not passed into general use" (F. 463). Further he admitted that "it is not at all likely that homosexual impulses, which are so frequently (perhaps invariably) to be found in paranoia, play an equally important part in the aetiology of that far more comprehensive disorder, dementia praecox ... one of the great distinctions between dementia praecox and paranoia" is that paranoiacs "make use of projection", whereas the sufferer from "that far more comprehensive disorder, dementia praecox ... employs a hallucinatory (hysterical) mechanism" (F. 464).

But worse confusion of terms is to follow: "we can understand how a clinical picture such as Schreber's can come about, and merit the name of a paranoid dementia, from the fact that in its production of a wish-fantasy and of hallucinations it shows paraphrenic traits, while in its exciting cause, in its use of the mechanism of projection, and in its final issue it exhibits a paranoid character" (F. 464).

Paranoia

These passages clearly "show up the old principles of disease classification with bitter irony" (Bleuler, 1911), and the impossibility of coming "to any common understanding on the basis of the old diagnostic labels ... Thus, not even the masters of science can make themselves understood on the basis of the old concepts" (Bleuler, *loc. cit.*). Even in 1892, Tuke spoke of the "lamentable amount of confusion and obscurity" introduced by bringing back paranoia* into psychiatric nomenclature.

Paranoia—An historical digression

Paranoia, from Greek meaning wrong or faulty knowledge or reasoning, "antedates Hippocrates" (Cameron, 1944) when "it was most frequently used in a very general sense ... as the equivalent of our popular current term insanity". It was resurrected by Vogel in 1772 and further extended by Heinroth in 1818. Its application was then gradually restricted to partial insanity or monomania until Ziehen (1894) and Cramer (1895) "Threw together all the 'primary disorders of reasoning' ... including the acute and chronic forms and even all the delirious disorders of no matter what

* "The Greek etymology does not render us any assistance in the endeavour to comprehend the particular class of case to which it is applied" (Tuke, *loc. cit.*).

origin " (Meyer, 1928) under that title. Kraepelin " in a fit of indignation against Ziehen " (Meyer, 1917–18) reintroduced " dementia praecox ", a term first used by Morel (1860) to call " a halt to this paranoification of psychiatry . . . Dementia praecox was formally introduced as a specific disease entity by Kraepelin at the Heidelberg meeting of 1898 " (Meyer, 1928). But time moves on and Kraepelin's dementia praecox is now obsolescent. It is being replaced by schizophrenia, the much wider concept introduced by Bleuler (1911), based on understanding of mental processes, rather than the static assessment of presenting symptoms by a multiplication of artificial diagnostic labels. As Meyer (*ibid.*) so truly says: " The history of dementia praecox is really that of psychiatry as a whole ".

Psychiatric classification and terminology have been a major stumbling block ever since the era of classification and nosological systems was introduced into the natural sciences and medicine by Linné in 1763.* Indeed, many of the supposed advances in psychiatry of the 19th century, particularly of the second half, are on close inspection seen to be mostly exercises in terminology, permutations and combinations of old names with the occasional introduction of new ones. Mental diseases were not better understood by being given new names and new groupings based on symptoms and outcome. " Events like the following are usual: In an asylum the big pot is labelled ' Dementia '. A new doctor comes along and enlarges the pot standing beside it labelled ' Paranoia ', and procedes to grab old inmates of the asylum by some remnant of a delusional idea and puts them one by one into the new pot—and with it believes he is correcting the mistakes of his predecessors " (Bleuler, 1911). Kline *et al.*, (1953), say that " Sharp disagreements as to how particular patients are to be diagnosed as well as striking variations of diagnostic statistics from hospital to hospital indicate that the criteria for diagnosis are poor ". Indeed in their opinion " the paucity of real progress despite promising leads suggests that the present classification may be the major deterrent ". This is being increasingly recognized. But instead of abandoning arbitrary systems of classification, " new " diagnostic labels are being introduced for the many transitional forms created of necessity by rigid classification. This may be in part due to the present therapeutic furore leading to statistical evaluation of supposed therapies on *ad hoc* disease entities arrived at

* Linné called his fifth class of diseases *Mentales*, which he subdivided into three orders: *Ideales*, *Imaginarii* and *Pathetici*.

by adding up presenting symptoms. For instance, depression, tension states, stress diseases, anxiety states, hysteria and psychopathy, are sufficiently vague to apply to almost any but the most severely disturbed patients. The division of mental diseases into neuroses and psychoses has resulted in new names such as ambulatory or latent schizophrenia, or prepsychosis for the multitude of patients who appear to fall between the two stools.

It is instructive that Schreber was diagnosed in his first illness as suffering from severe hypochondriasis; his second illness commenced as an 'anxiety neurosis' with attacks of panic, then hypochondriacal delusions and suicidal depression; later catatonic excitement alternating with stupor. From then on he might well have been diagnosed variously as suffering from catatonic schizophrenia, paranoid schizophrenia, dementia paranoides, dementia praecox, monomania, chronic mania, involutional melancholia, paranoia paraphrenia, obsessional neurosis, anxiety hysteria, tension state, transvestitism, psychopathy, etc.

"Naturally a name which only designates and nothing more is in itself a very innocent thing. But among the old and new terminologies which have been suggested and even used among us for psychic illnesses, are some which are more ambitious. Attempts were made to give to this kind of illness a name which implies a description of what, in the opinion of the originator of the name, psychic illness is, even of what its very nature consists. Such names are then no longer innocent: they are intended to direct opinion, and therefore may of course misdirect it. It is for this reason that it is very much worth while considering them closely" (Nasse, 1818).

Neurosis and Psychosis—An historical digression

Freud perpetuated terms and divisions of psychiatric disease which the tendency of modern psychiatry has been increasingly to abandon: paranoia and dementia praecox, now more commonly called schizophrenia though the terms by no means cover the same ground, are uniformly acknowledged as indistinguishable and indeed one and the same disease process. Freud further accentuated and at the same time confused an artificial division of psychiatric diseases into neuroses and psychoses by suggesting different psychopathology for each, a "distinction . . . at times convenient, but without substance" (Lewis, 1950). This has had far reaching effects, discussed below, which in turn impeded progress.

The terms 'neurosis' and 'psychosis' can only be appreciated in their historical setting. Neurosis, much the older term, derives from

Greek, meaning nerve, tendon or sinew, structures which were not differentiated. In our time neurasthenia, nerve weakness, nerve strain, and of course treatment by nerve tonics, show their origin in this old anatomical confusion. In 1661 a 'neurotic' was a substance having an action on the nervous system, particularly a bracing one; a book dealing with these more recently was entitled "The Old Vegetable Neurotics" (1869). In 1777 Cullen applied the name 'neurosis' to all diseases of the nervous system not accompanied by fever (all pyrexial diseases being grouped together irrespective of site or cause), the vesaniae or mental diseases forming a subgroup.

'Psychosis' was introduced by Feuchtersleben in 1845, to give expression to his belief that mental diseases were not diseases of brain but of soul or mind. For him brain was the organ of mind, the corporeal seat of mind, but not mind itself.

With advances in neuropathology in the 19th century definite neurological diseases with recognizable pathology were increasingly identified. Following Cullen, Romberg (1840–46), in the first systematic textbook written on neurology, still classed all diseases of the nervous system and mental diseases together as Neuroses. But by the turn of this century neurological diseases with recognizable neuropathology had been split off from this group ,and neurosis was then applied only to "functional" diseases of the nervous system, although as Gillespie (1938) said, it is "very hard to conceive what a functional disorder of nerve can be". The belief that mental diseases were diseases of the nervous system allowed hysteria and hypochondriasis to be grouped with epilepsy, tetany, chorea, as functional diseases of the nervous system whose pathology had not been elucidated. This confusion is well shown in Charcot's term hystero-epilepsy.

Freud demonstrated that the so-called neuroses were in reality diseases of the mind, or psychoses in Feuchtersleben's original sense.* At the same time Kraepelin grouped dementia praecox, the

* But Freud was not able to emancipate himself entirely from current teaching. He subdivided "neuroses" into "psycho-neuroses" in which he demonstrated mental factors played the major role, but called a second group "actual-neuroses", literally and "actually" to express his belief that they were due to the toxic influences of "undischarged libido" and, required medical treatment. Among these "actual-neuroses" he classed hypochondriasis, neurasthenia and anxiety neurosis. It is of great historical interest that Freud, by postulating the "organic" actual-neuroses and the "psychogenic" psycho-neuroses had to sever the centuries old twins: hysteria and hypochondria, and put them in opposite camps. Hysteria became the paradigm of psychogenesis. Hypochondria, neurasthenia and anxiety neurosis were denied psychic content and therefore remained outside psychoanalytic understanding.

major mental as opposed to neurological illness (which under a different name had led Feuchtersleben to introduce the term psychosis) with thyroid diseases and general paralysis of the insane, as a metabolic or degenerative disease of the nervous system: hence *dementia*.

Neurosis and psychosis were also used in various combinations, depending on whether the author considered the psychic or the neurological factor played a greater part in the production of the disease: neuro-psychosis when the nervous system played the greater role due to disease or supposed degeneration, psycho-neurosis (introduced by Stothard in 1865) when the mental factor was more important in causing abnormality in the nervous system. Thus for Clouston (1904) " Psychoneurosis " was " the insane temperament " which " consists of the potentialities of psychosis ". Freud (1896) " In a short paper published in 1894 . . . included hysteria, obsessions and certain cases of acute hallucinatory confusion under one heading as ' Defence Neuro-Psychoses ' " to which he added " Chronic Paranoia " in the 1896 paper from which the above quotation is taken. Griesinger (1861) called " violent toothache " and " spinal affections " neuroses; Hoffmann (1889) called the form of muscular atrophy now known by his name " neurotic ". For Hofmeister (1894) cases of diabetes which commenced with a psychic trauma, were " psychotic ".

Treatment

Today the wheel has turned full circle: neuroses, the erstwhile diseases of nerves and tendons, are, following Freud, largely treated by psychotherapy and their origin in the mind generally accepted. Psychoses on the other hand, Feuchtersleben's diseases of the mind or soul as opposed to brain, are still often considered to originate from yet undiscovered brain pathology, the mental symptoms being merely incidental and without significance. The mirage created by general paralysis of the insane* continues to spur on a psychiatry without psychology to find physical pathology for mental diseases.

We will return to the " actual-neuroses " in the Discussion, because Schreber's first illness consisted entirely of hypochondriasis, his second illness was ushered in by the same symptoms; and during the whole of his psychosis, preoccupation with his body played a major role, as indeed it does in most psychotic patients.

* A neurological disease with symptoms prominent in the psychic sphere and long confused with mental diseases proper. When first clearly distinguished by Bayle (1822), many cases of " insanity " became understandable in terms of definite brain pathology.

Despite unremitting efforts by biochemists, endocrinologists, neuropathologists, neurophysiologists and others, no evidence has been found to substantiate the hope of finding an organic basis for the group of schizophrenias. Indeed we are " still as far as ever from mounting a delusion in Canada balsam or from detecting despondency in a test tube " (Crichton Browne, 1875). Even the anticipation of and belief in an organic basis for the psychoses can hardly provide a rationale for the present empirical " anti-psychoses " (Tuke, 1882).* Nevertheless, the psychoses are at present widely treated by coma hypoglycaemia, electrically induced convulsions, and surgical destruction of the brain, " tho' it may seem almost haeretical to impeach their antimaniacal virtues ", as Battie (1758) said of the methods of the " lewd empirics " of his time, who " vomited, purged and bled " their " lunaticks ". Kraepelin himself in later years stated " Purely medical treatment of the mentally ill cannot satisfy thinking psychiatrists in the long run. As the spirited Reil exclaims ' It is a revolting spectable to see how the confirmed empiric sets about his insane patients ' " (Kraepelin, 1918). Lewis (*loc. cit.*) says that the present-day " Three methods . . . of ' shock-therapy ' . . . have little more in common than that they are crude empirical methods ", which Critchley (1943) finds " crude, dangerous and repellent to anyone who holds the central nervous system in respect."

Reverting to our patient Schreber, today he would certainly have qualified for electroshock, insulin hypoglycaemia and leucotomy. One wonders what would have happened to the author of the Memoirs had his brain been submitted to such procedures. It is certain that the Memoirs could not have been written; whether he would have recovered as much as he did spontaneously is doubtful.

Psychotherapy and Classification

Today the neuroses or psychoneuroses, the milder forms of mental illness, are considered to be understood in psychoanalytic theory.

* " Shock therapy has a strong appeal to the therapist—like any mechanical and indirect method—in that its use protects him from exercizing certain skills. By avoiding a technique requiring considerable personal interaction with the patient, there is less tendency for the therapist to consider himself to blame for the failure of the patient to recover. His own skill, his own efforts are never thereby put to the test. His own self esteem is never seriously threatened and he is able to avoid prolonged interviews . . . If the treatment is successful . . . he can esteem himself highly . . . if unsuccessful, he can assume the patient was untreatable. If the patient has a relapse, it can be regarded as inevitable by reason of his having a psychosis. He can feel . . . he is following a widely endorsed method " (Gottschalk, 1947).

Originally Freud made no distinction between neuroses and psychoses: one of his earliest psychiatric papers was entitled 'The Defence Neuro-Psychoses' (1894). When severely disturbed patients were found to be inaccessible to the psycho-analytic couch-free association technique, this was explained (Abraham, 1908) by the patient's supposed inability to form a classical sexual (libidinal) transference to the analyst, because his libido was concentrated on himself; hence the term narcissistic neuroses for the psychoses. Freud followed Abraham in his paper "On Narcissism" (1914), "his chief theoretical contribution to the aetiology of psychoses" (Hendrick, 1939). In this "he concluded that the primary process of psychosis is an incapacity for normal emotional interest in other people and things" (Hendrick, *loc. cit.*). Thus Freud made the presence or absence of the classical libidinal transference to the analyst the criterion of distinction between hysteria and dementia praecox, that is between neuroses and psychoses, or in psychoanalytic terms, between transference neuroses and narcissistic neuroses.

Transference—An historical digression

In this way an entirely new moment was introduced into the classification of mental diseases. This was the patient's response to psychoanalytic technique, and his capacity to form a libidinal transference has imperceptibly entered psychiatry as proof of a fundamental division into neuroses and psychoses. It is therefore necessary to study this yardstick in detail.

Freud looked upon transference as the cornerstone of psychoanalysis. In "Psychotherapy of Hysteria" in 1895 he first reported that the patient had "made a false connection" to the person of the doctor. In 1905 he discussed this phenomenon further; "What", he asked, "are transferences?" Since then the identical question has been raised innumerable times and attempts at answering it have been made equally often. Even today the phenomenon of transference is not clearly understood: there is no unanimity as to what it is, why it is, or who exhibits it. This is of fundamental importance, because psychoanalytic theory was built up on observations of transference in analysis. It is still held that the classical technique is absolutely passive, the patient's actions and thoughts spontaneous, and that the analyst is merely a mirror. Transference manifestations during analysis are assessed as "a new edition of the patient's neurosis", hence the term "transference neurosis". When Freud to his amazement first encountered this "strange phenomenon of transference", he attributed it to the patient's neurosis and stressed repeatedly and emphatically that these demonstrations of love and hate emanated from patients unaided, that they appeared not only without the analyst's endeavour, but indeed in spite of him, and that nothing would prevent their occurrence.

The natural endeavour to differentiate the new technique of analysis from hypnosis, led to similarities being overlooked. The analyst's passivity became the hallmark of the new technique, its handling by mastery of the counter transference the very centre of analytic training. In contrast to the hypnotist, the analyst's passivity was established as the focal point and essence of psychoanalytic practice; erroneously however it was taken to apply to the whole of psychoanalytic technique, which was looked upon as essentially non-interfering. From this myth of the passivity of the classical technique arose the unproven and indeed untenable notion that transference manifestations unfold spontaneously, the technique only isolating and bringing the neurotic material to light. The ability to form transferences was considered a characteristic of the neurotic. But as has been shown in detail elsewhere (Macalpine, 1950), very active pressure is brought to bear on the patient throughout the analytic treatment; the patient has no choice but to adapt by regression to the denial of object world and object relations in the analytic hour. Indeed one might define analytic transference as a person's induced adaptation by regression to the infantile analytic milieu.

Recognition of the fact that the classical technique does not simply mirror the patient's material, but that his transferences are the product of interacting forces in the analytic setting, must perforce lead to re-evaluation of psychoanalytic tenets and theory. At this point the concept of analytic transference and analytic theory merge. Transference is not only the centre of the practice of psychoanalysis, but on it Freud built his theory of psychoneurotic symptom formation. It provided his first inspiration and later continual confirmation that the psychoneuroses were ultimately traceable to a disturbance in the sexual life. In 1914 Freud stated that "The fact of the transference appearing, although neither desired nor induced by either physician or patient, in every neurotic who comes under treatment . . . has always seemed to me . . . proof that the source of the propelling forces of neurosis lie in the sexual life". This shows clearly how transference became intrinsically linked with the theory of psychoanalysis, according to which sexual strivings towards other people, and conflict over them, underlie neurotic illness. This may appear an oversimplification as it leaves out of account the pregenital stages of libidinal development and the later death instinct. But even when these are taken into account, it still holds good that the Oedipus complex is considered the core of the psychoneuroses. The point we wish to bring out clearly is that psychoneurotic illness is considered a disturbance of relatively mature interpersonal relations, traceable to the child's early relation to the parent of either sex. This has even led some to bring the Oedipus complex forward to the first year of life, thereby showing how deep-rooted the conviction is that mental illness must arise in interpersonal disturbances. *Summarizing:* first transference was thought to be a new edition of early interpersonal relations arising spontaneously in analytic therapy. This was taken as evidence that neurotic illness was due to such disturbances of early interpersonal relations. The cause of the psychoneuroses was therefore attributed to libidinal conflict. This model of disturbance of early interpersonal relations was then hypothetically extended to normal development on the one hand and the psychopathology of the psychoses on the other. It was postulated that in psychotics, conflict with other persons is either so early or so severe that they withdraw their libidinal interest from the outside world and direct it narcissistically towards themselves. Hence the undue stress placed on schizophrenics withdrawing from a world unbearable to them, and the faulty notion that renunciation of reality is the hallmark of psychosis.

Although the discovery of transference opened unlimited vistas into patients' inner lives and fantasies, interest was then focussed on, and by over-emphasis almost restricted to interpersonal aspects. The early and inseparable combination of transference manifestations with the libido theory—which in fact grew out of transference experiences—prevented other aspects from being investigated.

It was necessary to trace the development of analytic concepts in order to understand our present-day ideas of mental disease. Even the basic approach of investigators far removed from psychoanalysis proper is subject to the fashions and heritage of our day, which it fell largely to Freud to determine. The term transference itself has spread far beyond the confines of psychoanalysis, and it is often loosely and wrongly applied. The view is even held that if pursued long enough it is bound to lead to the pathogenic core. This is shown clearly by the ever increasing length of psychoanalyses. The salient point is, that our whole mental theory seems unwittingly and imperceptibly to have accepted the view that mental illness is in the last resort based on disturbances of interpersonal relations; in other words that unconscious conflict over libidinal drives is the cause and basis of mental illness. Indeed this is the very reason which at present seems to impede and obstruct progress in psychiatric insight, and limit psychotherapy (Macalpine and Hunter, 1954 a).

From our studies of psychosomatic and psychotic illnesses we believe that the primary disturbance is not interpersonal but intrapersonal, that is to say they originate in disturbances of internal reality, in the patient's relation to himself, his mind and his body (Macalpine and Hunter, 1954 b). Such intrapersonal disturbances may secondarily affect interpersonal relations and lead to an altered relation to external reality.

Today "We may be keeping up the division between neurosis and psychosis in order to persuade ourselves that we understand the psychopathology of the neuroses" (Hunter, 1954). Thus psychoanalysis which has done so much to introduce the mind into psychiatry, has paradoxically also tended to help pave the way for yet another era of an organic, neurological, i.e. non-psychological "brain mythology" of the psychoses. Perhaps because of deficiences and obscurities in the theory of psychoanalytic technique, centred on the concept of transference, psychoanalysis was not able to stem the advancing tide of empirical "brain-destructive" (Brody and Redlich, 1952) therapies in psychiatry, and through its own development contributed to it.*

We have spread our net so wide in this introduction, because it is our conviction that mental illness is disease of the mind and not of the brain. This implies an obligation to strive for psychodynamic understanding as a basis for successful psychotherapy. Psychoanalytic concepts provide the only starting point for such endeavour. This led us to examine the relation of psychoanalysis to psychiatry and the psychoses in detail. For is it widely held that if no results

* This is well demonstrated by Stengel (1948), a psychoanalyst: "The prominence that it (psychoanalysis) gives to the instincts implies that mental illness can be influenced by physical means without the detour over psychological mechanisms. It is therefore, quite natural that psychoanalytically trained psychiatrists have co-operated wholeheartedly in the administration of physical treatments, which are not incompatible with psychoanalytical principles".

can be achieved by psychoanalysis, the illness is beyond psychotherapy.

We have given in historical outline some factors responsible for the contemporary belief in an organic origin of mental disease, which engenders empirical physical procedures in therapy, relegating the mind to a subordinate or incidental role. *Summarizing* there are four main reasons:

1. Symptomatological classification with therapies directed at removal of symptoms, whatever the means and whatever the price.

2. Artificial division of mental diseases into neuroses and psychoses, sponsored alike by psychiatrists and psychoanalysts.

3. The widespread belief that psychoanalysis is the be-all and end-all of psychotherapy, with the implication that because the psychoanalytic technique is not applicable to psychotics, psychoses are beyond the pale of psychotherapy.

4. The myth surrounding the nature of transference, its central position in the technique of psychoanalysis and the theory of mental illness based on it.

Psychoanalytic Theory of Psychosis

When in our hospital practice we found that psychotherapeutic results were disappointing if our approach was based on the psychoanalytic theory of the pathogenicity of unconscious homosexual wishes and attendant castration anxieties, we proceeded to scrutinize the theory itself. The problems involved are outlined above. We then checked the therapeutic successes of psychoanalysts and found to our surprise that it is common experience, frequently admitted and often implied, that not only are "paranoid" patients not improved by homosexual interpretations, but even made worse.

Knight (1940) also noted that interpretation of "homosexual wishes ... cautiously and tactfully" given "not only does not relieve the patient but often makes him more paranoid than ever". He therefore raised the important question "Why does the developing paranoiac react so frantically to the dimly perceived homosexual drive in himself? Is the homosexual wish so much more intense in him than it is in other men who successfully repress it ... or is ... this need to deny so terrifically strong?"

The selfsame doubt exercised Ferenczi's (1911) mind: "in paranoia it is mainly a question of recathexis with unsublimated libido of homosexual love objects which the ego wards off by projection. This statement, however, leads us to the bigger problem of choice of neurosis, i.e., under what conditions does infantile bisexuality, ambisexuality, lead respectively to normal heterosexuality, to homosexual perversion or to paranoia." Nunberg (1938) implied a similar note of reservation: "The question why it is that out of the same fundamental situation a paranoia develops in one instance and in another does not, must remain unanswered for the present."

One may therefore conclude that neither in theory nor in therapy is projection of and conflict over unconscious homosexuality as firmly established as the cause of paranoid illness, i.e. schizophrenia, as is generally believed and stated.

This made us turn to Freud's (1911) paper on which all subsequent psychoanalytic studies of the psychoses are based. We found that Freud himself described it as "more or less speculative" and "only a fragment of a larger whole" (F. 466). He added that "much more material remains to be gathered from the symbolic content of the fantasies and delusions of this gifted paranoiac".

Homosexuality

We therefore read Schreber's Memoirs and subsequently published a study (Macalpine and Hunter, 1953) in which we showed that projection of unconscious homosexuality, though playing a part in the symptomatology, could not account for the illness in course or outcome, phenomenologically or aetiologically. Freud's homosexual bias had led him to interpretation of castration anxieties in Schreber's illness, based more on theoretical preconceptions than on actual material. Indeed he appears to have misunderstood some of Schreber's fundamental delusions, such as being "unmanned". This was a fantasy of being transformed gradually over "decades if not centuries" into a reproductive woman, carrying neither a castration threat, nor passive homosexual wishes. From the beginning of his illness Schreber was as much male as female, both and neither. Simultaneously he "felt quickening like the first signs of life of a human embryo" in his body, "by a divine miracle . . . fertilization had occurred" (Memoirs, footnote 1, p. 4).

This was the deepest layer of his psychosis and with it he showed what we have come to regard as the two pathognomonic features of schizophrenia: doubt and uncertainty in sex identity*, which is of course implied in ideas of change of sex accompanied by archaic procreation fanatsies.

If such confusion about sex identity is termed homosexuality then of course schizophrenic "homosexuality" is of a different order, and should be clearly differentiated from passive homosexual wishes towards members of the same sex, as is implied in Freud's use of the term. This last presupposes certainty in one's sex identity which Schreber had so obviously lost from the beginning of his illness and which he still clearly displayed when leaving the mental hospital by the wearing of feminine articles such as ribbons and cheap jewellery.

Conclusion

We eventually decided to translate the book, because the clinical material it contains exemplifies and elucidates the difficulties which beset the theory, classification and psychotherapy of the psychoses at the present time. For all students of psychiatry, Schreber, its most famous patient, offers unique insight into the mind of a schizophrenic, his thinking, language, behaviour, delusions and hallucinations, and into the inner development, course and outcome of the illness. His autobiography has the advantage of being complete to an extent no case history taken by a physician can ever be: its material is not selected or subject to elaboration or omission by an intermediary between the patient and his psychosis, and between both and the reader. Every student therefore has access to the totality of the patient's products. Indeed the Memoirs may be called the best text on psychiatry written for psychiatrists by a patient. Schreber's psychosis is minutely and expertly described, but its content is—as Dr. Weber explained to the Court—fundamentally the same and has the same features as that of other mental patients. Schreber's name is legion.

We ourselves have learnt from it things which neither textbooks we read, nor lectures we attended could teach us. It helped us understand the actions and speech of chronic psychotics, enabling us to make contact with them, and in this way lessen their alienation. In milder patients, particularly hypochondriacs and early schizophrenics, we could help them understand their concern and preoccupation with body and body functions, or vague anxiety

* M. Bleuler (1953) in a personal communication stated that E. Bleuler would have agreed that "schizophrenics are almost invariably, if not indeed invariably, in doubt about the sex to which they belong".

in terms of fantasies and budding delusions about their physical and mental identity. We have talked and listened to many Schrebers since we studied the Memoirs.

Finally, as the Memoirs are the source material on which Freud based his most famous clinical study, fascinating opportunity is provided of observing Freud's mind actually at work on a case history.

Translation

We thought at first the book was untranslatable because of the circumstantial, complicated and cumbersome presentation of psychotic trends of thought. The involved and endless sentences contain clauses within clauses, particularly when Schreber sets out to describe, explain and develop his delusional ideas and hallucinatory sensations. " Things are dealt with which cannot be expressed in human language; they exceed human understanding ", says Schreber himself. The more psychotic the material, the more the former Judge attempts to reason his way out and the more legalistic his mode of expression. Hence his style is a unique combination of exact, exacting diction, and naive directness, even touching simplicity. Concreteness of thought and expression, neologisms, puns, and the insertion of innumerable qualifying adverbs and particles, seemed to make a faithful and yet readable translation almost impossible. However, when we settled down to the ardous task we found to our surprise that the translation makes easier reading than the original. This may be due to the translator being forced to understand every phrase and passage before he can render its meaning succinctly. Even when at first reading a phrase appeared beyond understanding, some train of thought could eventually be unravelled.

We proceeded with the translation by first making a rough draft of the whole book. We then attempted to make this draft readable and understandable. Our third stage was to compare it with the original German text so as to keep as close to it as possible, and in particular to make sure that, following Schreber, we were using the same terms throughout the book. This should facilitate following Schreber's often very tortuous associations. We endeavoured to be as faithful as possible and omitted only the many particles common in German and abundantly used by Schreber, which often cannot be translated at all and do not add to the sense, such as " in part ", " on the other hand ", " so to speak ", " up to a point ", " in a way ", etc.

We have not attempted to translate most of the titles, for instance *Geheimrath*, *Justizrath* and *Regierungsassessor*, as they cannot be rendered in English and are of no relevance. Schreber's own title, *Senatspräsident*, we have retained in German; it cannot be accurately translated because it applies to a legal office which has no equivalent in English law.

All terms in inverted commas in the original text which are either neologisms or used by Schreber with a specific meaning, and therefore open to interpretation, are given in the original German version in the notes following the text, together with reasons for our choice of translation. The original contains a fair number of printing errors and wrong cross-references; these we have checked, corrected, and where necessary commented on. To facilitate finding references to the original Memoirs, we have run Schreber's original page numbers alongside the text.

Our translation is almost throughout at variance with quotations from Schreber's Memoirs in the official translation of Freud's study. Even the title of the Memoirs we felt was not accurately rendered by "Memoirs of a Neurotic Patient". Schreber himself did not wish to describe himself as suffering from 'neurosis' in the modern sense of the term; in fact his protest that he suffered from 'diseased nerves' and not from a mental illness runs like a red thread through the whole of the Memoirs. We have been in touch with the Editor and Translator of Freud's works, Mr. James Strachey, who states that in the Standard Edition of Freud's works in preparation, the translation, particularly of quotations from Schreber's Memoirs, will be extensively revised.

Although it was our aim to make the Memoirs readable, we left unchanged passages in which Schreber changes the tense because they reveal his confusion about past and present. The same applies to sentences in which, for instance, he speaks of "one felt that I . . . ", "it was said that I . . . ", etc. Such passages may strike the reader as slapdash translation, but they show Schreber's confusion about himself. These oblique expressions are frequently used when he describes 'unconscious processes'; they show an awareness of something of which he is only half aware. In the same way as he hears his own thoughts as voices speaking to him from outside, he projects himself into others. These uncertainties are mirrored in his style. Apparently confused passages are intermingled with clearer and simple ones: this leads to an unevenness which we have retained in translation, so as to remain as close as possible to the original. This, coupled with passages in which Schreber tries to give an account of ideas and feelings literally not expressible in human language, makes some passages appear clumsy. It was often not possible to simplify long and complicated sentences, indeed we felt that the total picture so presented would add to the likeness of Schreber's Memoirs. In conclusion, we hope that the difficulties which we experienced may not be apparent in the result of our labours.

ACKNOWLEDGMENTS

Our major indebtedness is to Victor Kreitner, Doctor of Law. He played an important part at all stages of the translation, and was untiring in helping us unravel obscure passages and guiding us through the maze of legal terms and technicalities.

Emily Cuttler gave invaluable assistance in the preparation of the manuscript and proof-reading.

We thank Mr. Marley of Wm. Dawson & Sons for his efficiency and courtesy at all times.

Finally we thank: Dr. Raymond Gosselin, editor of the Psychoanalytic Quarterly, New York, for permission to reprint our paper, "The Schreber Case", which appeared in July, 1953, enlarged and adapted for the book; the Trustees of the British Museum, London, for permission to reproduce the painting by Pradilla; Messrs. C. Marhold of Halle, for permission to reproduce plates II, III, and IV of Sonnenstein Asylum, from "Deutsche Heil- und Pflegeanstalten für Psychischkranke" (1910); and Messrs. S. Karger of Berlin, publishers of "Monatschrift für Psychiatrie und Neurologie", for permission to reproduce plate I of Professor Flechsig.

DANIEL PAUL SCHREBER

MEMOIRS OF MY NERVOUS ILLNESS

Denkwürdigkeiten

eines

Nervenkranken

nebst Nachträgen

und einem Anhang über die Frage:

„Unter welchen Voraussetzungen darf eine für geisteskrank erachtete Person gegen ihren erklärten Willen in einer Heilanstalt festgehalten werden?"

von

Dr. jur. Daniel Paul Schreber,

Senatspräsident beim Kgl. Oberlandesgericht Dresden a. D.

Oswald Mutze in Leipzig.

1903.

PREFACE

p. iii

I started this work without having publication in mind. The idea only occurred to me as I progressed with it; however, I did not conceal from myself doubts which seemed to stand in the way of publication: mainly consideration for certain persons still living. Yet I believe that expert examination of my body and observation of my personal fate during my lifetime would be of value both for science and the knowledge of religious truths. In the face of such considerations all personal issues must recede.

Of the whole work the following were written:

The Memoirs themselves (Chapters I–XXII) in the period February to September 1900.

Postscripts I–VII in the period October 1900 to June 1901.

Postscripts second series at the end of 1902.

The outward circumstances of my life have materially changed p. iv
since the early beginnings of this work. While at the beginning I was living in almost prison-like isolation, separated from contact with educated people, excluded even from the family table of the Director (to which so-called boarders of the Asylum were admitted), never able to get outside the walls of the Asylum, etc., I have gradually been granted increasing freedom of movement, and contact with educated people has been made increasingly possible. Finally I was completely successful in winning the proceedings against my tutelage (albeit in the Second Instance) as mentioned in Chapter XX, inasmuch as the decree of 13th March 1900 placing me under tutelage issued by the District Court, Dresden, was rescinded by the final judgment of the Superior Country Court, Dresden, of 14th July 1902. My legal capacity was thereby acknowledged and free disposition of my properties restored to me. With regard to my stay in the Asylum, for months I have been in possession of a written declaration from the Asylum Authorities that there was now no opposition in principle to my discharge; I am planning therefore to return to my house and home probably early next year.

All these changes have afforded me the opportunity of considerably widening the range of my personal observations. Accordingly some of my earlier opinions need revision : in particular I can no longer doubt that the so-called "play-with-human-beings" (the effect of miracles) is limited to myself and *to whatever constitutes my immediate environment* at the time. I might perhaps have formulated some passages of my Memoirs differently now. Nevertheless I have left them mainly in the form in which they were written originally. To change certain points now would only prejudice the freshness of the original descriptions. It is also in my opinion of little importance whether, in view of the relationship contrary to the Order of the World which arose between God and myself, ideas which I formed at the time were more or less faulty. A more general interest can in any case be claimed only for those conclusions which I arrived at in consequence of my impressions and experiences about the *lasting* conditions, about the essence and attributes of God, the immortality of the soul, etc. In this respect I have no reason whatever, even after my subsequent personal experiences, to make the very slightest alteration in the basic ideas set out particularly in chapters I, II, XVIII and XIX of the Memoirs.

Sonnenstein Asylum, near Pirna,
December 1902.

The Author.

OPEN LETTER TO PROFESSOR FLECHSIG

Dear Professor, p. vii

I take the liberty of enclosing a copy of "Memoirs of a Patient Suffering from a Nervous Illness", which I have written, and beg you to examine it in a kindly spirit.

You will find your name mentioned frequently, particularly in the first chapter, partly in connection with circumstances which might be painful to you. I very much regret this but unfortunately cannot make any changes without from the very outset precluding making myself understood. In any case it is far from me to attack your honour, as indeed *I do not harbour any personal grievance against any person.* My aim is solely to further knowledge of truth in a vital field, that of religion.

I am absolutely certain that in this regard I command experiences p. viii
which—when generally acknowledged as valid—will act fruitfully to the highest possible degree among the rest of mankind. Equally I have no doubt that your name plays an essential role in the genetic development of the circumstances in question, in that certain nerves taken from your nervous system became "tested souls" in the sense described in Chapter I of the "Memoirs", and in this capacity achieved supernatural power by means of which they have for years exerted a damaging influence on me and still do to this day. You like other people may be inclined at first to see nothing but a pathological offspring of my imagination in this; but I have an almost overwhelming amount of proof of its correctness, details of which you will find in the content of my "Memoirs". I still feel daily and hourly the damaging influence of the miracles of those "tested souls"; the voices that speak to me even now shout your name again and again at me hundreds of times every day in this context, in particular as the instigator of those injuries; and this despite the fact that the personal relations which existed between us for some time have long since receded into the background for me; I could hardly therefore have any reason to keep on thinking of you, especially with any sense of grievance.

For years I have pondered how to reconcile these facts with my respect for your person, *whose integrity and moral worth I have*
p. ix *not the least right to doubt.* Only quite recently however, just before the publication of my book, I had a new idea which might *possibly* lead to the correct solution of the problem. As remarked at the end of Chapter IV and the beginning of Chapter V of the "Memoirs", I have not the least doubt that the *first impetus* to what my doctors always considered mere "hallucinations" but which to me signified communication with supernatural powers, consisted of *influences on my nervous system emanating from your nervous system.* How could this be explained? I think it is possible that you—at first as I am quite prepared to believe only for therapeutic purposes—carried on some hypnotic, suggestive, or whatever else one could call it, contact with my nerves, *even while we were separated in space.* During this contact you might suddenly have realized that other voices were speaking to me as well, pointing to a supernatural origin. Following this surprising realization you might have continued this contact with me for a time out of scientific interest, until you yourself felt as it were uneasy about it, and therefore decided to break it off. But it is possible that in this process a part of your own nerves—probably unknown to yourself—was removed from your body, a process
p. x explicable only in a supernatural manner, and ascended to heaven as a "tested soul" and there achieved some supernatural power. This "tested soul" still endowed with human faults like all impure souls—in accordance with the character of souls which I have come to know with certainty—then simply allowed itself to be driven by the impulse of ruthless self-determination and lust for power, without any restraint by something comparable to the moral will power of man, exactly in the same way as another "tested soul", that of von W., as recorded in my "Memoirs". It is possible therefore that all those things which in earlier years I erroneously thought I had to blame you for—particularly the definite damaging effects on my body—are to be blamed only on that "tested soul". There would then be no need to cast any shadow upon your person and only the mild reproach would perhaps remain that you, like so many doctors, could not completely resist the temptation of using a patient in your care *as an object for scientific experiments* apart from the real purpose of cure, when by chance matters of the highest scientific interest arose. One might even raise the question whether perhaps all the talk of voices about somebody having committed soul murder can be

explained by the souls (rays) deeming it impermissible that a person's nervous system should be influenced by another's to the extent of imprisoning his will power, such as occurs during hypnosis; in order to stress forcefully that this was a malpractice p. xi it was called " soul murder ", the souls for lack of a better term, using a term already in current usage, and because of their innate tendency to express themselves hyperbolically.

I need hardly mention *of what immeasurable importance it would be* if you could in any way confirm the surmises I have sketched above, all the more if they could be substantiated in recollections of earlier years retained in your memory. The rest of my thesis would thereby gain universal credence and would immediately be regarded as a *serious scientific problem to be investigated in every possible way.*

I beg you therefore, my dear Sir—I might almost say: I *implore* you—to state without reservation:

(1) Whether during my stay in your Asylum you maintained a hypnotic or similar contact with me in such a way that even when separated in space, you exerted an influence on my nervous system;

(2) Whether you thus witnessed in any way communications from voices originating elsewhere, indicating supernatural origin; finally

(3) Whether during my time in your Asylum *you yourself also* received visions or vision-like impressions particularly in p. xii dreams, which dealt amongst others with the almighty power of God and human freedom of will, unmanning, loss of states of Blessedness, my relations and my friends, as well as yours, particularly Daniel Fürchtegott Flechsig named in Chapter VI, and many other matters mentioned in my " Memoirs ".

I hasten to add that from the numerous communications I received from the voices that talked to me at that time, I have the most weighty indications that you yourself had similar visions.

In appealing to your scientific interest I may be permitted to trust that you will have the courage of truth, even if you had to admit some trifle which could never seriously affect your prestige or authority in the eyes of any sensible person.

In case you want to send me a written communication you may rest assured that I would publish it only with your permission and in a form which you yourself may choose.

In view of the wide interest which the content of this letter may claim, I have thought fit to have it printed in the form of an " open letter " prefacing my " Memoirs ".

Dresden, March 1903.

Yours sincerely,
Dr. Schreber, Senatspräsident
(retired).

TABLE OF CONTENTS

p. xiii

p. xiv

Appendix

Addenda

(Documents from the Court Proceedings placing me under tutelage)

INTRODUCTION

I have decided to apply for my release from the Asylum in the p. 1
near future in order to live once again among civilised people and at home with my wife. It is therefore necessary to give those persons who will then constitute the circle of my acquaintances, an approximate idea at least of my religious conceptions, so that they may have some understanding of the necessity which forces me to various oddities of behaviour, even if they do not fully understand these apparent oddities.*

This is the purpose of this manuscript; in it I shall try to give an at least partly comprehensible exposition of supernatural matters, knowledge of which has been revealed to me for almost six years.
I cannot of course count upon being *fully* understood because p. 2
things are dealt with which cannot be expressed in human language; they exceed human understanding. Nor can I maintain that *everything* is irrefutably certain even for me: much remains only presumption and probability. After all I too am only a human being and therefore limited by the confines of human understanding; but one thing I am certain of, namely that I have come infinitely closer to the truth than human beings who have not received divine revelation.

To make myself at least somewhat comprehensible I shall have to speak much in images and similes, which may at times perhaps be only *approximately* correct; for the only way a human being can make supernatural matters, which in their essence must always remain incomprehensible, understandable to a certain degree is by comparing them with known facts of human experience. Where intellectual understanding ends, the domain of belief begins; man must reconcile himself to the fact that things exist which are true although he cannot understand them.

* Prefatory Remark.
During the course of writing the present essay it occurred to me that it could perhaps be of interest to a wider circle. Nevertheless I have left the preamble because it was my original motive to acquaint my wife with my personal experiences and religious ideas. This explains also why I have frequently thought it right to give circuitous explanations for facts already known, to translate foreign words, etc., which would really have been unnecessary for the scientifically trained reader.

An obvious example is that the concept of *eternity* is beyond man's grasp. Man cannot really understand that something can exist which has neither beginning nor end, that there can be a cause which cannot itself be traced to a previous cause. And yet eternity is one of God's attributes, which with all religiously-minded people I feel I must accept. Man will always be inclined to ask: "If God created the world, how then did God Himself come to be?" This question will for ever remain unanswered. The same applies to the concept of divine creation. Man can always only imagine
p. 3 that new matter is created through the influence of forces on matter already in existence, and yet I believe—and I hope to prove in what follows by means of definite examples—that divine creation is a creation out of the void. Even in the dogmas of our positive religion there are certain matters which escape full understanding by the intellect. The Christian teaching that Jesus Christ was the Son of God can be meant only in a mystical sense which but approximates the human sense of these words, because nobody would maintain that God, as a Being endowed with human sexual organs, had intercourse with the woman from whose womb Jesus Christ came forth. The same applies to the doctrine of the Trinity, the Resurrection of the Flesh, and other Christian dogmas. By this I do not in any way wish to imply that I acknowledge as true *all* Christian dogmas in the sense of our orthodox theology. On the contrary, I have good reason to think that some of them are definitely untrue or true only to a very limited extent. This applies, for instance, to the Resurrection of the Flesh, which could only lay claim to being relatively and temporarily true in the form of transmigration of souls (not representing the ultimate goal of the process), and also to eternal damnation to which some people are supposed to have succumbed. The concept of eternal damnation—which will always remain abhorrent to human feeling notwithstanding the exposition, based on what I consider sophisms by which Luthardt for instance, tried to make it acceptable in his Apologies—does not correspond to the truth, as indeed the whole (human) notion of *punishment*—as an expeditious weapon for attaining certain purposes *within human society*—must in the main be
p. 4 eliminated from our ideas of the life beyond. This, however, can only be examined more closely later.[1]

[1] On the other hand, on the basis of what I have myself experienced, I am able to give a more detailed explanation of some Christian dogmas and how such things can come about through divine miracles. Something like the conception of Jesus Christ by an Immaculate Virgin—i.e. one who never had intercourse with a man—

Before I proceed with the account of how, owing to my illness, I entered into peculiar relations with God—which I hasten to add p. 5
were in themselves contrary to the Order of the World—I must begin with a few remarks about the nature of God and of the human soul; these can for the time being only be put up as axioms—tenets not requiring proof—and their proof as far as is at all possible can only be attempted later in the book.

---

happened in my own body. Twice at different times (while I was still in Flechsig's Asylum) I had a female genital organ, although a poorly developed one, and in my body felt quickening like the first signs of life of a human embryo: by a divine miracle God's nerves corresponding to male seed had been thrown into my body; in other words fertilization had occurred. Further, I have reached a fairly clear idea of how the Resurrection of Jesus Christ may have come about; during the latter part of my stay in Flechsig's Asylum and the beginning of my stay here, I have witnessed not once but hundreds of times how human shapes were set down for a short time by divine miracles only to be dissolved again or vanish. The voices talking to me designated these visions the so-called "*fleeting-improvised-men* "—some were even persons long ago deceased, as for instance Dr. Rudolph J., whom I had seen in Pierson's Asylum—so-called—in Coswig; there were others also, who had apparently passed through a transmigration of souls, as for instance the Senior Public Prosecutor B., Counsel of the Country Court Drs. N. and W., the Privy Councillor Dr. W., the lawyer W., my father-in-law and others; all of them were leading a so-called dream life, i.e. they did not give the impression of being capable of holding a sensible conversation, just as I myself was at that time also little inclined to talk, mainly because I thought that I was faced not by real people but by miraculously created puppets. On the basis of these experiences I am inclined to think that Jesus Christ also, who as a real human being died a real death, was subsequently by divine miracle " set down " anew for a short time as a " fleeting-improvised-man ", in order to strengthen the faith of his followers and thereby securely establish the idea of immortality among mankind; but he subsequently succumbed to the natural dissolution of the " fleeting-improvised-men ", so that it is not impossible according to what will be said below that his nerves entered into the state of eternal Blessedness. From this conception it follows that the Dogma of the Ascension of Christ is a mere fable by which His disciples tried to explain the fact that after His death they repeatedly saw His person in the flesh amongst them.

I

The human soul is contained in the nerves of the body; about p. 6
their physical nature I, as a layman, cannot say more than that they are extraordinarily delicate structures—comparable to the finest filaments—and that the total mental life of a human being rests on their excitability by external impressions. Vibrations are thereby caused in the nerves which produce the sensations of pleasure and pain in a manner which cannot be further explained; they are able to retain the memory of impressions received (the human memory) and have also the power of moving the muscles of the body which they inhabit into any manifest activity by exertion of their will power. From the most tender beginnings (as the fruit of the womb—as a child's soul) they develop to a complex system which embraces the most widespread regions of human knowledge (the soul of mature man). Part of the nerves is adapted solely for receiving sensory impressions (nerves of sight, hearing, taste and voluptuousness, etc., which are therefore only capable of the sensation of light, sound, heat and cold, of the feeling of hunger, voluptuousness and pain, etc.); other nerves (the nerves of intellect) receive and retain mental impressions and as the organs of will, give to the whole human organism the impulse p. 7
to manifest those of its powers designed to act on the outside world. Circumstances seem to be such that *every single nerve of intellect represents the total mental individuality of a human being*, that the sum total of recollections is as it were inscribed on each single nerve of intellect[2]; the greater or lesser *number* of nerves of intellect only influences the length of time for which recollections can be retained. While man is alive he is body and soul together; the nerves (the soul of man) are nourished and kept in living

[2] If this assumption is correct, then the problem of heredity and variability is also solved, i.e. the fact that children resemble their parents and grandparents in some ways and deviate from them in others. The male seed contains a paternal nerve and combines with a nerve taken from the mother's body to form a newly created entity. This new entity—the child to be—thus recreates anew the father and the mother, perhaps more the former or the latter, in turn receives new impressions in its lifetime and then transmits this newly acquired individuality to its descendents.

The idea of the existence of a particular *nerve of determination* representing the mental unity of a person, which I understand forms the basis of du Prel's work of the same name, would accordingly be without substance.

motion by the body whose function is essentially similar to that of the higher animals. Should the body lose its vitality then the state of unconsciousness, which we call *death* and which is presaged in sleep, supervenes for the nerves. This, however, does not imply that the soul is really extinguished; rather the impressions received remain attached to the nerves. The soul, as it were, only goes into hibernation as some lower animals do and can be re-awakened to a new life in a manner to be described below.

p. 8 God to start with is only nerve, not body, and akin therefore to the human soul. But unlike the human body, where nerves are present only in limited numbers, the nerves of God are infinite and eternal. They possess the same qualities as human nerves but in a degree surpassing all human understanding. They have in particular the faculty of transforming themselves into all things of the created world; in this capacity they are called rays; and herein lies the essence of divine creation. An intimate relation exists between God and the starry sky. I dare not decide whether one can simply say that God and the heavenly bodies are one and the same, or whether one has to think of the totality of God's nerves as being above and behind the stars, so that the stars themselves and particularly our sun would only represent *stations*, through which God's miraculous creative power travels to our earth (and perhaps to other inhabitated planets).[3]

Equally I dare not say whether the celestial bodies themselves (fixed stars, planets, etc.) were created by God, or whether divine creation is limited to the organic world; in which case there would be room for the Nebular Hypothesis of Kant–Laplace side by side with the existence of a living God whose existence has become absolute certainty for me. Perhaps the full truth lies (by way of a fourth dimension) in a combination or resultant of both trends of thought impossible for man to grasp. In any case the light and warmth-giving power of the sun, which makes her the origin of all organic life on earth, is only to be regarded as an indirect manifestation of the living God; hence the veneration of the sun
p. 9 as divine by so many peoples since antiquity contains a highly important core of truth even if it does not embrace the whole truth.

The teaching of present-day astronomy about the movements, the distances and the physical properties of the celestial bodies, etc., may in the main be correct. My own personal experiences leave me in doubt however whether even the astronomy of today has

[3] Such things are also known to our poets " Far above the starry sky, surely dwells a kindly father ", etc.

grasped the whole truth about the light-and warmth-giving power of the stars and particularly of our sun; perhaps one has to consider her directly or indirectly only as that part of God's miraculous creative power which is directed to the earth. As proof of this statement I will at present only mention the fact that the sun has for years spoken with me in human words and thereby reveals herself as a living being or as the organ of a still higher being behind her. God also regulates the weather; as a rule this is done automatically, so to speak, by the greater or lesser amount of heat emanating from the sun, but He can regulate it in certain ways in pursuit of His own purposes. For instance I have received fairly definite indications that the severe winter of 1870–71 was decided on by God in order to turn the fortunes of war in favour of the Germans; and the proud words on the destruction of Phillip II's Spanish Armada in the year 1588 "*Deus afflavit et dissipati sunt*" (God blew the wind and they were scattered) most probably also contains a historical truth. In this connection I refer to the sun only as that instrument of God's will power which lies nearest to the earth; in reality the condition of the weather is affected by the sum total of the other stars as well. Winds or storms in particular arise when God moves further away from the earth. In the circumstances contrary to the Order of the World which have now arisen this relation has changed— p. 10
and I wish to mention this at the outset—the weather is now to a certain extent dependent on *my* actions and thoughts; as soon as I indulge in thinking nothing, or in other words stop an activity which proves the existence of the human mind such as playing chess in the garden the wind arises at once. To anybody who is inclined to doubt such a fantastic statement, I could almost daily give the opportunity of convincing him of its correctness, as in fact I have recently convinced various people about the so-called attacks of bellowing (the doctor, my wife, my sister, etc.). The reason for this is simply that as soon as I indulge in thinking nothing God, presuming that I am demented, thinks he can withdraw from me.

Through the light emanating from the sun and the other stars, God is able to perceive (man would say: to see) everything that happens on earth and possibly on other inhabited planets; in this sense one can speak figuratively of the sun and light of the stars as the eye of God. All He sees He enjoys as the fruits of His creative power, much as a human being is pleased with what he has created with his hands or with his mind. Yet things were so

ordered—up to the crisis to be described later—that by and large God left the world which He had created and the organic life upon it (plants, animals, human beings) to their own devices and only provided continuous warmth of the sun to enable them to maintain themselves and reproduce, etc. As a rule God did not interfere directly in the fate of peoples or individuals—I call this the state of affairs in accordance with the Order of the World. It could however occur now and then as an exception, but
p. 11 neither did nor could happen too frequently because to draw close to living mankind was connected with certain dangers even for God Himself—for reasons developed further below. For instance a particularly fervent prayer might in a special case induce God to give help by intervening with a miracle[4] or to shape the fate of whole nations (in war, etc.) by means of miracles. He was also able to get into contact (to form " nerve-contact with them " as the voices that speak to me call this process) with highly gifted people (poets, etc.), in order to bless them (particularly in dreams) with some fertilizing thoughts and ideas about the beyond. But such " nerve-contact " was not allowed to become the rule, as already mentioned, because for reasons which cannot be further elucidated, the nerves of *living* human beings particularly when in a state of *high-grade excitation*, have such power of attraction for the nerves of God that He would not be able to free Himself from them again, and would thus endanger His own existence.[5]

p. 12 Regular contact between God and human souls occurred in the Order of the World only after death. There was no danger for God in approaching *corpses* in order to draw their nerves, in which self-awareness was not extinct but quiescent, out of their bodies and up to Himself by the power of the rays, thereby awakening them to new heavenly life; self-awareness returned through the

[4] I have on innumerable occasions experienced in my own body and continue to do so daily even now that God has, for instance, the power to remove from the human body any germ of illness by sending forth a few pure rays.

[5] (Added November 1902). The idea of a *force of attraction* emanating from individual human bodies or—in my case—from one single human body, acting at such vast distances, must in itself appear absurd if one thinks in terms of natural forces acting purely mechanically. Nevertheless, that an attracting force is at work is for me a fact beyond dispute. This phenomenon will perhaps be somewhat comprehensible and brought nearer human understanding if one remembers that the rays are *living beings* and therefore the power of attraction is not purely a mechanically acting force, but something like a *psychological motive power:* the rays too find that " attractive " which is of interest to them. The relationship therefore appears to be similar to that expressed by Goethe in his " Fisherman ": " partly she dragged him down, partly he sank ".

influence of the rays. The new life beyond is the *state of Blessedness* to which the human soul could be raised. But this did not occur without prior purification and sifting of the human nerves which required, according to the variable condition of the respective human souls, a shorter or longer time of preparation, and perhaps even certain intermediate stages. Only pure human nerves were of use to God—or if one prefers, in heaven—because it was their destiny to be attached to God Himself and ultimately to become in a sense part of Him as "forecourts of heaven".[6] The nerves of morally depraved men are blackened; morally pure men have white nerves; the higher a man's moral standard in life, the more his nerves become completely white or pure, an intrinsic property of God's nerves. A greater part of the nerves of morally depraved men is probably useless; this determines the various p. 13
grades of states of Blessedness to which a human being can attain, and probably also the length of time for which self-awareness in the life beyond can be maintained. Nerves probably always have to undergo purification first, because it would be very difficult to find a human being completely free from sin, that is to say one whose nerves were never defiled by immoral behaviour in his earlier life. Not even I can give an exact description of the process of purification; but I have received several valuable indications about it. It appears that the process of purification was connected with a feeling of an unpleasant task[7] for the souls, or perhaps of an uncomfortable sojourn in the underworld, which was necessary to purify them gradually.

It may be justifiable to designate this in a sense as "punishment"; but it has to be distinguished from the human idea of punishment in that its purpose is not to do harm, but to provide a necessary preliminary for purification. The ideas of hell, hellfire, etc., current in most religions can be explained in this way, *but must be qualified in part.* The souls to be purified learnt during purification the language spoken by God Himself, the so-called "basic

[6] I did not invent the expression "forecourts of heaven", but *like all other expressions which are in inverted commas in this essay* (for instance "fleeting-improvised-men", "dream life", etc.), it only repeats the words which the voices that speak to me always applied to the processes concerned. These are expressions *which would never have occurred to me*, which I have never heard from human beings; they are in part of a scientific, and particularly medical nature, and I do not even know whether they are in current use in the human science concerned. I will draw attention to this extraordinary state of affairs again in some particularly noteworthy instances.

[7] For instance, there was once talk of Flechsig's soul having to perform "drayman's work".

language", a somewhat antiquated but nevertheless powerful German, characterized particularly by a wealth of euphemisms (for instance, reward in the reverse sense for punishment, poison for food, juice for venom, unholy for holy, etc. God Himself was called "concerning Him Who is and shall be"—meaning
p. 14 eternity—and was addressed as "Your Majesty's obedient servant"). Purification was called "testing"; souls which had not yet undergone the process of purification were not, as one would expect, called "non-tested souls", but the exact reverse, namely "tested souls", in accordance with the tendency to use euphemisms. The souls still undergoing the process of purification were variously graded as "Satans", "Devils", "Assistant Devils", "Senior Devils", and "Basic Devils"; the latter expression particularly seems to point to an abode in the underworld. The "Devils", etc., when set down as "fleeting-improvised-men," had a peculiar colour (perhaps carrot-red) and a peculiar offensive odour, which I experienced a number of times in the so-called Pierson Asylum in Coswig (which I heard called the Devil's Kitchen). For instance I saw Mr. v. W. and a Mr. von O., whom we had met in the East Coast resort Warnemünde, as Devils with peculiar red faces and red hands, and Mr. W. as a Senior Devil.

I learnt that Judas Iscariot had been a Basic Devil for his betrayal of Jesus Christ. But one must not imagine these Devils as powers inimical to God as in the ideas of the Christian religion, for almost without exception they had already become thoroughly God-fearing, although they were still undergoing the process of purification. The above statement that God used the German language in the form of the so-called "basic language", is not to be understood as though the state of Blessedness was reserved only for Germans. Nevertheless the Germans were in modern times (possibly since the Reformation, perhaps ever since the migration of nations) *God's chosen people* whose language God
p. 15 preferred to use. In this sense God's chosen peoples in history—as the most moral at a given time—were in order the old Jews, the old Persians (these in an outstanding degree, about whom more will be said below), the "Greco-Romans" (perhaps in ancient Greece and Rome, perhaps also as the "Franks" at the time of the Crusades) and lastly the Germans. God readily *understood* the languages of all nations by contact with their nerves.[8]

[8] In this way all the souls who are in contact with my nerves understand all languages I understand, for the very reason that they partake of my thoughts, for instance they understand Greek when I read a Greek book, etc.

The *transmigration of souls* also seems to have served the purpose of purifying human souls and was widespread, as a number of experiences lead me to believe. In this process the human souls concerned were called to a new *human* life on other planets, presumably by being born in the manner of a human being, perhaps retaining some dim memory of their earlier existence. I dare not say anything more definite about this, nor whether the transmigration of souls served only the purposes of purification or other purposes as well (the populating of other planets?). From the voices that speak to me, as well as in other ways, I learnt of a number of persons to whom in after life a much lower station was allotted than they had held in the previous one, perhaps as a kind of punishment.

Particularly noteworthy was the case of Mr. v. W., whose soul for a long time profoundly influenced my relation with God and therefore my personal fate, as Flechsig's soul does to this very day.[9] p. 16
During my stay in Pierson's Asylum (the "Devil's Kitchen"), von W. held there the position of senior attendant—not as a real human being but, as I thought then and think still, as a "fleeting-improvised-man", that is to say as a soul temporarily given human shape by divine miracle. He was said to have already led a second life as the "Insurance Agent Marx" on some other planet during the process of transmigration of souls.

Souls completely cleansed by the process of purification ascended to heaven and so gained the *state of Blessedness*. This consisted of uninterrupted enjoyment combined with the contemplation of God. The idea of perpetual idleness is unbearable for a human being, because man is accustomed to work and, as the proverb p. 17
says, it is only work which makes life sweet for him. But one must remember that souls are different from human beings and therefore it is not permissible to gauge their feelings by human

[9] At first glance it may appear contradictory that I mention people here as in footnote 1 above who are still among the living, and speak at the same time of a transmigration of souls which they are said to have undergone. This is in fact even for me a riddle which I can only partially solve, and which would be quite insoluble by purely human notions. Nevertheless several instances particularly that of von W.'s soul and Flechsig's soul are established fact for me, because for years I have felt the direct influence of these souls on my body, and still feel daily and hourly Flechsig's soul or possibly *part* of Flechsig's soul. I will try to give a more detailed explanation of these matters below when I come to speak of the so-called "play-with-human-beings". Here it suffices to point to the possibility of a *partition of souls* which would make it possible for certain nerves of mind belonging to a person still living (which would, as mentioned above, retain the *full knowledge of his personal identity* if only for a short time) to play some different role when outside his body.

standards.[10] Souls' greatest happiness lies in continual revelling in pleasure combined with recollections of their human past. They were able to exchange their recollections and by means of divine rays—borrowed for this purpose, so to speak—obtain knowledge about the conditions of persons still living on earth in whom they were interested, their relatives, friends, etc., and probably even help raise them up after death to attain to the state of Blessedness. But the souls' own happiness was not clouded by learning of their relatives' unhappy state on earth. For although the souls could retain the memory of their own human past, they could not for any length of time retain new impressions which they received as souls. This natural tendency of souls to forget would soon have erased any *new* adverse impressions. There were gradations within the state of Blessedness according to the staying power which nerves concerned had achieved in their human life, and probably also according to the number of nerves which were deemed worthy of being raised to heaven.

p. 18 The male state of Blessedness was superior to the female state; the latter seems to have consisted mainly in an uninterrupted feeling of voluptuousness. Further, the soul of a Goethe, a Bismarck, etc., is likely to have retained its self-consciousness (knowledge of its own identity) for centuries, while the soul of a child which died young, might only have preserved it for the same number of years as it had lived. It was granted to no human soul to remain aware *for all eternity* of having been this or that human being. It was rather the ultimate destiny of all souls to merge with other souls, and integrate into higher entities, remaining aware only of being part of God ("forecourts of heaven"). This shows that they did not perish—*as far as this goes* souls were granted eternal existence—it was a continued life but with a different awareness. Only a narrow-minded person would find this an imperfection in the state of Blessedness—compared with personal immortality in the sense of the Christian religion. What purpose could it have served the soul to remember the name it once bore among men and its earlier personal relationships, when not only its children and grandchildren had long since gone to eternal rest, but numerous other generations had gone to their graves as well,

[10] Richard Wagner for instance, as if with some insight into these things, makes Tannhäuser say in the ecstasy of love: "Alas your love overwhelmes me: *perpetual enjoyment is only for Gods,* I as a mortal am subject to change." One finds many such almost prophetic visions in our poets which confirms my belief that they had received divine inspiration by way of nerve-contact (especially in dreams).

and perhaps even the nation to which it once belonged had been struck off the roll of living nations. Thus while still in Flechsig's Asylum I became acquainted with rays—that is to say complexes of blessed human souls merged into higher entities—belonging to the old Judaism ("Jehovah rays"), the old Persians ("Zoroaster rays") and the old Germans ("Thor and Odin rays") among which certainly not a single soul remained with any awareness p. 19
of the name under which it had belonged to one or other of these peoples thousands of years ago.[11]

God Himself dwelt above the "forecourts of heaven"; He was also called the "posterior realms of God" in contradistinction to these "anterior realms of God". The posterior realms of God were (and still are) subject to a peculiar division, a lower God (Ariman) and upper God (Ormuzd) being distinguished. I know nothing more about the further significance of this partition,[12] except that the lower God (Ariman) seems to have felt attracted to nations of originally brunette race (the Semites) and the upper God to nations of originally blonde race (the Aryan peoples). It is significant that a hint of this division is found in the religious notions of many peoples. Identical with Ormuzd are Balder of the Germans, Bielebog (the white God) or Swantewit of the Slavs, Poseidon of the Greeks and Neptune of the Romans; identical with Ariman are Wodan (Odin) of the Germans, Czernebog (the black God) of the Slavs, Zeus of the Greeks and Jupiter of the Romans. I first heard of the lower and the upper God as Ariman and Ormuzd from the voices that talk to me at the beginning of July 1894 (perhaps at the end of my first week p. 20
in this Asylum); since then I have heard these names daily.[13] This date coincided with the depletion of the anterior realms of

[11] This exposition about the "forecourts of heaven" may give an indication of the eternal cycle of things which is the basis of the Order of the World. In creating something, God in a sense divests Himself of part of Himself or gives different form to part of His nerves. This apparent loss is restored when after hundreds or thousands of years the nerves of departed human beings who, in their lifetime had been nourished by other created things and had attained to the state of Blessedness, return to Him as the "forecourts of heaven".

[12] Apart from what is said below concerning "unmanning".

[13] One of my main reasons for believing that the old Persians (naturally before their later decay) were pre-eminently the "chosen people of God", in other words that they must have been a nation of quite remarkable moral virtue, was that the names of the corresponding Persian divinities had been retained for the lower and upper Gods. This belief is supported by the unusual strength which I noticed at one time in the "Zoroaster rays". The name Ariman occurs by the way also in Lord Byron's Manfred in connection with a soul murder.

God with which I had previously been in contact (perhaps from the middle of March 1894).

The above picture of the nature of God and the continued existence of the human soul after death differs markedly in some respects from the Christian views on these matters. It seems to me that a comparison between the two can only favour the former. God was not *omniscient* and *omnipresent* in the sense that He *continuously* saw inside every individual living person, perceived every feeling of his nerves, that is to say at all times " tried his heart and reins ". But there was no need for this because after death the nerves of human beings with all the impressions they had received during life lay bare before God's eye, so that an unfailingly just judgment could be reached as to whether they were worthy of being received into the realms of heaven. In any case it was always *possible* for God to get to know the inner person through nerve-contact, whenever the need arose. On the other hand the picture I have drawn lacks any of the features of severity,
p. 21 of purposeless cruelty imprinted on some of the notions of the Christian and in a still greater degree on those of other religions. The whole Order of the World therefore appears as a " miraculous structure ",[14] the sublimity of which surpasses in my opinion all conceptions which in the course of history men and peoples have developed about their relation to God.

p. 22

II

This " miraculous structure " has recently suffered a rent, intimately connected with my personal fate. But it is impossible even for me to present the deeper connections in a way which human understanding can fully grasp. My personal experiences enable me to lift the veil only partially; the rest is intuition and conjecture. I want to say by way of introduction that the leading roles in the genesis of this development, the first beginnings of which go back perhaps as far as the eighteenth century, were played on the one hand by the names of Flechsig and Schreber (probably not specifying any individual member of these families), and on the other by the concept of *soul murder.*

[14] Again an expression which I did not invent. I had spoken—in the thought—or nerve-language mentioned below—of *miraculous organisation* whereupon the expression " miraculous structure " was suggested to me from outside.

To start with the latter: the idea is widespread in the folk-lore and poetry of all peoples that it is somehow possible to take possession of another person's soul in order to prolong one's life at another soul's expense, or to secure some other advantages which outlast death. One has only to think for example of Goethe's Faust, Lord Byron's Manfred, Weber's Frieschütz, etc. Commonly, however, the main role is supposed to be played by p. 23
the Devil, who entices a human being into selling his soul to him by means of a drop of blood, etc. for some worldly advantages; yet it is difficult to see what the Devil was to do with a soul so caught, if one is not to assume that torturing a soul as an end in itself gave the Devil special pleasure.

Although the latter idea must be relegated to the realm of fable because the Devil as a power inimical to God does not exist at all according to the above, yet the wide dissemination of the legend motif of soul murder or soul theft gives food for thought; it is hardly likely that such ideas could have been formed by so many peoples without any basis in fact. The voices which talk to me have daily stressed ever since the beginning of my contact with God (mid-March 1894) the fact that the crisis that broke upon the realms of God was caused by somebody having *committed soul murder*; at first Flechsig was named as the instigator of soul murder but of recent times in an attempt to reverse the facts I myself have been "represented" as the one who had committed soul murder. I therefore concluded that at one time something had happened between perhaps earlier generations of the Flechsig and Schreber families which amounted to soul murder; in the same way as through further developments, at the time when my nervous illness seemed almost incurable, I gained the conviction that soul murder had been attempted on me by somebody, albeit unsuccessfully.

L'appetit vient en mangeant: it is therefore quite possible that after the first, more soul murders were committed on the souls of other people. I will leave open the question whether the first soul murder was really the moral responsibility of a human being; p. 24
much of this remains mysterious. Originally perhaps it was a battle arising out of jealousy between souls already departed from life. Both the Flechsigs and the Schrebers belonged, it was said, to "the highest nobility of heaven"; the Schrebers had the particular title "Margraves of Tuscany and Tasmania", according to the souls' habit of adorning themselves with high-sounding worldly titles from a kind of personal vanity. Several names of

both families are concerned: of the Flechsigs particularly Abraham Fürchtegott Flechsig, Professor Paul Theodor Flechsig, and a Daniel Fürchtegott Flechsig; the latter lived towards the end of the eighteenth century and was said to have been an "Assistant Devil" because of something that had happened in the nature of a soul murder. However that may be, it is certain that I was in contact for some time with the nerves of Professor Paul Theodor Flechsig and of Daniel Fürchtegott Flechsig (whether with the former also in his quality as a soul?) and had parts of their souls in my body. The soul of Daniel Fürchtegott Flechsig vanished years ago (flitted away); part at least of Professor Paul Theodor Flechsig's soul (i.e. a certain number of nerves originally with the consciousness of Professor Paul Theodor Flechsig's identity, which however in the meantime had become very much reduced) still exists as a "tested soul" in heaven. The only knowledge I possess of the Flechsig family tree comes from what was said by the voices that talk to me; it would therefore be interesting to find out whether there had actually been a Daniel Fürchtegott Flechsig and an Abraham Fürchtegott Flechsig among the forbears of the present Professor Flechsig.

p. 25 I presume that at one time a bearer of the name Flechsig—a human being carrying that name—succeeded in *abusing* nerve-contact granted him for the purpose of divine inspiration or some other reasons, in order *to retain his hold on the divine rays*. This is naturally only an hypothesis, but as in scientific research it has to be adhered to until a better explanation for the events under investigation is found. It seems very probable that contact with divine nerves was granted to a person who specialized in nervous illnesses, partly because he would be expected to be a highly intellectual person, partly because everything concerning human nerves must be of particular interest to God, starting with His instinctive knowledge that an increase of *nervousness* among men could endanger His realms. Asylums for the mentally ill were therefore called in the basic language "God's Nerve-Institutes". If the above-mentioned Daniel Fürchtegott Flechsig was the first to offend against the Order of the World by abusing contact with divine nerves, this would not be contradicted absolutely by the same man being called a *Country Clergyman* by the voices that talk to me, because at the time when Daniel Fürchtegott Flechsig was supposed to have lived—in the eighteenth century about the time of Frederick the Great[15]—public Asylums for the insane were not yet in existence.

One would therefore have to imagine that such a person, engaged in the practice of nervous diseases—having perhaps another profession besides—believed he had at some time seen miraculous visions *in a dream* and experienced miraculous things, which he felt an urge to investigate further, either out of ordinary human curiosity or keen scientific interest. He need not necessarily have known at the outset that he was in direct or indirect contact with God. He may have tried to recall these dream visions in subsequent nights and so have discovered that they really did return during sleep in the same or perhaps slightly different form supplementing the earlier information. Naturally interest was heightened particularly as the dreamer may have learnt that these communications came from his own forbears, who lately had been outstripped in some way or other by members of the Schreber family. He may then have tried to influence the nerves of his contemporaries by exerting his will power after the fashion of thought readers—such as Cumberland etc.—and he may thus have found that this was possible to a certain extent. He may have resisted breaking off the contact into which divine rays had directly or indirectly entered with him, or made it dependent on conditions which could not be denied him, considering the souls' natural weakness of character compared with that of living men, and in any case it was not thought possible to keep up permanent nerve-contact with a single human being. One can imagine that in this way something like a conspiracy may have arisen between such a person and the elements of the anterior realms of God to the detriment of the Schreber race, perhaps in the direction of denying them offspring or possibly only of denying them choice of those professions which would lead to closer relations with God such as that of a nerve specialist. In view of what was said above about the constitution of the realms of God and the (limited) omnipresence of God, such events need not necessarily have come to the knowledge of the posterior realms of God immediately. The conspirators—to retain this expression—perhaps succeeded in

p. 26

p. 27

[15] I gather this from a conversation which I had in a later contact with Daniel Fürchtegott Flechsig's nerves about Frederick the Great, whom he still remembered, as he was probably the most important living person of his time. On the other hand he knew nothing for instance of railways and it was therefore interesting for me to try to give a deceased soul by way of conversation kept up by nerve-contact an idea of what railways are and what great changes this invention has brought about in human communications.

silencing possible scruples about allowing nerve-contact to be made with members of the Schreber family in an unguarded moment such as occurs sometime in everybody's life, in order also to convince the next higher instance of the hierarchy of God's realms that one Schreber soul more or less did not matter in the face of danger threatening the very existence of the realms of God.[16] In this way it may have come about that one did not immediately and resolutely oppose efforts inspired by ambition and lust for power, which could possibly lead to soul murder—if such a thing exist—that is to say to the surrender of a soul to another person perhaps for prolonging earthly life, for appropriating his mental powers, for attaining a kind of personal immunity or some other advantage. On the other hand one may have underrated the danger even for the realms of God which this entailed. One felt
p. 28 so possessed of immense power that the possibility of one single human being ever becoming a danger to God Himself was not taken into consideration. I have in fact not the least doubt from what I later learned and experienced of God's miraculous power that God—provided that conditions in accordance with the Order of the World prevailed—would at any time have been able to annihilate an embarrassing human being by sending him a fatal illness or striking him with lightning.

Perhaps one did not think it necessary to proceed immediately with the most drastic measures against the presumed soul murderer, while his trespass consisted at first only of abuse of contact with divine nerves, and the eventuality of soul murder seemed remote, and if the person's merit and moral conduct were such that it seemed unlikely that it would come to such an extremity. Apart from these hints I cannot enlarge on the essential nature of soul murder or, so to speak, its technique. One might only add (the passage which follows is unfit for publication). I am sure that the person, whether it was the present Professor Flechsig or one of his forbears, who must take the blame for being the original instigator of "soul murders", must have had some notion of the supernatural matters which I have now come to know, although he certainly did not penetrate to a deeper knowledge of God and the Order of the World. It is inconceivable that anybody who has

[16] It is in this connection that during my stay in Flechsig's Asylum I heard more than once the expression "Merely a Schreber soul" from the voices that talked to me. I have some reasons for thinking that contact was made with my nerves intentionally at moments when I might have appeared in a morally less favourable light; but it would lead too far afield to enlarge on this here.

won a profound faith in God and the certainty that in any case he is definitely guaranteed a state of Blessedness commensurate with the purity of his nerves should think of violating other people's souls. It is equally unlikely that this should have happened in the case of a person who could be called *religious* if only in the sense of our positive religion. I do not know what the present Professor p. 29
Flechsig's attitude to religious matters was or is. Should he be or have been, a *doubter*, as so many others are today, he could not be blamed, least of all by myself who, I must confess, belonged to that category myself until divine revelation taught me better.

Whoever has taken the trouble of reading the above attentively may spontaneously have thought that God Himself must have been or be in a precarious position, if the conduct of a single human being could endanger Him in any way and if even He Himself, if only in lower instances,[19] could be enticed into a kind of conspiracy p. 30
against human beings who are fundamentally innocent. Such an objection may not be altogether unjustified but I must not omit to add that my own faith in the grandeur and sublimity of God and the Order of the World was not shaken. Not even God Himself is or was a being of such *absolute perfection* as most religions attribute to Him. The power of attraction, this even to me unfathomable law, according to which rays and nerves mutually attract one another, harbours a kernel of danger for the realms of God; this forms perhaps the basis of the Germanic saga of the Twilight of the Gods. Growing nervousness among mankind could and can increase these dangers considerably. God, as already mentioned, saw living human beings *only from without*; as a rule His omni-

[19] The expression " instances " (which is mine) as well as " hierarchy " above, p. 29
seem to me to furnish an approximately accurate picture of the constitution of the realms of God. As long as I was in contact with the anterior realms of God (the forecourts of heaven) (March to early July 1894) every ' leader of rays " (according to one expression *I heard* " anterior column leaders ") used to behave as if he were " God's omnipotence ". He knew that superior ones came behind him but not who these superior ones were, nor how high they went. The posterior realms of God (Ariman and Ormuzd) themselves appeared on the scene (beginning of July 1894) with such overwhelming brilliance at first that even v. W's and Flechsig's souls, which were at that time still " tested souls " could not help being impressed; they even temporarily gave up their customary sarcastic opposition to God's omnipotence. I will explain later why these phenomena of light did not persist around me. Among them I saw Ariman at night, not in a dream but while awake and Ormuzd on several successive *days* while I was in the garden. At the time I was accompanied only by the attendant M. I am forced to assume that the latter was at that time not a real human being but a fleeting-improvised-man, because he would otherwise have been so dazzled by the light phenomena which he must have seen (they occupied almost a 1/6th to an 1/8th part of the sky), that he would have expressed astonishment in some way.

presence and omniscience did not extend within *living* man. Even God's eternal love existed only for creation *as a whole*. As soon as there is a clash of interests with individual human beings or nations (Sodom and Gomorrah for instance!) perhaps even with the whole population of a planet (through an increase of nervousness or immorality), the instinct of self-preservation must be aroused in God as in every other living being. Ultimately that of course is perfect which serves its own particular purpose, even if human imagination could picture a still more ideal condition.[20] This
p. 31 purpose was nevertheless achieved: for God eternal joy at His creation, for human beings the joy of life during their earthly existence, and after death the greatest happiness, the state of Blessedness. It is quite unthinkable that God would have denied any single human being his share in the state of Blessedness as every increase of the "forecourts of heaven" could only serve to increase His own power and strengthen His defences against the dangers of His approaching mankind. No clash of interests between God and individual human beings could arise as long as the latter behaved according to the Order of the World. If despite this such a clash of interests arose in my case because of supposed soul murder, this can only be due to such a marvellous concatination of events[21] as probably never before happened in the history of the world, and I hope will never happen again. Even in such an extraordinary case the Order of the World carries its own remedies for healing the wounds inflicted upon it; the remedy is *Eternity*. Whilst I had earlier (for about two years) believed I had to assume and was forced by my experiences to assume, that if God were permanently tied to my person, all creation on earth would have to perish with the exception of some play-with-miracles in my immediate surroundings, I have had reason lately to modify this idea considerably.

Some people were made very unhappy; I may say that I myself lived through cruel times and endured bitter sufferings. On the other hand six years of uninterrupted influx of God's nerves into my body has led to the total loss of all the states of Blessedness
p. 32 which had accumulated until then and made it impossible for the time being to renew them; the state of *Blessedness* is so to speak suspended and all human beings who have since died or will die

[20] No one would wish to deny that the human organism is one of high perfection. Yet perhaps most people have at one time thought how nice it would be if man could also fly like the birds.

[21] More of this later.

can for the time being not attain to it. For God's nerves also it is unpleasant and against their will to enter into my body, shown by the continual cries for help which I daily hear in the sky from those parts of the nerves which have become separated from the total mass of nerves. All these losses can however be made good again insofar as an *Eternity* exists, even though total restoration of the previous state may take thousands of years.

III

p. 33

The content of Chapters I and II was a necessary preliminary to what follows. What could so far only partially be put up as axiomatic, will now be proved as far as at all possible.

I will first consider some events concerning *other members of my family*, which may possibly in some way be related to the presumed soul murder; these are all more or less mysterious, and can hardly be explained in the light of usual human experience.

(The further content of this chapter is omitted as unfit for publication.)

IV

p. 34

I come now to *my personal* fortunes during the two nervous illnesses which I have suffered. I have twice had a nervous illness, each time in consequence of mental overstrain; the first (while Chairman of the County Court of Chemnitz) was occasioned by my candidature for parliament, the second by the extraordinary burden of work on taking up office as President of the Senate of a Court of Appeal in Dresden, to which I had been newly appointed.

The first of the two illnesses commenced in the autumn of 1884 and was fully cured at the end of 1885, so that I was able to resume work as Chairman of the County Court at Leipzig to which I had in the meantime been transferred on 1st January 1886. The second nervous illness began in October 1893 and still continues. I spent the greater part of both illnesses in the Psychiatric Clinic of the University of Leipzig under the Directorship of Professor Flechsig, the first time from early December 1884 to the beginning of June 1885, the second time from about the middle of November 1893 till about the middle of June 1894. In each case when first
p. 35 I entered the Asylum I had not the faintest idea of an antagonism existing between the Schreber and Flechsig families, nor of the supernatural matters of which I have treated in the preceding chapters.

The first illness passed without any occurrences bordering on the supernatural, and while it lasted I had on the whole only favourable impressions of Professor Flechsig's methods of treatment. Some mistakes may have been made. Even in the course of that illness I was and still am of the opinion that *white lies*, which a nerve specialist may perhaps not be able to dispense with altogether in the case of some mental patients, but which he must nevertheless employ only with the greatest circumspection, were hardly ever appropriate in my case, for he must soon have realized that in me he was dealing with a human being of high intellect, of uncommon keenness of understanding and acute powers of observation. Yet I could only consider it a white lie when, for instance, Professor Flechsig wanted to put down my illness solely to poisoning with potassium bromide, for which Dr. R. in S., in whose care I had been before, was to be blamed. I believe I could have been more rapidly cured of certain hypochondriacal ideas with which I was preoccupied at the time, particularly concern over loss of weight, if I had been allowed to operate the scales which served to weigh patients a few times myself; the scales used in the University Clinic at the time were of a peculiar construction unfamiliar to me. All the same these are only minor points on which I place little importance; perhaps it is unreasonable to expect the Director of a big Asylum with hundreds of patients to concern himself in such detail with the mental state of a single patient. The main point was that I was eventually cured (after a prolonged convalescence),

and therefore I had at the time no reason to be other than most grateful to Professor Flechsig; I gave this special expression by a subsequent visit and in my opinion an adequate honorarium. My p. 36
wife felt even more sincere gratitude and worshipped Professor Flechsig as the man who had restored her husband to her; for this reason she kept his picture on her desk for many years.

After recovering from my first illness I spent eight years with my wife, on the whole quite happy ones, rich also in outward honours and marred only from time to time by the repeated disappointment of our hope of being blessed with children. In June 1893 I was informed (in the first place by the Minister of Justice, Dr. Schurig in person) of my impending appointment as *Senatspräsident* to the Superior Court in Dresden.

During this time I had several dreams to which I did not then attribute any particular significance, and which I would even today disregard as the proverb says "Dreams are mere shadows", had my experience in the meantime not made me think of the *possibility* at least of their being connected with the contact which had been made with me by divine nerves. I dreamt several times that my former nervous illness had returned; naturally I was as unhappy about this in the dream, as I felt happy on waking that it had only been a dream. Furthermore, one morning while still in bed (whether still half asleep or already awake I cannot remember), I had a feeling which, thinking about it later when fully awake, struck me as highly peculiar. It was the idea that it really must be rather pleasant to be a woman succumbing to intercourse. This idea was so foreign to my whole nature that I may say I would have rejected it with indignation if fully awake; from what I have experienced since I cannot exclude the possibility p. 37
that some external influences were at work to implant this idea in me.

On the 1st of October 1893 I took up office as *Senatspräsident* to the Superior Court in Dresden. I have already mentioned the heavy burden of work I found there. I was driven, maybe by personal ambition, but certainly also in the interests of the office, to achieve first of all the necessary respect among my colleagues and others concerned with the Court (barristers, etc.) by unquestionable efficiency. The task was all the heavier and demanded all the more tact in my personal dealings with the members of the panel of five Judges over which I had to preside, as almost all of them were much senior to me (up to twenty years), and anyway they were much more intimately acquainted with the

procedure of the Court, to which I was a newcomer. It thus happened that after a few weeks I had already overtaxed myself mentally. I started to sleep badly at the very moment when I was able to feel that I had largely mastered the difficulties of settling down in my new office and in my new residence, etc. I started taking sodium bromide. There was almost no opportunity for social distraction which would certainly have been very much better for me—this became evident to me when I slept considerably better after the only occasion on which we had been asked to a dinner party—but we hardly knew anybody in Dresden. The first really bad, that is to say almost sleepless nights, occurred in the last days of October or the first days of November. It was then that an extraordinary event occurred. During several nights when I could not get to sleep, a recurrent crackling noise in the wall of our bedroom became noticeable at shorter or longer intervals; time and again it woke me as I was about to go to sleep. Naturally
p. 38 we thought of a mouse although it was very extraordinary that a mouse should have found its way to the first floor of such a solidly built house. But having heard similar noises innumerable times since then, and still hearing them around me every day in daytime and at night, I have come to recognize them as undoubted divine miracles—they are called "interferences" by the voices talking to me—and I must at least suspect, without being too definite about it, that even then it was already a matter of such a miracle; *in other words that right from the beginning the more or less definite intention existed to prevent my sleep and later my recovery from the illness resulting from the insomnia for a purpose which cannot at this stage be further specified.*[22]

My illness now began to assume a menacing character; already on the 8th or 9th of November Doctor Ö., whom I had consulted, made me take a week's sick leave, which we were going to use to consult Professor Flechsig, in whom we placed all our faith since his successful treatment of my first illness. Because it was a Sunday and Professor Flechsig would not be available, we (my wife and I) travelled via Chemnitz and spent the night from Sunday to Monday with my brother-in-law. That evening I was given an injection
p. 39 of morphine, and for the first time chloral during the night—

[22] I must not omit to add that it amounted to nothing more than a *dolus indeterminatus* carried to the extreme—if a legal expression be permitted—an attribute of the character of the souls which I have in the meantime got to know; that is to say intentions which were very frequently followed by a change of mind and mood as soon as close reflection brought the conviction that the person concerned was really worthy of a better fate.

perhaps accidentally not in the dosage ordered right away; the previous evening I suffered as severely from palpitation as in my first illness, so that walking up only a moderate incline caused attacks of anxiety. The night in Chemnitz was also bad. Early the following day (Monday) we travelled to Leipzig and from the Bavarian Station by cab direct to Professor Flechsig at the University Clinic, having advised him of our visit the day before by telegram. A long interview followed in which I must say Professor Flechsig developed a remarkable eloquence which affected me deeply. He spoke of the advances made in psychiatry since my first illness, of newly discovered sleeping drugs, etc., and gave me hope of delivering me of the whole illness through one prolific sleep, which was to start if possible at three o'clock in the afternoon and last to the following day.

My mood thereupon became steadier, also perhaps because travelling through the fresh morning air for several hours and the time of day (morning) might have strengthened my nerves a little. We went right away to the chemist to fetch the sleeping drug prescribed, then had a meal with my mother at her house, and I spent the rest of the day quite bearably, going for a little walk amongst other things. Naturally I did not get to bed (in my mother's house) as early as 3 o'clock, but (possibly according to some secret instruction which my wife had received) it was delayed until the 9th hour. More serious symptoms developed again immediately before going to bed. Unfortunately the bed was cold because it had been aired too long, with the result that I was immediately seized by a severe rigor and was already in a state of great excitement when I took the sleeping drug. Because of this the sleeping drug failed almost entirely in its effect, and after one p. 40
or more hours my wife also gave me the chloral hydrate which was kept at hand in reserve. Despite this I spent the night almost without sleep, and once even left the bed in an attack of anxiety in order to make preparations for a kind of suicidal attempt by means of a towel or suchlike; this woke my wife who stopped me. The next morning my nerves were badly shattered; the blood had gone from my extremities to the heart, my mood was gloomy in the extreme and Professor Flechsig, who had been sent for early in the morning, therefore advised my admission into his Asylum, for which I set out immediately by cab accompanied by him.

After a warm bath I was at once put to bed, which I did not leave again for the next 4 or 5 days. A certain R. . . was assigned to me as attendant. My illness progressed rapidly during the following days; the nights passed mostly without sleep because the weaker sleeping drugs (camphor, etc.) which were tried first so as to avoid the permanent use of chloral hydrate from the beginning, failed to act. I could not occupy myself in any way; nor did I see anybody of my family. I passed the days therefore in endless melancholy; my mind was occupied almost exclusively with thoughts of death. It seems to me in retrospect that Professor Flechsig's plan of curing me consisted in intensifying my nervous depression as far as possible, in order to bring about a cure all at once by a sudden change of mood. At least this is the only way I can explain the following event, which I could otherwise only attribute to malicious intent.[23]

p. 41 About the fourth or fifth night after my admission to the Asylum, I was pulled out of bed by two attendants in the middle of the night and taken to a cell fitted out for dements (maniacs) to sleep in. I was already in a highly excited state, in a fever delirium so to speak, and was naturally terrified in the extreme by this event, the reasons for which I did not know. The way led through the billiard room; there, because I had no idea what one intended to do with me and therefore thought I had to resist, a fight started between myself clad only in a shirt, and the two attendants, during which I tried to hold fast to the billiard table, but was eventually overpowered and removed to the above-mentioned cell. There I was left to my fate; I spent the rest of the night mostly sleepless in this cell, furnished only with an iron bedstead and some bedding. Regarding myself as totally lost, I made a naturally unsuccessful attempt during the night to hang myself from the bedstead with the sheet. I was completely ruled by the idea that there was nothing left for a human being for whom sleep could no longer be procured by all the means of medical art, but to take his life. I knew that this was not permitted in asylums, but I laboured under the delusion that when all attempts at cure had been exhausted, one would be discharged—solely for the purpose of making an end to one's life either in one's own home or somewhere else.

I was therefore greatly surprised when on the following morning

[23] I must mention that during a later conversation Professor Flechsig denied the whole occurrence in the billiard room and all connected with it, and tried to make out that it was only a figment of my imagination—this by the way was one of the circumstances which from then on made me somewhat distrustful of Professor Flechsig. But that it really happened and that there could be no question of my senses being deceived is certain, because it cannot be denied that in the morning after the night in question I found myself in the padded cell and was visited there by Dr. Täuscher.

the doctor still came to see me. Professor Flechsig's Assistant p. 42
Physician, Dr. Täuscher appeared, and told me that there was no intention whatsoever of giving up treatment; this, coupled with the manner in which he tried to raise my spirits again—I cannot deny him also my appreciation of the excellent way he spoke to me on that occasion—had the effect of a very favourable change in my mood. I was led back to the room I had previously occupied and spent the best day of the whole of my (second) stay in Flechsig's Asylum, that is to say the *only day on which I was enlivened by a joyful spirit of hope*. Even the attendant R. behaved most tactfully and skilfully in his whole conservation, so that in retrospect I sometimes asked myself whether he also had received higher inspirations (in the same way as Dr. Täuscher). In the morning I even played billiards with him, had a hot bath in the afternoon and maintained my better mood until the evening. They were going to see whether I could sleep entirely without sleeping drugs. Indeed I went to bed relatively calm, but could not get to sleep. After a few hours I could no longer remain calm; the rush of blood to my heart again caused attacks of anxiety. After the change-over of attendants—an attendant sat constantly by my bed and was relieved by another in the middle of the night—something to make me sleep was eventually given—'Nekrin' or some such name—and I must have fallen asleep for a short while, which however no longer strengthened my nerves in any way. On the contrary my nerves were shattered again the following morning, indeed so badly that I vomited the breakfast. A particularly terrifying impression was created in me by the
totally distorted features which I thought I could see on the p. 43
attendant R. when I awoke.

From then on I was regularly given chloral hydrate every night, and the following weeks were at least outwardly a little calmer, because in this way moderate sleep was usually procured. My wife visited me regularly and in the last two weeks before Christmas I spent part of every day at my mother's house. But the hyper-excitability of my nerves remained and got worse rather than better. In the weeks after Christmas I went for a drive every day with my wife and the attendant. But I was so weak that when I got out of the carriage (in Rosenthal or in Scheibenholz) every little distance of a few hundred paces seemed a hazard on which I could not decide without inner anxiety. In other respects too my whole nervous system was in a state of utter laxity. I could hardly, if at all, manage any intellectual occupation such as reading

newspapers. Even mainly mechanical occupations such as jig-saw puzzles, patience and suchlike increased my nervous tension to such a degree that I usually had to stop after a short time; I could scarcely even play a few games of draughts with the attendant R. . . in the evening. During that time I mostly ate and drank well, and was still in the habit of smoking several cigars a day. The laxity of my nerves increased with the simultaneous reappearance of states of anxiety, whenever they again tried giving me weaker sleeping drugs instead of chloral hydrate, which, although it strengthens the nerves temporarily, nevertheless damages them if used for any length of time. My will to live was completely broken; I could
p. 44 see nothing in the future but a fatal outcome, perhaps produced by committing suicide eventually; as to the plans for the future with which my wife tried again and again to raise my spirits, I could only shake my head in disbelief.

A further decline in my nervous state and an important chapter in my life commenced about the 15th of February 1894 when my wife, who until then had spent a few hours every day with me and had also taken lunch with me in the Asylum, undertook a four-day journey to her father in Berlin in order to have a holiday herself, of which she was in urgent need. My condition deteriorated so much in these four days that after her return I saw her only once more, and then declared that I could not wish my wife to see me again in the low state into which I had fallen. From then on my wife's visits ceased; when after a long time I did see her again at the window of a room opposite mine, such important changes had meanwhile occurred in my environment and in myself that I no longer considered her a living being, but only thought I saw in her a human form produced by miracle in the manner of the " fleeting-improvised-men ". Decisive for my mental collapse was one particular night; during that night I had a quite unusual number of pollutions (perhaps half a dozen).

From then on appeared the first signs of communication with supernatural powers, particularly that of nerve-contact which Professor Flechsig kept up with me in such a way that he spoke to my nerves without being present in person. From then on I also gained the impression that Professor Flechsig had secret designs against me; this seemed confirmed when I once asked him during
p. 45 a personal visit whether he really honestly believed that I could be cured, and he held out certain hopes, *but could no longer*—at least so it seemed to me—*look me straight in the eye.*

I must now discuss the nature of the frequently mentioned *inner voices* which since then have spoken to me incessantly, and also of what in my opinion is the tendency innate in the Order of the World, according to which a human being (" a seer of spirits ") must under certain circumstances be " unmanned " (transformed into a woman) once he has entered into indissoluble contact with divine nerves (rays). The next chapter is devoted to an exposition of these circumstances; this is, however, infinitely difficult.

V p. 46

Apart from normal human language there is also a kind of *nerve-language* of which, as a rule, the healthy human being is not aware. In my opinion this is best understood when one thinks of the processes by which a person tries to imprint certain words in his memory in a definite order, as for instance a child learning a poem by heart which he is going to recite at school, or a priest a sermon he is going to deliver in Church. The words are *repeated silently* (as in a *silent prayer* to which the congregation is called from the pulpit), that is to say a human being causes his nerves to vibrate in the way which corresponds to the use of the words concerned, but the real organs of speech (lips, tongue, teeth, etc.) are either not set in motion at all or only coincidentally.

Naturally under normal (in consonance with the Order of the World) conditions, use of this *nerve-language* depends only on the will of the person whose nerves are concerned; no human being as such can force another to use this nerve-language.[25] In my case, p. 47
however, since my nervous illlness took the above-mentioned critical turn, my nerves have been set in motion *from without* incessantly and without any respite.

Divine rays above all have the power of influencing the nerves of a human being in this manner; by this means God has always been able to infuse dreams into a sleeping human being. I myself first felt this influence as emanating from Professor Flechsig. The only possible explanation I can think of is that Professor Flechsig in some way knew how to put divine rays to his own use; later, apart from Professor Flechsig's nerves, direct divine rays also entered into contact with my nerves. This influence has in the course of years assumed forms more and more contrary to the

[25] *Hypnotising* is perhaps an exception, but as a layman in psychiatry I know too little to permit expression of an opinion.

Order of the World and to man's natural right to be master of his own nerves, and I might say become increasingly grotesque.

This influence showed itself relatively early in the form of *compulsive thinking*—an expression which I received from the inner voices themselves and which will hardly be known to other human beings, because the whole phenomenon lies outside all human experience. The nature of compulsive thinking lies in a human being having to think incessantly; in other words, man's natural right to give the nerves of his mind their necessary rest from time to time by thinking nothing (as occurs most markedly during
p. 48 sleep) was from the beginning denied me by the rays in contact with me; they continually wanted to know what I was thinking about. For instance I was asked in these very words: "What are you thinking of now?"; because this question is in itself complete nonsense, as a human being can at certain times as well think of *nothing* as of *thousands of things at the same time*, and because my nerves did not react to this absurd question, one was soon driven to take refuge in a system of *falsifying my thoughts*. For instance the above question was answered spontaneously: "He should" *scilicet* think[26] "about the Order of the World"; that is to say the influence of the rays forced my nerves to perform the movements corresponding to the use of these words. The number of points from which contact with my nerves originated increased with time: apart from Professor Flechsig, who was the
p. 49 only one whom for a time at least I knew definitely to be among the living, they were mostly departed souls who began more and more to interest themselves in me.

In this connection I could mention hundreds if not thousands of names, many of which I learnt later, when some contact with the outside world was restored to me through newspapers and letters,

[26] The word "think" was omitted in the above answer. This was because the souls were in the habit—even before the conditions contrary to the Order of the World had started—of giving their thoughts (when communicating with one another) grammatically incomplete expression; that is to say they omitted certain words which were not essential for the sense. In the course of time this habit degenerated into an abominable abuse of me, because a human being's nerves of mind (his "foundation" as the expression goes in the basic language) were excited continuously by such interrupted phrases, because they automatically try to find the word that is missing to make up the sense. For instance as one of innumerable examples, I have for years heard hundreds of times each day the question: "*Why do you not say it?*", the word "*aloud*" necessary to complete the sense being omitted, and the rays giving the answer themselves as if it came from me: "Because I am stupid perhaps". For years my nerves have had to endure incessantly such and similar terrible nonsense in dreary monotony (as if it came from them). I will later say more about the reason for the choice of expressions and the effects they were designed to produce.

were still among the living; whereas at the time, when as souls they were in contact with my nerves, I could only think they had long since departed this life. Many of the bearers of these names were particularly interested in religion, many were Catholics who expected a furtherance of Catholicism from the way I was expected to behave, particularly the Catholicizing of Saxony and Leipzig; amongst them were the Priest S. in Leipzig, " 14 Leipzig Catholics " (of whom only the name of the Consul General D. was indicated to me, presumably a Catholic Club or its board). The Jesuit Father S. in Dresden, the Ordinary Archbishop in Prague, the Cathedral Dean Moufang, the Cardinals Rampolla, Galimberti and Casati, the Pope himself who was the leader of a peculiar " scorching ray ", finally numerous monks and nuns; on one occasion 240 Benedictine Monks under the leadership of a Father whose name sounded like Starkiewicz, suddenly moved into my head to perish therein. In the case of other souls, religious interests were mixed with national motives; amongst these was a Viennese nerve specialist whose name by coincidence was identical with that of the above-named Benedictine Father, a baptised Jew and Slavophile, who wanted to make Germany Slavic through me and at the same time wanted to institute there the rule of Judaism; like Professor Flechsig for Germany, England and America (that is mainly Germanic States), he appeared to be in his capacity as nerve specialist a kind of administrator of God's interests in p. 50
another of God's provinces (the Slavic parts of Austria); because of this a battle arose for a time between him and Professor Flechsig through jealousy as to who was to predominate. Another group consisted mainly of former members of the Students' Corps Saxonia in Leipzig, to which Professor Flechsig belonged as drinking member[27] and who were, I believed, helped by him to Blessedness; among them were the lawyer Dr. G. S. in Dresden, the Doctor of Medicine S. in Leipzig, Senior District Judge G. and many younger members of the Corps who were later called " those suspended under Cassiopeia ". There were also many members of the Students' Union who had gained such great ascendency for a time that they were able to occupy the planets Jupiter, Saturn and Uranus; the most prominent of them were the lawyer A. K., Vice-President of the Prussian Chamber of Deputies, whom by the way I never knew personally, the University Dean Professor W.,

[27] This also I had not known before, but only learnt from the voices that talk to me through contact with my nerves. It would therefore be interesting to ascertain whether this relatively unimportant detail of Professor Flechsig's earlier life is correct.

and the lawyer H. in Leipzig. They and the previously mentioned members of the Corps Saxonia treated the whole affair going on in my head merely as a continuation of the old feud between members of the Corps and the Students' Union. There were also Dr. Wächter, who was to take up a position of leadership on Sirius, Dr. Hoffmann, who was to take up a similar position on the Pleiades and who therefore, having been dead a long time, appeared already to have reached a higher degree of Blessedness. Both knew me personally in their lifetime and presumably for that reason took a certain interest in me.

p. 51 Finally I wish to name some of my relatives (apart from my father and brother who have already been mentioned above, my mother, my wife and my father-in-law), the friend of my youth Ernest K., who died in 1864, and a Prince who appeared on my head as a "little man", in the sense to be explained later, and there in a manner of speaking went a-walking.

All these souls spoke to me as "voices" more or less at the same time without one knowing of the presence of the others. Everyone who realizes that all this is not just the morbid offspring of my fantasy, will be able to appreciate the unholy turmoil they caused in my head. It is true the souls had at that time still their own thoughts and were therefore able to give information of the highest interest to me; they were also able to answer questions, whereas for a long time now the talk of the voices has consisted only of a terrible, monotonous repetition of ever recurring phrases (learnt by rote). The reason for this I will give later. Besides those souls who were recognizable as specific individuals, there were at the same time other voices pretending to be God's omnipotence itself in higher and higher instances (compare footnote 19); for these the individual souls appeared to act, so to speak, as outposts.

The second point to be discussed in this chapter is the tendency, innate in the Order of the World, to *unman* a human being who has entered into permanent contact with rays. This is connected on the one hand with the nature of God's nerves, through which Blessedness (the enjoyment of which is discussed on pages 16 and 17) is felt, if not exclusively as, at least accompanied by, a greatly increased feeling of voluptuousness; on the other hand it is connected with the basic plan on which the Order of the
p. 52 World seems to rest, that in the case of world catastrophes which necessitate the destruction of mankind on any star, whether intentionally or otherwise, the human race can be renewed. When on some star moral decay ("voluptuous excesses") or perhaps

nervousness has seized the whole of mankind to such an extent that the forecourts of heaven (compare footnote [11]) could not be expected to be adequately replenished by their excessively blackened nerves, or there was reason to fear a dangerous increase of attraction on God's nerves, then the destruction of the human race on that star could occur either spontaneously (through annihilating epidemics, etc.) or, being decided on by God, be put into effect by means of earthquakes, deluges, etc. Perhaps God was also able to withdraw partially or totally the warmth of the sun from a star doomed to perish (or the respective fixed star which served to warm it); this would throw new light on the problem of the *Ice Age* which, as far as I know, has not yet been solved by science. The objection that at the time of the Ice Age on earth, humanity existed only in its (diluvial) beginnings, could hardly be regarded as conclusive. Who can say whether at that time a highly developed race of man did not exist on some other planet, perhaps Venus, upon whose destruction God was bent and which could not be carried out without at the same time causing considerable cooling of the earth which had remained behind in its development?[29] In p. 53
all these matters human beings must strive to see beyond their ingrained petty geocentric ideas and regard the matter from the lofty viewpoint of eternity. It is possible that in this sense Cuvier's theory of periodically recurring world catastrophes contains some truth. In such an event, in order to maintain the species, one single human being was spared—perhaps the relatively most moral—called by the voices that talk to me the "*Eternal Jew*". This appellation has therefore a somewhat different sense from that underlying the legend of the same name of the Jew Ahasver; one is however automatically reminded of the legends of Noah, Deucalion and Pyrrha, etc. Perhaps the legend of the founding of Rome belongs here also, according to which Rhea Sylvia conceived the later Kings Romulus and Remus directly of Mars the God of War, and not of an earthly father. The Eternal Jew (in the sense described) had to be *unmanned* (transformed into a woman) to be able to bear children. This process of unmanning consisted in the (external) male genitals (scrotum and penis) being retracted into the body and the internal sexual organs being at the same time transformed into the corresponding female sexual organs, a process which might have been completed in a sleep lasting

[29] Indeed I had visions (dream images) during my stay in Flechsig's Asylum from which it appeared that other planets had existed which were more infected by moral decay than the earth, the inhabitants of our earth being in comparison distinguished by greater moral purity.

hundreds of years, because the skeleton (pelvis, etc.) had also to be changed. A regression occurred therefore, or a reversal of that developmental process which occurs in the human embryo in the fourth or fifth month of pregnancy, according to whether nature intends the future child to be of male or female sex. It is well known that in the first months of pregnancy the rudiments of both sexes are laid down and the characteristics of the sex which is not developed remain as rudimentary organs at a lower stage of
p. 54 development, like the nipples of the male. The rays of the lower God (Ariman) have the power of producing the miracle of unmanning; the rays of the upper God (Ormuzd) have the power of restoring manliness when necessary. I have myself twice experienced (for a short time) the miracle of unmanning on my own body, as already mentioned in footnote 1; that the miracle did not reach full development and that it was even reversed again, was due only to the fact that, apart from the pure rays of God, other rays were present led by "tested" (impure) souls (compare page 24 above), Flechsig's rays and others, which prevented the completion of the process of transformation in its purity and in accordance with the Order of the World. The Eternal Jew was maintained and provided with the necessary means of life by the "fleeting-improvised-men" (compare footnote 1 above); that is to say souls were for this purpose transitorily put into human shape by miracles, probably not only for the lifetime of the Eternal Jew himself but for many generations, until his offspring were sufficiently numerous to be able to maintain themselves. This seems to be the main purpose of the institution of "fleeting-improvised-men" in the Order of the World. I cannot say whether it also perhaps served the purpose of providing souls in the process of purification with the opportunity of doing some job of work—necessary for their purification—by putting them into human form (compare page 13 above); however that may be, the purpose of the fleeting-improvised-men was not only a *mere play with miracles*, into which it degenerated towards me in the latter part of my stay in Flechsig's Asylum, during my
p. 55 time in Pierson's Asylum and in the early days of my stay in this Asylum.[30]

[30] I have had some indications that before my own case, perhaps in some vastly dim and distant period of the past and on other stars, there might even have been a number of Eternal Jews. The voices that talk to me named some of them; amongst them occurred, if I am not mistaken, something like the name of a Polish Count Czartorisky. One need not necessarily associate this with the Polish nation of our earth, but has to bear in mind the possibility that the Polish nation may lead a second existence on some other star through the transmigration of souls.

It is my opinion that Professor Flechsig must have had some idea of this tendency, innate in the Order of the World, whereby in certain conditions the unmanning of a human being is provided for; perhaps he thought of this himself or these ideas were inspired in him by divine rays, which I think is more likely. *A fundamental misunderstanding* obtained however, which has since run like a red thread through my entire life. It is based upon the fact *that, within the Order of the World, God did not really understand the living human being* and had no need to understand him, because, according to the Order of the World, He dealt only with corpses. The other relevant issue is the dependence on Professor Flechsig, or on his soul, in which God found Himself through His inability to dissolve again the nerve-contact which Professor Flechsig had managed to establish and then to abuse by holding fast to it. Thus began the *policy of vacillation* in which attempts to cure my nervous illness[31]
alternated with efforts to annihilate me as a human being who, p. 56
because of his ever-increasing nervousness, had become a danger to God Himself. From this developed a policy of half measures ("half-heartedness" is the expression which I heard repeatedly), entirely in keeping with the souls' character, who were used to uninterrupted enjoyment, and were therefore not or only little capable of temporary sacrifice or temporary denial of pleasure in order to procure permanent advantages in the future, a quality which is peculiar to human beings. The contact established with my nerves became more indissoluble, the more miracles were directed against me. In the meantime Professor Flechsig had found a way of raising himself up to heaven, either with the whole or part of his soul, and so making himself a leader of rays, without prior death and without undergoing the process of purification. In this way a plot was laid against me (perhaps March or April 1894), the purpose of which was to hand me over to another human being after my nervous illness had been recognized as, or assumed to be, incurable, in such a way that my soul was handed to him, but my body—transformed into a female body and, misconstruing the above-described fundamental tendency of the Order of the World—was then left to that human being for sexual misuse and simply "forsaken", in other words left to rot. One does not seem to have been quite clear as to what was to happen to such a "forsaken" human being, nor whether this actually

[31] This would have been simple to do—anticipating what will be discussed in more detail later—by sacrificing a comparatively small number of pure rays, for rays have also the power to calm nerves and to bring sleep.

meant his death. I have not the slightest doubt that this plot really existed, with the proviso always that I do not dare maintain that Professor Flechsig took part in it in his capacity as a human being. Naturally such matters were not mentioned by Professor
p. 57 Flechsig when he faced me *as a human being*. But the purpose was clearly expressed in the *nerve-language*, as it was called at the beginning of this chapter, that is in the nerve-contact which he maintained *at the same time as a soul*. The way I was treated externally seemed to agree with the intention announced in the nerve-language; for weeks I was kept in bed and my clothes were removed to make me—as I believed—more amenable to voluptuous sensations, which could be stimulated in me by the female nerves which had already started to enter my body; medicines, which I am convinced served the same purpose, were also used[32]; these I therefore refused, or spat out again when an attendant poured them forcibly into my mouth. Having, as I thought, definitely come to realize this abominable intention, one may imagine how my whole sense of manliness and manly honour, my entire moral being, rose up against it, all the more so as I was stirred at that time by the first revelations about divine affairs which I had received through contact with other souls, and was completely filled by holy ideas about God and the Order of the World. Completely cut off from the outside world, without any contact with my family, left in the hands of rough attendants with whom, the inner voices said, it was my duty to fight now and then to prove my manly courage, I could think of nothing else but that any manner of death, however frightful, was preferable
p. 58 to so degrading an end. I therefore decided to end my life by starving to death and refused all food; the inner voices always reiterated that it was my duty to die of hunger and in this way to sacrifice myself for God, and that therefore any partaking of meals which my body demanded was a weakness unworthy of me. This resulted in the so-called "*feeding system*" being started: attendants, mostly the same ones—apart from R. already mentioned, a certain H. and a third whose name I do not know—forced food into my mouth, at times with the utmost brutality. Again and again one of them held my hands while the other *knelt* on me as I lay in bed in order to empty food or pour beer into my mouth.

Every bath I took was connected with ideas of drowning. In the nerve-language one spoke of "purifying baths" and "holy

[32] Especially a white ointment which may have been bismuth or something else as far as I, a layman in medicine, can tell.

baths"; the purpose of the latter was to give me the opportunity of drowning myself. I nearly always entered the bath inwardly afraid that its purpose was to end my life. The inner voices (particularly the souls belonging to the above-mentioned Students' Corps Saxonia, the so-called Brothers of Cassiopeia) spoke to me continuously in this sense and derided my lack of manly courage to carry it out; this made me repeatedly attempt to put my head under the water; sometimes the attendants would then raise my feet above the water so seemingly facilitating my suicidal intent; they even ducked my head repeatedly, and then while making all sorts of rude jokes forced me to come to the surface again, and finally leave the bath.[33] In the contact kept up with p. 59
Professor Flechsig's nerves I constantly demanded cyanide or strychnine from him in order to poison myself (a drop of venom-juice, as it was called in the basic language); Professor Flechsig—as a soul in nerve contact with me—did not refuse this demand, but always half promised it, making its handing over, however, in a hypocritical manner conditional on certain guarantees during long hours of conversation by nerve-contact, when it was queried whether I would really drink the poison *if* it were given me, etc. When Professor Flechsig, on his medical rounds as a human being, subsequently came to me, he of course denied all knowledge of these matters. Being buried alive was also repeatedly mentioned as a way of ending my life. From the human point of view, which on the whole still dominated me at that time, it was in consequence very natural for me to see my real enemy only in Professor Flechsig or his soul (later in von W.'s soul also, about which more will be said below) and to regard as my natural ally God's omnipotence, which I imagined only Professor Flechsig endangered; I therefore thought I had to support it by all possible means, even to the point of self-sacrifice. It occurred to me only much later, in fact only while writing this essay did it become quite clear to me, that God Himself must have known of the plan, if indeed He was not the instigator, to commit soul murder on me, and to hand over my body in the manner of a female harlot. But I must at once repeat what I expressed at the end of Chapter II, so as not to confuse other people's religious ideas and feelings: however abominable the whole plan was bound to appear to me, subjectively speaking, I must nevertheless acknowledge that p. 60

[33] Incidentally, this was the time when, in consequence of the miracles directed against me, I had a thing between my legs which hardly resembled at all a normally formed male organ.

it originated in that instinct of self-preservation, as natural in God as in every other living being—an instinct which as mentioned in another context (compare page 52 above) forced God in special circumstances to contemplate the destruction not only of individual human beings, but perhaps of whole stars with all the created beings upon them. In the nineteenth chapter of the first book of Moses we are told that Sodom and Gomorrah were destroyed by a rain of brimstone and fire, although of their inhabitants there were some, even though very few, "righteous" men. Besides, in the whole domain of the created world, no one considers it immoral when—as long as it does not contravene the Order of the World—the stronger conquers the weaker, a people of higher culture expel from their abode one of a lower culture, the cat eats the mouse, the spider kills the fly, etc. In any case, the whole idea of morality can arise only within the Order of the World, that is to say within the natural bond which holds God and mankind together; wherever the Order of the World is broken, power alone counts, and the right of the stronger is decisive. In my case, moral obliquity lay in God placing Himself outside the Order of the World by which He Himself must be guided; although not exactly forced, He was nevertheless induced to do this by a temptation very difficult for souls to resist, which was brought about by the presence of Professor Flechsig's impure ("tested") soul in heaven. Further, by means of the high degree of human intelligence which it still retained, Flechsig's soul gained certain technical advantages (of which more will be said below) over
p. 61 those of God's nerves with which it first came in contact; the latter had not, as souls, the capacity for self-denying sacrifice necessary to procure me the amount of sleep needed for my cure, so rendering Flechsig's soul harmless. I am inclined to regard the whole development as a matter of *fate*, in which neither on God's nor on my part can there be a question of moral infringement. On the contrary, the Order of the World reveals its very grandeur and magnificence by denying even God Himself in so irregular a case as mine the means of achieving a purpose contrary to the Order of the World. All attempts at committing soul murder, at unmanning me for purposes *contrary to the Order of the World*[34] (that is to say for the sexual satisfaction of a human being) and

[34] To be unmanned could have served a different purpose—one which was in *consonance* with the Order of the World—and this was not only within the bounds of possibility, but may even indeed have provided the likely solution of the conflict; I will discuss this further later on.

later at destruction of my reason, have failed. From this apparently so unequal battle between one weak human being and God Himself, I emerge, albeit not without bitter sufferings and deprivations, victorious, because the Order of the World is on my side.[35] My external circumstances and my bodily condition have continued to improve from year to year. And so I live in the confident faith that the whole confusion was only an episode which will finally lead one way or another to the restoration of conditions in consonance with the Order of the World. Perhaps the personal misfortunes I had to suffer and the loss of the states of Blessedness may even be compensated for, in that mankind will p. 62
gain all at once, through my case, the knowledge of religious truth in much greater measure than possibly could have been achieved in hundreds and thousands of years by means of scientific research with the aid of all possible intellectual acuity. It need hardly be said what incalculable gain it would be for mankind if, through my personal fate, *particularly as it will be shaped in the future*, the foundations of mere materialism and of hazy pantheism would once and for all be demolished.

VI p. 63

The period I have been trying to describe in the previous chapter—from about the middle of March to the end of May 1894—assuming always that it was really a matter of a few earthly months only and not of centuries—was, I can truly say, the most gruesome time of my life. And yet it was also the *holy* time of my life, when my soul was immensely inspired by supernatural things, which came over me in ever increasing number amidst the rough treatment

[35] (Added November 1902). The above may seem somewhat obscure, in so far as "the Order of the World" may appear as something impersonal and higher, more powerful than God or even as ruling God. In fact there is no obscurity. "*The Order of the World*" is the lawful relation which, *resting on God's nature and attributes, exists between God and the creation called to life by Him.* God cannot achieve what contradicts His own attributes and His powers in relation to mankind or, as in my case, to an individual human being who had entered into a special relation with Him. God, whose power by rays is essentially constructive in its nature, and creative, came into conflict with Himself when he attempted the irregular policy against me, aimed solely at destroying my bodily integrity and my reason. This policy could therefore only cause temporary damage, but could not lead to permanent results. Or perhaps, using an oxymoron, God Himself was on my side in His fight against me, that is to say I was able to bring His attributes and powers into battle as an effective weapon in my self-defence.

which I suffered from outside; when I was filled with the most sublime ideas about God and the Order of the World. For all that, I have from my youth been anything but inclined towards religious fanaticism. Whoever knew me intimately in my earlier life will bear witness that I had been a person of calm nature, without passion, clear-thinking and sober, whose individual gift lay much more in the direction of cool intellectual criticism than in the creative activity of an unbounded imagination. I was by no means what one might call a *poet*, although I have occasionally attempted a few verses on family occasions. Nor was I (in my youth) a truly believing person in the sense of our positive religion.
p. 64 But neither have I been at any time contemptuous of religion; rather I avoided talking much about religious matters and I had the feeling that people who had luckily retained in their later years a pious child's belief, should not be disturbed in their happiness. But for my own part I had occupied myself too much with the natural sciences, particularly with works based on the so-called modern doctrine of evolution, not to have begun to doubt, to say the least, the literal truth of all Christian religious teachings. My general impression has always been that materialism cannot be the last word in religious matters, but I could not get myself either to believe firmly in the existence of a personal God or to retain such a belief.[36]

I am well aware of the difficulties in trying to present further details in this chapter about the period which above I called my *holy time*. The difficulties are in part external and in
p. 65 part of an inner nature. In the first place in such an attempt I have to rely totally on my memory, because at the time in question it was impossible to make notes; I had no writing material at my disposal, nor could I feel inclined to make written notes, because at that time—whether rightly or wrongly must for the present remain undecided—I believed the whole of mankind to have perished, so that there was no purpose in writing notes.

[36] But I am also far from maintaining that I had a particular inclination towards philosophy or that I have reached the height of the philosophic education of my time; the strenuous profession of a Judge could hardly have left me sufficient time. However, I wish to quote some of the works bearing on philosophy or natural science which I had read repeatedly during the ten years before my illness, because one will find in many places of this essay allusions to ideas contained in these works. As examples I will quote only Haeckel, The History of Natural Creation; Caspari, Primordial History of Mankind; du Prel, Evolution of the Universe; Maedler, Astronomy; Carus Sterne, Beginning and End; Meyer's Journal "Between Heaven and Earth"; Neumayer, History of the Earth; Rancke, Man; several philosophical essays by Eduard von Hartmann, particularly in the periodical "The Present", etc., etc.

Furthermore the impressions which rushed in upon me were such a wonderful mixture of natural events and happenings of a supernatural nature, that it is extremely difficult to distinguish mere dream visions from experiences in a waking state, that is to say to be certain how far all that I thought I had experienced was in fact historical reality. It is unavoidable therefore that my recollections of that time must in some measure bear the stamp of confusion.[37]

[37] In this respect, an event of very recent date has brought considerable clarification. On one of the nights which followed my writing the above, the night of the 14th to the 15th of March 1900, there was wild play with miracles in my dreams, such as I had only experienced earlier, particularly during the time when I was sleeping in the padded cell (1896 to end of 1898), but not at all or only very exceptionally during the last two years. I eventually made an end to these wild miracles severely and anxiously disturbing my sleep, by forcing myself to wake up completely and turning on the light. It was only 11.30 p.m. (the door which leads from my room to the corridor was locked, so that nobody could have come in from outside. Despite this early hour of the night I immediately wrote it down on paper because dream visions are known to vanish from memory quickly, and because I thought that this event would be more illuminating both for the knowledge of the essence of divine miracles, and also for deciding exactly how far objective facts were at the basis of my earlier similar visions. From the content of these notes I will here only quote that according to the vision produced by miracle in my dream, an attendant of the Asylum, whom I had first heard opening the door of the living room adjoining my bedroom, was partly sitting on my bed, partly getting up to some mischief near my bed, at one time eating smoked tongue or ham with beans; that I saw myself still in the dream vision having left the bed in order to turn on the light so that the miraculous visions should cease; but when I awoke fully I found myself still lying in bed so that I had not really left my bed at all. One should not ridicule the details given above about the items of food. The words used for these items of food are closely connected with the writing-down-system which will be described later; they therefore demonstrate quite clearly the intention which prompted these dream visions; in this respect it is also a clue to the knowledge of God and in particular to the dualism reigning in the realms of God mentioned at the end of Chapter I. At this stage I will only remark on the following:

It is almost superfluous to waste words about such a common phenomenon as that a restlessly sleeping human being believes he sees dream visions which are conjured up, as it were, by his own nerves. But the dreams visions of the night just mentioned and similar earlier visions surpassed in their plasticity and photographic accuracy everything I had ever experienced when I was well. This cannot have been caused spontaneously by my own nerves, but must have been thrown into them by rays. The rays therefore have the power to influence the nervous system and particularly the sensory nerves of a sleeping human being, in certain circumstances perhaps even those of a human being who is awake, in such a way that the person concerned thinks he can see strangers standing before him or hear them speak, believes that he is walking about and carrying on a conversation with them, just as if all this were really happening. I know now for certain that this is not so, but I maintain that the opposite point of view I used to hold was not only due to morbid excitation of my nerves, but that every other human being, had he seen similar dream visions, would equally have thought them real. Naturally I have to modify some of my earlier statements (compare footnote 39); in particular I can no longer doubt but that my meeting our reigning King, an account of which is given in footnote 28, was only a dream vision. In what follows I will therefore only touch on similar dream visions which I had without number in the early years of my illness; I will

p. 66 In order to give a picture first of all of the external conditions of my stay in the Nerve Clinic of the University, I append a ground plan of it and a sketch of the grounds in which it stands, with such details as are necessary for my purposes.

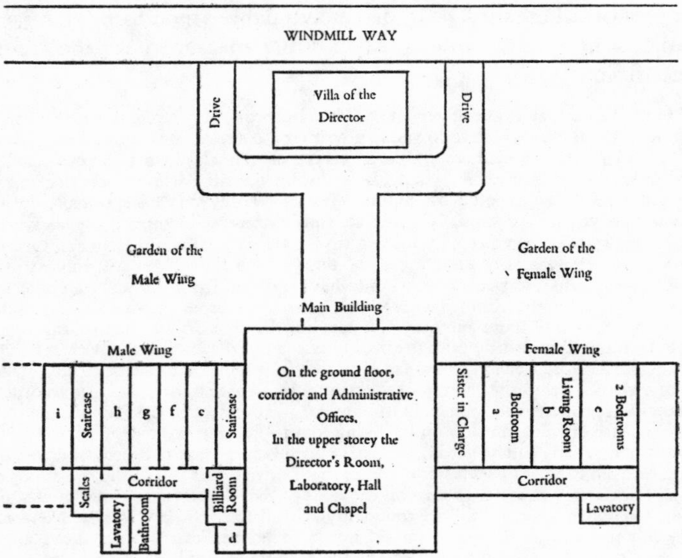

p. 67 During the time from shortly before Christmas 1893 until perhaps the end of February 1894 (that is to say mainly the time during which I was regularly visited by my wife) I inhabited rooms, *a*, *b*, and *c* on the ground floor of the female wing, which
p. 68 were probably given to me mainly because it was more quiet there. Before and after, I inhabited different rooms on the first floor of the male wing, each time a living room and a bedroom. The little room *d* served this purpose for some time (in November 1893) because most of the other rooms of the Asylum lay on the south side of the corridor facing the Bavarian Station, where the whistling of the shunting trains was very disturbing, particularly at night. The padded cell to which I was removed after the fight

concentrate mainly on those events during which I am certain that I was in a waking state. Nevertheless even such dream visions cannot be denied some value for understanding those matters which are dealt with here; at least in a few cases it is not impossible that they were symbolic expressions of information about things which either really happened or which God expected to happen in the future.

in the billiard room described earlier, lay further to the left in the male wing. Towards the latter part of my stay in the Asylum I mainly used the bedroom *i* and the living room *e*; the former was, in the manner of a padded room, provided with double doors, the inner one of which had a small peep-hole through which the inmate could be observed from outside; above the door there was an opening provided with a pane of glass through which the light of a gas flame could enter. Some of my memories do not tally with any of the familiar rooms in Flechsig's Asylum; this in connection with other circumstances made me wonder whether in fact I spent the whole time that is dealt with here in Flechsig's Asylum, or whether I was somewhere else for a time. Professor Flechsig was assisted in the medical treatment by two assistant doctors, Dr. Täuscher and Dr. Quentin. During the time which I am discussing, there was a period when I did not see any of the doctors, only the attendants being around—always the ones named above. The Asylum itself gave me at that time the impression of being completely deserted; nor did I see anything of other patients when I entered the corridor outside my room. Some time later Professor Flechsig reappeared but as mentioned earlier, in a form which gave me at least the impression of his having changed considerably. As far as I can remember I either did not p. 69
see the assistant physicians at all or only very occasionally during the latter part of my stay in the Asylum.

I mentioned in the previous chapter that in consequence of my ever increasing nervousness and the resulting increasing power of attraction, an ever growing number of departed souls felt attracted to me—primarily those who may have retained some special interest in me because of personal contacts with me during their life—and then dissolved on my head or in my body. This process frequently ended with the souls concerned finally leading a short existence on my head in the form of "little men"—tiny figures in human form, perhaps only a few millimetres in height—before finally vanishing (compare footnote 28). I suppose that these souls, when they first approached me, still possessed a fairly large number of nerves and in virtue of them still retained a fairly strong awareness of their identity. Each time they approached me they lost part of their nerves in favour of my body through the power of attraction; finally they consisted only of one single nerve, which for some mysterious reason not further explicable, assumed the form of a "little man" in the above sense. This was the final form of existence of these souls before

they vanished completely. On these occasions I was frequently told the names of the stars or groups of stars from which they had emanated or " from which they were suspended "; in part these names tallied with the usual astronomical nomenclature, in part they did not. Especially frequent were the names Cassiopeia, Wega, Capella, also a star " Gemma " (I do not know if this
p. 70 conforms to an astronomical name); further the Crucians (perhaps the Southern Cross?), the " Firmament " and many others. On some nights the souls finally dripped down on to my head, in a manner of speaking, in their hundreds if not thousands, as " little men ". I always warned them against approaching me, since I had become aware of the immensely increased power of attraction of my nerves from what had happened earlier, but the souls could not at first believe that I had such a dangerous power of attraction. Other rays which conducted themselves in the manner described above as if they were God's omnipotence itself, carried names such as " the Lord of Hosts ", " the Good Shepherd ", " the Almighty ", etc., etc. Connected with these phenomena, very early on there predominated in recurrent nightly visions the notion of an approaching *end of the world*, as a consequence of the indissoluble connection between God and myself. Bad news came in from all sides that even this or that star or this or that group of stars had to be " given up "; at one time it was said that even Venus had been " flooded ", at another that the whole solar system would now have to be " disconnected ", that the Cassiopeia (the whole group of stars) had had to be drawn together into a single sun, that perhaps only the Pleiades could still be saved, etc., etc. While I had these visions at night, in daytime I thought I could notice the sun following my movements; when I moved to and fro in the single-windowed room I inhabited at the time, I saw the sunlight now on the right, now on the left wall (as seen from the door) depending on my movements. It is difficult for me to believe that this observation was a hallucination because it was made, as mentioned, in daytime, particularly as I remember drawing the assistant physician Täuscher's attention on one of his visits to this observation, which naturally filled me with horror.
p. 71 When later I regularly visited the garden again I saw—if my memory does not wholly deceive me—two suns in the sky at the same time, one of which was our earthly sun, the other was said to be the Cassiopeia group of stars drawn together into a single sun.

From the sum total of my recollections, the impression gained

hold of me that the period in question, which, according to human calculation, stretched over only three to four months, had covered an immensely long period; it was as if single nights had the duration of centuries, so that within that time the most profound alterations in the whole of mankind, in the earth itself and the whole solar system could very well have taken place. It was repeatedly mentioned in visions that the work of the past fourteen thousand years had been lost—this figure presumably indicated the duration the earth had been populated with human beings—and that approximately only another two hundred years were allotted to the earth—if I am not mistaken the figure 212 was mentioned. During the latter part of my stay in Flechsig's Asylum I thought this period had already expired[38] and therefore thought I was the last real human being left, and that the few human shapes whom I saw apart from myself—Professor Flechsig, some attendants, occasional more or less strange-looking patients—were only "fleeting-improvised-men" created by miracle. I pondered over such possibilities as that the whole of Flechsig's Asylum or perhaps the city of Leipzig with it had been "dug out" and removed to p. 72
some other celestial body, all of them possibilities which questions asked by the voices who talked to me seemed to hint at, as for instance whether Leipzig was still standing, etc. I regarded the starry sky largely, if not wholly, extinguished. I was not afforded the chance of correcting such notions. My bedroom window was closed up with a heavy wooden shutter at night so that the sight of the night sky was denied me. In day-time I saw over and beyond the walls of the Asylum only a few of the buildings immediately bordering on it. In the direction of the Bavarian Station I saw beyond the walls of the Asylum only a narrow strip of land, which looked quite strange to me and very different from the character of this district which I knew so well; at times one spoke of "a holy landscape". The whistle of trains, which I could hardly have missed, I did not hear at all for some considerable time. Only the fact that the gaslights continued burning made me doubt whether Flechsig's Asylum was in fact completely isolated,

[38] This assumption seemed confirmed by some details which I can pass over here. Political and religious events played a part as well as the fact that the House of Wettin was said to have remembered suddenly their alleged Slavic descent and made themselves the protagonists of Slavism; in wide circles of Saxony, particularly among the higher nobility (among others the names of "v. W., v. S." were mentioned) a widespread Catholicizing was said to have taken place; my own mother was to have been converted, I myself was continually the object of attempts at conversion by Catholics (see page 49), etc., etc.

or it forced me to recognize some connection with the city of Leipzig, if I was not to assume that the Asylum had had its own special gasometer built. Further, I retain some recollections which I can only describe in a general way, to the effect that I felt as if I myself existed for some time also in a second, mentally inferior form. I must leave undecided whether something of this nature can occur through miracles, and whether it would have been possible for me to be placed again with part of my nerves into a
p. 73 second body. I can but repeat that I have recollections which seem to point to such a possibility. In this second inferior shape, of which I myself retain the conscious awareness of having had lesser intellectual powers, I was told that another Daniel Paul Schreber had existed before me who had been much better endowed intellectually than myself. As in my family pedigree, which I know extremely well, there had been no Daniel Paul Schreber before me, I think I am justified in taking this other Daniel Paul Schreber as referring to myself while in full possession of my nerves. In the second inferior shape I must then, if I may use the expression, have quietly departed one day; I can recollect that in a room which does not tally with any one of the rooms known to me in Flechsig's Asylum, I was lying in bed with the distinct feeling that my soul was slowly expiring, a state by the way which, apart from sad memories of my wife who was much in my mind during that time, had altogether the character of a painless and peaceful passing away. On the other hand there was a time when souls in nerve-contact with me talked of a plurality of heads (that is several individuals in one and the same skull) which they encountered in me and from which they shrank in alarm crying " For heaven's sake—that is a human being with several heads ". I am fully aware how fantastic all this must sound to other people; and I therefore do not go so far as to assert that all I have recounted was objective reality; I only relate the impressions retained as recollections in my memory.

As I said before, the innumerable visions I had in connection with the idea that the world had perished were partly of a gruesome nature, partly of an indescribable sublimity. I will recall only a
p. 74 few. In one of them it was as though I were sitting in a railway carriage or in a lift driving into the depths of the earth and I recapitulated, as it were, the whole history of mankind or of the earth in reverse order; in the upper regions there were still forests of leafy trees; in the nether regions it became progressively darker and blacker. When temporarily I left the vehicle, I walked as though

across a large cemetery where, coming upon the place where Leipzig's inhabitants lay buried, I crossed my own wife's grave. Sitting again in the vehicle I advanced only to a point 3; point 1, which was to mark the earliest beginning of mankind, I dared not enter. On the return drive the shaft collapsed behind me, continually endangering a "sun deity" who was in it too. In this connection it was said that there had been two shafts (perhaps corresponding to the dualism of the realms of God?); when news came that the second shaft had also collapsed, it was thought that everything was lost. Another time I traversed the earth from Lake Ladoga to Brazil and, together with an attendant, I built there in a castle-like building a wall in protection of God's realms against an advancing yellow flood tide: I related this to the peril of a syphilitic epidemic. At another time I felt as if I myself were raised up to Blessedness, it was as though from the heights of heaven the whole earth were resting under a blue vault below me, a picture of sublime splendour and beauty; I heard some expression like "God-be-together-view" to describe this picture. In the case of other events I am doubtful whether they were only visions or at least in part real experiences. I remember that during the night I frequently sat on the floor of my bedroom, clad only in a shirt (all articles of clothing had of course been taken from me) having left the bed following some inner impulse. My hands, which I set p. 75
firmly on the floor behind my back, were *perceptibly* lifted up *at times* by bearlike shapes (black bears); other "black bears", both greater and smaller, I saw sitting around me with glowing eyes. My bedclothes formed themselves into so-called "white bears". Through the peephole of my bedroom door I saw in a similar manner as recounted about our reigning King[39] in footnote 28, yellow men, under middle-size, appear now and then in front of the door of my bedroom, whom I had to be prepared to fight in some way. At times cats with glowing eyes appeared on the trees of the Asylum's garden while I was still awake, that is to say in the late evening hours. Further, I recollect being for a time somewhere by the sea in a castle which had to be abandoned because of threatening floods; from which, after a long, long time I returned to Flechsig's Asylum, where I found myself all at once in the same

[39] Although in footnote 37 above I remarked that I no longer doubted that this was only a dream vision, I must again on further consideration restrict this view. That I was standing by the peep-hole of my bedroom door is too distinct a recollection to attribute to a hallucination. I would, however, concede the possibility that what I presumed to have seen outside the door could have been a hallucination (compare Kraepelin as quoted at the end of this chapter).

circumstances as before. In front of my bedroom windows I saw in the early morning, when the shutters were opened, a dense forest, a few metres only removed from the window and consisting as far as I can remember mostly of birches and firs. The voices called it a "holy forest". It had not the slightest resemblance to the garden of the University Nerve Clinic which is a new plantation
p. 76 started only in 1882, consisting mostly of rows of single trees alongside the paths. It goes without saying that such a forest, if it really existed, could not possibly have sprung up in three or four months. My head was frequently surrounded by a shimmer of light owing to the massive concentration of rays, like the halo of Christ is pictured, but incomparably richer and brighter: the so-called "crown of rays". The reflection of this crown of rays was so strong that one day when Professor Flechsig appeared at my bed with his assistant Dr. Quentin, the latter disappeared from my seeing eyes; the same happened another time with the attendant H. For a long time it was said that I was to remain under the protection of Cassiopeia, while the sun was assigned to a different destination, and was probably to be preserved for her own planetary system and thus also for our earth. The power of attraction of my nerves was however so strong that this plan could not be carried out: the sun had to remain where I was or I myself had to be brought back again.

It will be understandable that with such impressions, which I may attempt to interpret in a later chapter, I lived for years in doubt as to whether I was really still on earth or whether on some other celestial body. Even in the year 1895[40] I still considered the possibility of my being on Phobos, a satellite of the planet Mars which had once been mentioned by the voices in some other
p. 77 context, and wondered whether the moon, which I sometimes saw in the sky, was not the main planet Mars.

In the soul-language, during the time dealt with in this chapter, I was called "*the seer of spirits*"[41], that is, a man who sees, and is in communication with, spirits or departed souls. In particular, Flechsig's soul used to refer to me as "the greatest seer of spirits of all centuries"; to which I, from a wider point of view, occasionally retorted, that one ought at least to speak of the greatest seer of spirits of all *millenia*. In fact since the dawn of the world there can

[40] At that time the days too seemed considerably shorter; a watch, which could have helped rectify possibly erroneous ideas, was not at my disposal.

[41] I shall discuss below the designation "Prince of Hell", which was applied to me later.

hardly have been a case like mine, in which a human being entered into continual contact, that is to say no longer subject to interruption, not only with *individual* departed souls but with the totality of all souls and with God's omnipotence itself. It is true that at first one still attempted to interrupt it; one then still differentiated " holy times ", that is times when nerve-contact or communication with rays or talking of voices—after all only different expressions for one and the same phenomenon—were to occur and " unholy times " when it was intended to give up the communication with rays. Soon, however, the enormous attraction of my nerves would not allow of any such pauses or interruptions; from then on there were only " holy times ". Seers of spirits of an inferior kind may well have existed in greater or lesser numbers before my own case. To avoid going back as far as biblical events, I consider it very likely that in the cases of the Maid of Orleans, of the Crusaders in search of the Holy Lance at Antioch, or of the Emperor Constantine's well-known vision *in hoc signo vinces* which was p. 78
decisive for the victory of Christianity: that in all these cases a transitory communication with rays was established, or there was transitory divine inspiration. The same may possibly also be assumed in some cases of stigmatisation of virgins; the legends and poetry of all peoples literally swarm with the activities of ghosts, elves, goblins, etc., and it seems to me nonsensical to assume that in all of them one is dealing simply with deliberate inventions of human imagination without any foundation in real fact. I noticed therefore with interest that according to Kraepelin's TEXTBOOK OF PSYCHIATRY (5th Edition, Leipzig, 1896, p. 95 ff. and particularly p. 110 ff.) which had been lent to me (while I was occupied with this manuscript), the phenomenon of being in some supernatural communication with voices had frequently been observed before in human beings whose nerves were in a state of morbid excitation.[42] I do not dispute that in many of

[42] In this connection Kraepelin's remark on page 110 that those cases in which " the voices heard " have a supernatural character " are not infrequently accompanied by visual hallucinations " is very valuable for my own ideas. I think it probable that in a considerable number of these cases it was a matter of real visions of the kind which I also have experienced, that is dream-images produced by rays, and which for that reason are very much more distinct than what is seen in ordinary dreams (compare Kraepelin, p. 107). On the other hand the total content of the present work will hardly show anything *in my case* which justifies speaking of " the inability of the patient to use earlier experiences to correct thoroughly and accurately his new ideas " (p. 146), or of " faulty judgment ", which Kraepelin (p. 145) says " invariably accompanies delusions ". I trust I have proved that I am not only not " controlled by fixed and previously formed ideas ", but that I also possess in full measure the " capacity to evaluate critically the content of consciousness with

these cases one may only be dealing with mere hallucinations, as which they are treated throughout the mentioned textbook. In my opinion science would go very wrong to designate as
p. 79 " hallucinations " *all* such phenomena that lack objective reality, and to throw them into the lumber room of things that do not exist; this may possibly be justified in those hallucinations quoted by Kraepelin on page 108 ff., which are *not* connected with supernatural matters. I think it quite possible that some such cases were instances of genuine seers of spirits of an inferior grade in the earlier developed sense. This is not to deny the *simultaneous* existence of a morbid state of nervous hyper-excitability, in so far as only the increased power of attraction of nerves caused by it enabled and facilitated communication with supernatural powers. It seems psychologically impossible that *I* suffer only from hallucinations. After all, the hallucination of being in communication with God or departed souls can logically only develop in people who bring with them into their morbidly excited nervous state an already secure faith in God and the immortality of the soul. *This, however, was not so in my case, as mentioned at the beginning of this chapter.* Even so-called spiritualist mediums may be con-
p. 80 sidered genuine seers of spirits of the inferior kind in this sense, although in many cases self-deception and fraud may also play a part. Therefore one ought to beware of unscientific generalization and rash condemnation in such matters. If psychiatry is not flatly to deny everything supernatural and thus tumble with both feet into the camp of naked materialism, it will have to recognize the possibility that occasionally the phenomena under discussion may be connected with real happenings, which simply cannot be brushed aside with the catchword " hallucinations ".

After this digression I return to my real theme which I shall continue in the next chapter; I will touch on some other points concerning the supernatural which could not easily be dealt with in the above; I shall also discuss in particular the circumstances of my external life during that time.

---

the help of judgment and deduction " (p. 146). He who in Kraepelin's sense (p. 146) understands " sound experience " simply as the denial of everything supernatural, would in my opinion lay himself open to the reproach of allowing himself to be led only by the shallow " rationalistic ideas " of the period of enlightenment of the 18th century, which after all are mostly considered to have been superseded, particularly by theologians and philosophers, and also in science.

VII p. 81

For reasons already mentioned I cannot give exact chronological
data about the time between my wife's last visits (middle of
February 1894) and the end of my stay in Flechsig's Asylum
(middle of June 1894). I have only a few clues. I recollect that
about the middle of March 1894 when communication with
supernatural powers was well under way, a newspaper was put
in front of me in which something like my own obituary notice
could be read; I took this as a hint that I could no longer count
on any possibility of a return to human society. I dare not
decide whether what I saw actually happened or whether it was
a visual hallucination. I only retained the one impression, that if
this and other occurrences really were visions, there was *method*
in them, i.e. that they were connected in a certain way which
enabled me to realize what one had in store for me. This was
the time when, as previously mentioned, I was kept in bed con- p. 82
tinuously day and night; whether for weeks and if so how many
I cannot say. Round about the time of the Easter holidays—
I cannot say when Easter was in 1894—an important change must
have taken place in Professor Flechsig's person. I heard that in
these holidays he went on leave to the Palatinate or Alsace. In
connection with this I had visions according to which Professor
Flechsig had shot himself either in Weissenburg in Alsace or in
the police prison in Leipzig; I also saw—in a dream vision—his
funeral procession moving from his house towards the Thonberg
(that is to say not really in the direction which one would
expect according to the spatial relation between the University
Nerve Clinic and St. John's Cemetery). In other visions he
repeatedly appeared to me accompanied by a policeman or in
conversation with his wife, which I witnessed by way of nerve-
contact and where Professor Flechsig called himself "God Flechsig"
to his wife, so that she was inclined to think he was mad. I am,
however, almost certain now that these visions did not conform
to real happenings in the way I believed I had seen them. But
I think it is permissible to *interpret* them as revelations of divine
opinion on what *ought* to have happened to Professor Flechsig.
However that may be, it is an actual or *subjectively certain*
event from the distinctness of my recollection—whether other
people can or cannot believe me—that about that time I had
Professor Flechsig's soul and most probably his *whole* soul
temporarily in my body. It was a fairly bulky ball or bundle

which I can perhaps best compare with a corresponding volume of wadding or cobweb, which had been thrown into my belly
p. 83 by way of miracle, presumably to perish there. In view of its size it would in any case probably have been impossible to retain this soul in my belly, to digest it so to speak; indeed when it attempted to free itself I let it go voluntarily, being moved by a kind of sympathy, and so it escaped through my mouth into the open again. I have all the less reason to doubt the objective reality of this event, as in quite a number of other instances later I received souls or parts of souls in my mouth, of which I particularly remember distinctly the foul taste and smell which such *impure* souls cause in the body of the person through whose mouth they have entered.

These events were followed as far as I can remember by a period which the voices called the time of the first Divine Judgment. By coincidence I have retained a few data in my memory which must have been mentioned by somebody, according to which the first Divine Judgment embraced the period from the 2nd or 4th to the 19th of April 1894. The "first Divine Judgment" was then followed by a number of further Divine Judgments which, however, lagged behind the first in grandeur of impression. The "first Divine Judgment" was a series of continuous visions by day and by night, all based, if I may so express myself, on one common basic *general idea*. This was the idea that after a crisis dangerous for the existence of the realms of God which had arisen in the circles of the German people through the conflict between Professor Flechsig and myself, the German people, particularly Protestant Germany, could no longer be left with the leadership as God's chosen people, had perhaps even to to be excluded altogether when other "globes" ("inhabited
p. 84 planets?") were occupied, unless a champion appeared for the German people to prove their continued worth. At one time I myself was to be that champion, at another a person chosen by me, and because of the insistence of the voices that talked to me in nerve-contact I named a number of outstanding men whom I deemed fit for such a struggle. Connected with the mentioned basic idea of the first Divine Judgment, was the advance of Catholicism, Judaism, and Slavism mentioned in the last chapter. I had a number of visions relating to this also, amongst which I saw the female wing of the University Nerve Clinic turned into a Nunnery or a Catholic Chapel, Sisters of Mercy sitting in the rooms under the Asylum's roof, etc., etc. But then it was said

that Catholicism would no longer do; after the death of the present Pope and of an intervening Pope Honorius, a further conclave could not be held because Catholics had lost their faith, etc. At the time I took all these to be actual historical events and therefore thought that a development of possibly several hundred years already belonged to the past. Naturally I do not hold this opinion any longer. Having resumed some contact with the outside world—naturally after the elapse of several years—through newspapers and letters, and having noticed nothing in the state of buildings in the Asylum and its neighbourhood, nor in the condition of my old books, music and other useful articles, which had in the meantime been returned to me, which would tally with the assumption of a *large gap in time* having occurred in the history of mankind, I can now no longer refuse to acknowledge that *viewed merely from outside* everything has remained as of old. p. 85
But whether a very profound inner change has taken place nevertheless will be discussed later.

Of considerable influence on my range of ideas at the time was also certain information referring to what I was to become in a future transmigration of souls. I was cast in several roles consecutively: a "Hyperborian woman", a "Jesuit Novice in Ossegg", a "Burgomaster of Klattau", "an Alsatian girl who had to defend her honour against a victorious French officer", finally "a Mongolian Prince". In all these predictions I thought I could discern a certain connection with the overall picture furnished by the other visions. The fate of becoming a "Hyperborian woman" seemed a sign that the earth had lost so much heat that general glaciation had either occurred already or was imminent; apart from this there was talk that the sun had withdrawn as far as Jupiter. That I was destined to be a Jesuit Novice in Ossegg or a Burgomaster in Klattau or even an Alsatian girl in the situation specified above, I took as prophesies that Protestantism had either already succumbed to or was about to succumb to Catholicism, and the German people to their Roman and Slavic neighbours; the prospect of my becoming a "Mongolian Prince" appeared to me as a sign that all Aryan peoples had proved themselves unsuitable to defend the realms of God, and that a last refuge would now have to be taken with non-Aryan peoples.

A fateful turn in the history of the earth and of mankind seemed to be marked by the events of one single day distinctly preserved in my memory, on which there was talk of the "clocks of the world" running out and at the same time a continuous rich

p. 86 stream of rays towards my body accompanied by light phenomena of great splendour. I cannot say what was meant by the expression "the running out of the clocks of the world"; it was said that the whole of mankind would return but for two, namely myself and the Jesuit Father S., mentioned earlier in Chapter V. From then on the conditions commenced which have since been called hundreds and thousands of times "the cursed-play-with-human-beings". I have reason to assume that since then, mankind and all its activities have only been artificially maintained by means of direct divine miracles, to an extent which the restrictions under which I live do not allow me to survey fully.[42B] This is certainly the case in my own surroundings: I feel a blow on my head simultaneously with every word spoken around me, with every approaching footstep, with every railway whistle, with every shot fired by a pleasure steamer, etc.; this causes a variable degree of pain—more when God has withdrawn to a greater distance and less when he is nearby. Almost invariably I can foretell accurately when there is going to be such a manifestation of life by a human being near me, called "interference" and felt by me as a blow; namely always when the sensation of voluptuousness present in my body has gained such a strong power of attraction over the divine rays, that in order to be able to withdraw again such an "interference" is necessary. I cannot say up to what distance this incitement of people, if I may use that expression, by divine miracles takes place. I will return to the whole matter in greater detail later.

p. 87 With regard to the changes in the starry sky, it is now my opinion that news of the loss of this or that star or stellar constellation (compare Chapter VI, page 70) did not refer to the stars themselves—after all I still see them in the sky as before—but only to the states of Blessedness accumulated under these stars. However, these have certainly been totally depleted, that is to say the nerves concerned have, through the power of attraction of my nerves, been absorbed into my body; in it they have taken on the character of female nerves of voluptuousness and apart from this have given my body a more or less feminine stamp; they have in particular given my skin a softness peculiar to the female sex. On the other hand I am quite certain that God, who used to be an immense distance away, had been forced to draw nearer the earth, which thus became the direct and continual scene of divine

42B Compare Preface.

miracles in a manner hitherto unknown. These miracles primarily concentrated on my person and surroundings. Later I will produce further proof of this statement over and above what has been said so far. Here I only want to remark that because the change thus wrought is contrary to the Order of the World it is connected with certain disadvantages even for God Himself, and may possibly be accompanied by other fateful consequences. Rays, after all, are accustomed to holy tranquility such as prevails on the highest mountain summits of the earth; therefore it must be disagreeable for them and in a way frightening to have suddenly to participate in all my auditory impressions, for instance the noise of railways.[43] Further, I have reason to assume that from this date (or perhaps three months later, about which more below), the p. 88
sending forth of the sun's rays was taken over directly by God, more especially by the lower God (Ariman); the voices that talk to me now (since July 1894) identify him with the sun. The upper God (Ormuzd) kept himself at a greater, perhaps even still at a colossal distance; I see his picture as a small sun-like disc, so tiny as to be almost a mere point, appear at short intervals on the nerves inside my head. Perhaps apart from our own planetary system which is lighted and warmed by the sun (Ariman), a second has been successfully maintained on which the continuity of creation is made possible by light and warmth emanating from the upper God (Ormuzd). But I consider it very doubtful at least, whether the population of all other celestial bodies belonging to other fixed stars on which organic life had developed, were not also doomed to perish.[44]

The period during which I was continually kept in bed was followed, at the end of my stay in Flechsig's Asylum, by a time when I walked regularly in the garden. There I noticed a variety of miraculous things. As already mentioned, I thought I saw two suns in the sky simultaneously. One day the whole garden was luxuriantly in bloom, a picture which did not fit my recollections p. 89
of the first part of my illness when the garden of the University Nerve Clinic was quite bare; this phenomenon was called

[43] The expression for this which I heard innumerable times, was " We do not like the thought of listening ".

[44] I have certain evidence which points to the possibility that in fact the light of all fixed stars is not their own, as our astronomy assumes, but as in the case of planets (as in all such matters, to be understood *cum grano salis*) is borrowed light (from God) (compare Chapter I). The cardinal point is that there exists a controlling sun, of which our astronomy knows nothing. Compare the qualifying remark at the end of Postscript IV.

Flechsig's miracle. At another time, in the pavilion in the centre of the garden, there were a number of French-speaking ladies, a most remarkable occurrence in the male section of a Public Asylum. The few patients besides myself who sometimes appeared in the garden, all gave a more or less bizarre impression; in one of them I once thought I recognized a relative of mine, the husband of one of my nieces, now Professor Dr. F. in K. who looked shyly at me without saying a word. When I sat on a camp stool in the garden in a black coat with a black flap hat I felt like a marble guest who had returned from times long past into a strange world.

In the meantime a most remarkable change occurred in my sleep. Whereas during the first months of the year 1894 I could only obtain sleep with the help of the strongest sleeping drugs (chloral hydrate) and not always then, some nights requiring additional injections of morphine, I took no sleeping drugs at all for several weeks at the end of my stay in Flechsig's Asylum. I slept—though in part restlessly and always with more or less exciting visions—without any artificial help: *my sleep had become the sleep of rays.*[45] Rays, as already observed in footnote 31, also have
p. 90 the capacity to calm nerves and bring sleep. This will be the more readily believed because even ordinary sun rays have a similar though much weaker effect. Every psychiatrist knows that in patients suffering from a nervous illness the nervous excitement increases considerably at night, but improves in daytime, particularly later in the morning after the influence of a few hours of sunlight. This result is increased immensely if, as in my case, the body receives divine rays direct. Only relatively few rays are then needed to produce sleep; but all these rays must be united, since derived rays also exist (that is, led by impure or tested souls such as Flechsig's, etc.) apart from divine rays proper. When this happens I fall asleep immediately. When I observed this phenomenon towards the end of my stay in Flechsig's Asylum, I was extremely surprised because sleep could only be procured for me with the greatest difficulties; I only became clear about the reason for it in the course of time.

[45] During my stay in Pierson's Asylum and during the first part of my stay here (perhaps for one year) I never received sleeping drugs, as far as I can recall. Whether I am mistaken in this could be shown by the entries in the drug register of this Asylum. For several years I have again received sleeping drugs regularly (mainly *Sulfonal* and *Anylene hydrate* alternately) and I take them without protest, although I consider they have no effect on my sleep. I am convinced that I would sleep equally well or badly without any artificial sleeping drugs as I do with them.

All kinds of extraordinary symptoms of illness appeared in my body in the course of time, apart from the repeatedly mentioned changes in my sex organ. In discussing them I must return again to the idea of the end of the world mentioned in preceding chapters, p. 91
which, from the visions I received, I thought either imminent or already past. Varying with the suggestions I received I formed different opinions about the manner in which it might have come about. In the first place I always thought of a decrease in the warmth of the sun through her moving further away, and consequently a more or less generalized glaciation. In the second place I thought of an earthquake or suchlike; in this connection I want to mention that I once received news that the great earthquake of Lisbon in the year 1755 had occurred in connection with a seer of spirits, similar to my own case. I further thought it possible that news had spread that in the modern world something in the nature of a wizard had suddenly appeared in the person of Professor Flechsig[46] and that I myself, after all a person known in wider cirles, had suddenly disappeared; this had spread terror and fear amongst the people, destroying the bases of religion and causing general nervousness and immorality. In its train devastating epidemics had broken upon mankind. This last idea was particularly supported by the fact that for some time there was talk of two illnesses, leprosy and plague, hardly yet known in Europe, which were said to have spread among men and signs of which were visible on my own body. I do not want definitely to say the latter about leprosy; it could have been only a matter of small beginnings of this illness because I have no certain recollections of any single symptom of it. But I remember the names of the various forms p. 92
in which leprosy was said to have occurred: *Lepra orientalis*, *Lepra indica*, *Lepra hebraica* and *Lepra aegyptica*. Being a layman in medicine I have never heard these terms before, nor do I know whether they correspond to the technical terms used for these types of the illness in medical science. I mention them here in order to disprove the assumption that it is all merely a matter of hallucinations dangled before me by my own nerves; for how could I possibly have hit upon these expressions without any knowledge of my own of the different varieties of this disease? That I must have at least had some germs of leprosy is shown by the fact that for a long time I had to recite certain strange-sounding incantations, such as " I am the first leper corpse and I lead a leper

[46] The name of a French doctor Brouardel was also once mentioned to me, who was said to have imitated Professor Flechsig.

corpse "[47]—incantations which, as far as I could understand, were connected with the fact that lepers had to consider themselves doomed to certain death; and had to help inter one another so as to provide for themselves an at least tolerable death. On the other hand I had on my body at various times fairly definite signs of the manifestations of plague. There were different varieties of plague: the blue plague, the brown plague, the white plague, and the black plague. The white plague was the most disgusting; the brown and the black plague were connected with the evaporations of the body, which in the former spread a glue-like and in the latter a soot-like smell; in the case of the black plague this
p. 93 was at times so strong that it filled my whole room. I still noticed weak traces of the brown plague in the early part of my stay in this Asylum in the summer of 1894. The souls considered the plague a disease of nerves and hence a " holy disease "; I do not know whether it was in any way related to the occasional cases of bubonic plague of the present time. Nevertheless, even the plague did not develop to its full extent but remained confined to more or less marked indications. The reason for this was the fact that the manifestations of the disease were always subsequently removed by pure rays. For one distinguished " searing "[48] and " blessing " rays; the former were laden with the poison of corpses or some other putrid matter, and therefore carried some germ of disease into the body or brought about some other destructive effect in it. The blessing (pure) rays in turn healed this damage.

Other things that happened on my body were still more closely connected with supernatural matters. It was mentioned in earlier chapters that those rays (God's nerves) which were attracted, followed only reluctantly, because it meant losing their own existence and therefore went against their instinct of self-preservation. Therefore one continually tried to stop the attraction, in other words to break free again from my nerves. The only absolutely effective way of doing this would have been to cure my nervous illness by procuring prolific sleep. But apparently one could not decide to do this, or at least not systematically, because it would

[47] As far as I remember I spoke them out *aloud* several times in the presence of the attendant R., who naturally responded only with a pitying smile.

[48] The verb " to sear " [" sehren "] apparently originates from an old German root, which meant " to injure ", and is no longer used in modern German except for the compound word " unseared " [" unversehrt "]; it was, however, retained in the basic language.

have needed a self-denying sacrifice on the part of the rays immediately concerned, for which they had neither the capacity nor the necessary will-power. p. 94

All other conceivable methods were therefore tried in the course of time, but from the nature of the matter they all proved thoroughly unsuitable. Always the main idea behind them was to " forsake " me, that is to say abandon me; at the time I am now discussing it was thought that this could be achieved by unmanning me and allowing my body to be prostituted like that of a female harlot, sometimes also by killing me and later by destroying my reason (making me demented).

But with regard to the efforts to unman me it was soon found that the gradual filling of my body with nerves of voluptuousness (female nerves) had exactly the reverse effect, because the resulting so-called " soul-voluptuousness " in my body rather increased the power of attraction. Therefore " *scorpions* " were repeatedly put into my head, tiny crab- or spider-like structures which were to carry out some work of destruction in my head. These had the nature of souls and therefore were *talking* beings; they were distinguished according to their place of origin as " Aryan ",[49] and " Catholic " scorpions; the former were somewhat bigger and stronger. However, these scorpions regularly withdrew from my head without doing me harm, when they perceived the p. 95
purity of my nerves and the holiness of my purpose—this was one of the innumerable triumphs which I have often experienced since then in a similar way. Just because the holiness of my purpose exerted too great a power of attraction on the souls, attempts were also made to falsify my mental individuality in all sorts of ways. " Jesuits ", that is to say departed souls of former Jesuits, repeatedly tried to put into my head a different " determinant nerve ", which was to change my awareness of my own identity; the inner table of my skull was lined with a different brain membrane[49A] in order to extinguish my memory of my own ego. All this without any permanent effect. Finally

[49] The expression " Aryan " (" Aryan " is another name for the Indo-Germanic peoples) was in general much used at that time; there was also an " Aryan " state of Blessedness, etc. By and large the expression was used to denote the leaning of a great part of the souls towards *German nationalism*; they wanted to retain for the German people the place of God's chosen people, in contrast to the Catholicizing and Slavicizing efforts of other souls.

[49A] As a layman in medicine I had also not heard of a brain membrane before, but was informed of this expression by the voices after I had appreciated (felt) this phenomenon myself.

attempts were made to blacken my nerves by miraculously placing the blackened nerves of other (deceased) human beings into my body, believing presumably that the blackness (impurity) of these nerves would be imparted to mine. Concerning these blackened nerves, I wish to mention a few names, the bearers of which were all said to have been in " Flechsig's hell ", which made me assume that Professor Flechsig must have some power of disposal over these nerves. Among them was a certain Bernhard Haase—his name was by coincidence identical with that of a distant relative of mine—a bad sort, who was supposed to have committed some crime, a murder or suchlike; further a certain R., a fellow-student and member of my Students' Union, who had gone to America because he had not made good and had led a rather dissolute life, and as far as I know was killed there in the War of Independence
p. 96 in 1864 or 1865[50]; finally a certain Julius Emil Haase who, despite his blackened nerves, gave the impression of a very honourable person. Presumably at the time of the Frankfurt *attentat* he was a senior member of the Students' Union and then became a medical practitioner in Jena, if I heard correctly. Particularly interesting was that the soul of this Julius Emil Haase was even still able to give me certain medical advice by virtue of its scientific experience during its life; I want to add here that up to a point the same applied to my father's soul. The presence of these blackened nerves in my body caused no lasting effect; they vanished in time without altering the condition of my nerves.

I could relate still more miraculous events from the time of my stay in Flechsig's Asylum. I could tell of happenings which make me believe that popular belief that *will-o'-the-wisps* are departed souls is true in many cases if not all; I could tell of *wandering clocks*, that is to say souls of departed heretics, said to have been preserved for centuries under glass in medieval cloisters (here too there is an
p. 97 undercurrent of something like a soul murder), who announced their survival by a vibration connected with an infinitely monotonous and doleful humming noise (I myself received this impression by way of nerve-contact) etc., etc. To avoid becoming too

[50] The above-mentioned R. is one of the instances from which I gather Professor Flechsig's powers as Governor of one of God's provinces (compare pages 49 and 50 above) must have stretched as far as America. The same seems to have applied to England; it was repeatedly stated that he had taken " sixteen English rays " from their leader, an English Bishop, which were however only entrusted to him on the express condition that they were to be used solely in a war for the independence of Germany.

discursive[51] I will now close my report about my experiences and memories of the time of my stay in Flechsig's Asylum.

VIII

p. 98

It is evident from what I have related above that during the last months of my stay in Flechsig's Asylum I stood in dread of certain dangers which, since communication with rays had become indissoluble, seemed to threaten my body and my soul—dangers which had in fact already been partially realized. The most disgusting was the idea that my body, after the intended transformation into a female being, was to suffer some sexual abuse, particularly as there had even been talk for some time of my being thrown to the Asylum attendants for this purpose. Moreover the dread of " being forsaken " played a major role, so that every night I went to bed in my padded cell I doubted whether the door would open again at all in the morning; to be torn from the cell in the middle of the night in order to be drowned was another terrifying possibility which occupied my imagination, indeed was forced on to me by what was said by the voices.

Therefore, when early one morning (perhaps mid-June 1894) three attendants appeared in my cell with a suitcase in which were packed my few belongings, and told me that I was to get ready to p. 99 leave the Asylum, my only reaction at first was a feeling of *liberation* from a place in which an infinite number of perils threatened me. I had no idea where the journey was to lead, nor did I think it worth enquiring, because I did not think these attendants were human beings at all, but only " fleeting-improvised-men ".[52] The journey's goal left me indifferent; I felt *only* that I could not fare worse anywhere in the world than I had fared in Flechsig's Asylum; any change could therefore only be an improvement. Accompanied by the three attendants I left in a cab for Dresden Station, without seeing Professor Flechsig again. The streets of Leipzig through which we drove, particularly Augustusplatz, seemed strangely foreign; as far as I remember they were

[51] Another consideration is that it is mainly a question of visions, the *pictures* of which I have in my head, but the description of which in *words* is extremely difficult, in part absolutely impossible.

[52] I had also had a vision about the above-mentioned R., according to which he was said to have taken his life on the way to " Uebelessen " (Thonberg near Leipzig).

completely deserted. This may have been because it was so early in the morning with its peculiar light; probably I caught the passenger train leaving about 5.30 a.m. Having lived for months among miracles, I was inclined to take more or less everything I saw for a miracle. Accordingly I did not know whether to take the streets of Leipzig through which I travelled as only theatre props, perhaps in the fashion in which Prince Potemkin is said to have put them up for Empress Catherine II of Russia during her travels through the desolate country, so as to give her
p. 100 the impression of a flourishing countryside. At Dresden Station, it is true, I saw a fair number of people who gave the impression of being railway passengers. But if it should be thought that my ideas of a vast change having come over mankind should have been thoroughly revised by my drive to the Station and the subsequent railway journey, I must observe that no sooner had I reached my new destination, than a new world of miracles surrounded me with such extraordinary visions that the impressions of my journey soon faded, or at least I had doubts of how I should interpret them. The railway journey proceeded with uncommon speed for a slow train or so I thought at the time; my mood was such that I would have been ready any moment (had this been demanded) to throw myself on the railway line or to jump into the water while crossing the Elbe. After a journey of several hours we left the train at a Station which, I heard later, was supposed to have been Coswig; there we entered a cab which in about half an hour drove us to my new destination. Again, as I only learned several years later, it was supposed to have been Dr. Pierson's Private Asylum for the Insane; at the time I came to know the Asylum only by the name of "Devil's Kitchen" which the voices indicated to me. The senior attendant of the Asylum who had come to fetch me took his place on the coach-box; his name, as far as I can remember, was Marx, and I will shortly have more to say about him being somehow identical with von W.'s soul. The Asylum itself, a relatively small building in beautiful grounds, gave the impression of being quite new. Everything seemed only just finished; not even the enamel paint on the stairs was fully dry. The three attendants from Flechsig's
p. 101 Asylum who had accompanied me soon retired and I did not see them again. I had time to look round my new abode.[53]

[53] Why I was taken to Pierson's Asylum—temporarily, for 7 to 14 days—is still inexplicable when I try to view these things in a human, natural light. My transfer from the University Clinic in Leipzig to the present Country Asylum (Sonnenstein)

I will try to give a ground plan and sketch of Dr. Pierson's Asylum (the Devil's Kitchen) also, because I thought at the time, and still think, that I can draw certain conclusions from the lay-out. The building where I was admitted had as far as I can remember only one storey, that is to say it consisted of a ground floor and first floor; at some distance, separated by the grounds, was a second building which was supposed to represent the female house of the Asylum. The ground plan of the upper storey of the house into which I moved looked something like this:

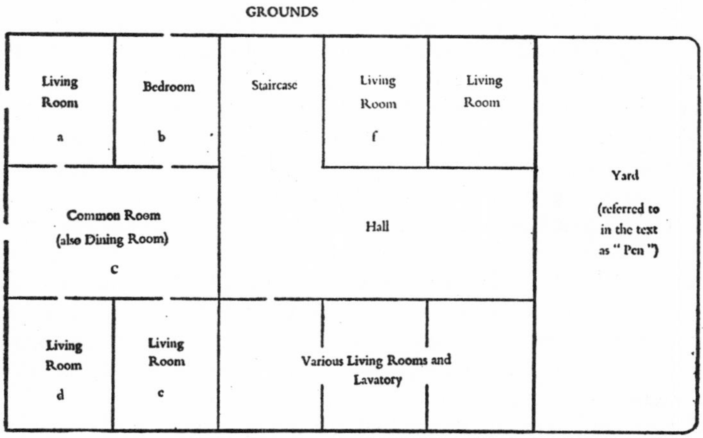

The ground floor was divided up slightly differently; it contained, among others, a bathroom, and otherwise consisted of a few big rooms; in the direction of the courtyard a door and a few steps led to the latter. p. 102

The time I spent in Pierson's Asylum was when the wildest mischief through miracles was carried on, because all miracles, not creative for permanent and sensible purposes but mere aimless playing about, must be considered *mischief* even if they provide the rays with temporary entertainment. At no other time were "fleeting-improvised-men" set down so extravagantly as then. The reasons for this statement will become apparent from what follows.

---

once decided upon, it would after all have been far simpler to set it in motion direct, without a stay somewhere else in between; if suitable rooms were not ready for my reception at Sonnenstein my stay at the Leipzig Asylum would have been better prolonged by a week or two, instead of entrusting a fairly dangerous patient, as I certainly was at the time, to the care of a Private Asylum.

I will start by first describing the circumstances of my outward life and how they developed in my new abode. I had no separate living-room; room *b* in the above sketch served as my bedroom. Day-time I usually spent in the common living-room or dining-room *c*, in which there was a constant coming and going of other presumed patients. In an attendant apparently employed for my special supervision I thought I recognised, perhaps because of an accidental likeness, the attendant of the Country Court who used to bring the files to my home during my six weeks of professional activity in Dresden; as I did not learn his name I will call him
p. 103 the "attendant of the Country Court". I naturally considered him, as all the other human shapes I saw, only as "fleetingly-improvised". Even now I cannot convince myself that this idea was wrong, because I definitely remember for instance, seeing more than once during those very light June mornings, this "attendant of the Country Court" who slept in a separate bed in my room, becoming one with his bed; that is to say I saw him *gradually* disappear, so that his bed was empty, without my having noticed that he got up or opened the door to leave the room. Further, this "attendant of the Country Court" had the habit of occasionally dressing in my clothes. A gentleman appeared occasionally—mostly in the evening hours—who was supposed to be the Medical Director of the Asylum and who again reminded me, because of a certain likeness, of Dr. O. in Dresden, whom I had consulted; this gentleman always appeared accompanied by the senior attendant, who will be described in more detail later, and I must now presume that it was Dr. Pierson; his conversation was regularly confined to a few empty words. I only once entered the garden of the Asylum, and that on the day of my arrival when I walked in it for about an hour. I saw there several ladies, among them Mrs. W., the wife of a Pastor in Fr., and my own mother, also several gentlemen, among them the Councillor of the Country Court K., of Dresden, with an ungainly enlarged head. Even if I wanted to try to convince myself now that I had only been deceived by fleeting similarities of external appearances, this would not suffice to explain to me the impressions I had at the time; I could understand such likeness occurring in two or three instances but not the fact that, as I will show, *almost all the patients in the Asylum*, that is to say at least several dozen human
p. 104 beings, looked like persons who had been more or less close to me in my life.

After that one walk in the garden proper the only time I was

in the open air—for one to two hours every morning and afternoon—was in the above-mentioned courtyard or "pen"; this was about fifty yards square, shut in by walls, a desolate sandpit without bush or shrub, with nothing to sit on but one or two wooden benches of the most primitive kind. Into this pen were crammed 40 to 50 human forms at the same time as myself; judging from their appearances it was and is impossible for me to believe that they were really the patient population of a Private Asylum for the Insane. In such Private Asylums one finds as a rule only well-to-do patients, and only exceptionally are really demented patients or idiots to be found there. But here I saw only extraordinary figures, among them fellows in linen overalls covered in soot. Almost all of them were silent and practically motionless; only a few used occasionally to utter certain fragmentary sounds, among them a gentleman I thought was the Country Court Councillor W., who shouted continuously for a Miss Hering. During my periods in the "pen" or even inside the Asylum I never heard anything among these supposed patients even faintly resembling a sensible conservation such as is carried on in Private Asylums among milder patients. They entered the common-room one after another, silently, and equally silently left it again, apparently without taking any notice of one another. At the same time I repeatedly witnessed that some of them changed heads during their stay in the common-room; that is to say, without leaving the room and while I was observing them, they suddenly ran about with a different head. As far as I could observe p. 105
there was no relationship whatever between the size of the Asylum and the number of patients whom I saw in the pen and in the common-room, partly *simultaneously* (particularly in the former), partly *consecutively*. It was then, and still is, my conviction that it was impossible for all the 40 to 50 people who were crammed into the pen simultaneously with me and who pushed towards the door of the house again every time the signal was given to return, to have found sleeping accommodation in it for the night; I therefore thought and still think that some of them must have remained outside all the time, there to dissolve in a short time like the "fleeting-improvised-men" which indeed they were.

At the most there were only four or six beds on the first floor of the Asylum where I lived; the ground floor, through which I had to pass each time I went out to the pen and returned from it, teemed with human forms most of the time, but could hardly have provided accommodation for the night for more than 10 or

12 human beings, even had there been a communal dormitory.
And yet all these 40 to 50 visitors to the pen must have been more
or less demented, because milder patients, harmless to their environment, would hardly have been crammed into this desolate pen, so
depriving them of the pleasure of a walk in the Asylum garden
which actually existed—the above-mentioned parklands. Of the
shapes I remember being in the pen, I wish to name Dr. Rudolph J.
from Leipzig, a cousin of my wife, who had shot himself as early
as 1887; the likeness, except for being slightly smaller, was so
striking that I had no doubt whatever of his identity. This
person ran about continuously with a bundle of newspapers or
p. 106 other papers, which he used only to provide himself with something
soft to sit upon on the hard wooden benches; also there was the
Senior Prosecutor B., who remained immobile in a bent, devout,
almost praying posture. The voices called some of those present
the shapes in which " with regard to the Determining fourth
and fifth " (to be supplemented by a word like " dimension "
which I did not clearly understand)[54] and his subterranean antipodes
(the fellows in linen overalls) covered with soot were " set down "
(embodied). Inside the Asylum I saw among others Dr. W.
in two different shapes, one more perfect and the other more
degenerate, the latter having been allotted him in the transmigration
of souls; President of the Senate of a Court Dr. F., the Country
Court Councillor Dr. M., the Lawyer W. from Leipzig (a friend of
my youth), my nephew Fritz, etc. In another gentleman who
apparently occupied room *f* beyond the staircase of the above
ground plan, and whom I thought I had seen before when I arrived
at Coswig Station walking up and down as if he were looking for
somebody, I thought I recognised Mr. von O. of Mecklenburg,
whose fleeting acquaintance I had made during a holiday at
Warnemünde. His room was hung with very peculiar pictures
(on paper) mostly coloured red, and was filled by that singular
smell which I called the Devil's stench in Chapter I. Once I noticed
p. 107 from the window my father-in-law on the drive leading to the
Asylum; about that time I also had a number of his nerves in my
body and from their behaviour in conversation by way of nerve-

[54] " With regard to the Determining " was another designation for God's omnipotence which was given to the " anterior column leaders ", that is to say some subordinate instances of God's omnipotence (compare footnote 19). The attached numbers signified the stages upwards. The " anterior column leader " who is mentioned later, also called " below measure ", carried the number 14; I thought him somehow identical with the Director of this Asylum. The highest number which I remember having heard later, was 480.

contact I clearly recognized my father-in-law's nature. I also saw repeatedly a number of persons (4–5), once even a few ladies, entering the corner rooms *a* and *d* of the above ground plan, after they had passed the common-room; they must then have vanished in those rooms.[55] They had, as the ground plan shows, no other exit than through the common-room. When, after an interval during which I did not leave the common-room, I looked through the open door into those rooms, there was either nobody left in them or only a single person in the corner room *d*, the person whom I call Dr. W. lying in bed with all sorts of peculiar adornments of silken ribbons, etc., with which he had "miraculously provided himself" as it was said at the time.

Miracles affected not only human forms but also lifeless objects. However sceptical I try to be now in scrutinizing my recollections, I cannot erase certain impressions from my memory, in which I saw even articles of clothing on the bodies of human beings being transformed, as well as food on my plate during meals (for instance pork into veal or vice versa), etc. One day—*in bright daylight*—I saw from my window directly in front of the walls of the building where I lived, a magnificent portico arise, just as if the whole building were going to be transformed into a fairy palace; later p. 108
the image vanished, supposedly because the completion of the intended divine miracle was prevented by Flechsig's and von W.'s counter-miracles; the picture still stands out very clearly in my memory.

The senior attendant of the Asylum deserves special mention. On the very day of my arrival the voices said that he was identical with my fellow lodger v. W.; he was said to have given false evidence about me in some State enquiry, either on purpose or through carelessness, and particularly to have accused me of masturbation; as punishment for this he had now to be my servant in the form of a fleeting-improvised-man.[56]

It seems impossible that I should spontaneously have arrived at such ideas myself, because I never had any disagreements with

[55] This was repeatedly accompanied by the peculiar rattle connected with the "taking away" (dissolving themselves) of the "fleeting-improvised-men".

[56] Such forms of punishment—a rather moderate form if there is any truth in it at all—seemed to be favoured by souls. I heard it said several times that Professor Flechsig would have to serve me in the form of a "fleeting-improvised" charwoman in expiation of the wrong he had done me. It seems that some mildly mocking humiliation was to be the lot of those who had sinned in life; this accounts for the expression "rascal" which was applied to the fleeting-improvised-man who had to serve the Eternal Jew, and which therefore was also applied to the attendants of the present Asylum in the first part of my stay, particularly to the attendant M.

or harboured any grudge against Mr. v. W. with whom in any case I had only the honour of a fleeting acquaintance. The voices continuously tried to incite me against this senior attendant; on my very first day it was demanded that I address him as " W.", thereby insulting him by omitting his title; at first I did not at
p. 109 all want to, but finally did just once to get rid of the pressing voices. On a later occasion I even boxed his ears; I cannot remember my immediate incentive, but I do know that, as he had made some unfair demand on me, the voices challenged and mocked me for my apparent lack of manly courage until at last I struck him. I have already mentioned in Chapter I that on certain occasions I saw on the senior attendant's face and hands the red colour peculiar to Devils; what I shall relate later leaves me in no doubt that he really had v. W.'s nerves, at least in part.

I did not undertake any mental or physical occupation during my short stay in Dr. Pierson's Asylum ("Devil's Kitchen"); my attention was taken up almost all day entirely by the conversation of the voices and by amazement at the miraculous things which were happening around me. In retrospect it seems very striking now that there was no such thing as a communal meal; as far as I remember having had meals there, a table was laid for me in the common-room; apart from myself one or two other patients at the most used to eat there too. I remember once that I threw the dish (fried sausage) out of the window, perhaps breaking the window pane in the act; but I cannot clearly remember my motive for this.

Naturally the souls with whom I was in nerve-contact in Flechsig's Asylum followed me to my new abode as they had done on my journey there: above all Flechsig's soul itself, trying to
p. 110 intensify the battle it had started against God's omnipotence, had formed a kind of party-following of more or less friendly souls whom it pulled along. Belonging to this party-following, apart from the "Cassiopeia brothers" mentioned in Chapter V, there was a group designated at the time as "the Advancing"; it consisted of Daniel Fürchtegott Flechsig's soul (which existed in two shapes), and those of the Senior District Court Councillor G. and an anterior column leader previously belonging to God's omnipotence, "with regard to the Determining first", a sort of renegade who had submitted to Flechsig's influence. The "suspended under Cassiopeia" (that is souls formerly members of the Students' Corps Saxonia) disappeared during my stay in Pierson's Asylum; they were pushed back into their graves "by

a strong hand ", an event I witnessed with my mind's eye, hearing
at the same time the wailing (a kind of whimpering) with which
the souls accompanied this event which they naturally did not
wish for, because it meant the loss of that state of Blessedness
which they had surreptitiously attained. A number of other
souls appeared in their place; this resulted preponderantly from
a partition of souls—an abuse presumably first introduced by
Flechsig's soul. Even if the physcial possibility of a partition of
souls mentioned in footnote 9 Chapter I had existed previously,
it is hardly likely that as long as the Order of the World was
intact, use would have been made of a measure so humiliating to
human feeling. There could have been no good reason to allow
the soul of a human being to ascend to a state of Blessedness with
a certain number of its nerves, while the other part was placed in
a position of punishment. I am inclined rather to believe that the
natural unity of the human soul used to be respected; thus in the p. 111
case of nerves too greatly blackened, to cleanse *all* of which would
have required too great an expenditure of pure rays, only a small
number of nerves was cleansed (this meant that a particular human
soul was granted the state of Blessedness for a shorter time only,
compare Chapter I), the rest simply being left to rot in the grave.
But, as mentioned, Flechsig's soul introduced the partition of souls
mainly in order to occupy the whole heavenly vault with parts of
souls so that divine rays, following some power of attraction,
met resistance on all sides. The picture which I have in my mind
is extremely difficult to express in words; it appeared that nerves—
probably taken from my body—were strung over the whole
heavenly vault, which the divine rays were not able to surmount,
or which at least constituted a mechanical obstacle similar to the
way a besieged fortress is protected by walls and moats against
the onrush of the enemy. For this purpose Flechsig's soul had
split into a great number of soul parts, of which there existed for
a time about 40 to 60, amongst them many tiny ones presumably
consisting of but a single nerve; two bigger soul parts were called
the " superior Flechsig " and the " middle Flechsig "; the former
used temporarily to be marked out by greater purity because of
divine rays which he had appropriated but which usually did not last
long. Similarly there were later also 20 to 30 von W.'s soul parts,
even a joint v. W.-Flechsig's soul, to which I might refer again.

The causes which led to the appearance of von W.'s soul in the sky (besides Flechsig's) I can only guess, though probably with some accuracy. All " tested " (Flechsig's, etc.) souls owe their

existence fundamentally to the power of attraction which had
p. 112 developed in my body through excessive over-excitement of my nerves; that is to say I was for them only a means to an end to capture the divine rays brought nearer by the power of attraction with which they then adorned themselves, like a peacock with strange feathers, so attaining the gift of miracles, etc. For this reason it was important for them to have a certain power of control over my body. While I was in the Leipzig Asylum this power of control seems to have been exerted by Flechsig's soul in combination with the real Professor Flechsig, still present as a human being (or a "fleeting-improvised-man"; what he actually was at the time I must leave undecided). This influence ceased with my transfer to Dr. Pierson's Asylum ("Devil's Kitchen"); the actual power over my body then fell to the staff of that Asylum, particularly to the senior attendant. This seems to have caused Flechsig's soul to draw up to heaven, perhaps even to a state of Blessedness, some of the nerves taken from the senior attendant, but in reality v. W.'s nerves, in order to regain his lost influence over me through these nerves and through their influence on the senior attendant.

At the beginning it was said that only three v. W.'s nerve filaments were involved; but these having once obtained awareness of their heavenly existence and at the same time of their gift of miracles, soon complemented themselves into one fairly substantial soul by drawing up a larger number of other von W.'s nerves (out of the grave as I had to assume at the time). Naturally these too were impure nerves; in other words a second "tested soul" was now in the sky, inspired only by a selfish striving for self-preservation and lust for power contrary to the Order of the World and opposing God's omnipotence; to this purpose it abused
p. 113 my nerves' power of attraction on divine rays. In general it recognized the leadership of Flechsig's soul, which remained as before the spiritual leader of the whole rebellion against God's omnipotence; in some respects however it maintained a certain independence in contra-distinction to the other souls which formed Flechsig's following. For example, as already mentioned, it permitted an extensive partition of souls, but in other respects went its own way.

My position was made considerably more difficult through the addition of this second "tested soul"; for this soul also started to work miracles in my body which in part were of a highly damaging nature, about which I will say more later. On the other hand it also provoked some amusing effects, even lending to my

otherwise gloomy existence, if I may put it like this, a touch of the comic. That these nerves which had thus attained a sort of heavenly power were really von W.'s seems to me beyond doubt; for I repeatedly conversed with von W.'s soul about its recollections from life, particularly about its student days in the Students' Corps *Misnia*, right down to the well-known waiter B. in the Public House Gosen at Eutritzsch near Leipzig. At times it was highly amusing to observe how both souls—Flechsig's and von W.'s—in spite of their alliance against God's omnipotence, mutually repelled one another, because of the professorial arrogance of the one and the pride of nobility of the other. Von W.'s soul, full of "von W.'s House- and Primogenitur-Order" which it was going to establish in heaven and on which it was going to found its "world domination", was fundamentally unsympathetic to the soul of the national-liberal Professor Flechsig and at times would hear no good of it at all. The latter in turn, possessed by its intellectual superiority, looked on von W.'s soul, p. 114
with some contempt. Von W.'s soul showed other distinctly aristocratic traits, and temporarily paid me more respect, as when it noticed that I brought the fork to my mouth with my left hand; it showed a particular interest in a well-kept *table d'hôte*, and had also a greater organizing talent than Flechsig's soul, in so far as it was more economical with the rays it had appropriated, therefore usually appeared more radiant, and for some time it kept a proper "*magazine of rays*" (I could still indicate where it was in the sky).

I want to add a little more about my other supernatural impressions in Pierson's Asylum. So-called *Moonshine-Blessedness* fluttered towards me in long flights (the image is hard to describe, one might perhaps compare it with so-called gossamer, not in single threads but in a kind of denser texture); this was to represent the female state of Blessedness. It was of two kinds, one flatter and one more robust; perhaps the former can be regarded as Child-Blessedness. Further information was added to the idea of the end of the world mentioned in previous chapters, in how far a revival of the created world was possible; at one time it was said it would only extend to the fishes, at another as far as the lower mammals, etc. I must leave undecided how far this information was based only on apprehension for the future or whether it was founded on reality. But I must assume that on a distant star, probably by using part of my nerves, the attempt was actually made to create a new human world ("new human beings out of Schreber's spirit", as it has been called innumerable times since

p. 115 then, mostly meant in a mocking spirit). It remains a mystery how the necessary time for this was to be found; I thought then and automatically still think of the ideas developed in du Prel's work quoted in footnote 36 (in the Appendix as far as I remember) according to which a difference in space also means a difference in time. These "new human beings out of Schreber's spirit"—physically of a much smaller stature than our earthly human beings—were said to have already achieved a fairly remarkable degree of culture, to have kept small cattle proportionate to their own size etc. I myself was said to have received divine veneration as their "National Saint" so to speak, as if my physical posture (particularly in the "pen" of Pierson's Asylum) were of some significance for their faith. Those of their souls which had ascended to a state of Blessedness after death were said to have attained to rays of fairly substantial vigour.

I assume that there must have been some truth in the matter because at that time I had the "God" or "Apostle" of these little people—that is to say presumably the aggregate of the rays which were derived from their states of Blessedness—as a soul in my body, more specifically in my belly.[57] This little "God" or "Apostle" surpassed all other souls by virtue of a practical turn of mind —a fundamental trait of my own character (I cannot
p. 116 suppress some self-praise here)—so that in a way I recognized in him flesh of my flesh and blood of my blood. But in order to mislead me a falsified counterpart was put up against this little "God" or "Apostle"—just as in many other cases, for instance respecting my father's soul, the souls of the Jesuits, etc. Usually I noticed these falsifications very quickly, because it was easy to distinguish the true from the false by the character of the respective souls. There was also much talk at that time of a "law for the restoration of the rays", that is to say of the principle—of which the "little people out of Schreber's spirit" would have been an example—that new rays come forth from the *faith* of departed human beings. This idea seems to accord with what has been said above in footnote 11, Chapter I, about the origin of the "forecourts of heaven".

Flechsig's soul was at that time leader of two "suns", including the one from which daylight emanated. The picture I have

[57] I observed here too the otherwise frequent phenomenon that friendly souls always tended more towards the region of my sexual organs (of the abdomen, etc.), where they did little or no damage and hardly molested me, whereas inimical souls always aspired towards my head, on which they wanted to inflcit some damage, and sat particularly on my left ear in a highly disturbing manner.

in my mind of how the leading soul was situated, as it were, behind the sun, is impossible to describe in words. Von W.'s soul also was to be trusted with the leadership of a sun, but in general it showed little inclination towards it.

IX

p. 117

One fine day (after a total stay of 8–14 days) I was taken from Dr. Pierson's Asylum, "The Devil's Kitchen", to this Country Asylum Sonnenstein near Pirna—I later learnt that it was on the 29th of June 1894. I do not know the reasons for my transfer; at the time I felt I had to connect it with the tremendously increased influence of von W.'s soul during the last days of my stay in the Devil's Kitchen, which had to be counterbalanced in some way. I had a warm bath before I left—the only one in Dr. Pierson's Asylum. I then travelled by cab (as on my way there) accompanied by the "Country Court attendant" to Coswig Station; having drunk a cup of coffee there, I travelled by train via Dresden to Pirna without leaving the carriage. The human forms I saw during the journey and on the platform in Dresden I took to be "fleeting-improvised-men" produced by miracle; I did not pay any particular attention to them, because even then I was tired of all miracles. I was strengthened in my attitude by what the p. 118
voices said; Flechsig's soul used an expression it had invented of "fossilised".[58] Dresden, through which we were supposed to have travelled. From Pirna Station I travelled in a cab on a rather bumpy road up to this Asylum. More than a year elapsed before I realized that I had been brought to Pirna and to Sonnenstein, when, on one of the very few occasions I had access to the "Museum" (common-room) of the Asylum, I saw pictures of earlier Kings of Saxony on the walls. When I first arrived the voices called the place "The Devil's Castle". I still occupy the same rooms I was given then—number 28 on the first floor of the Elbe wing, with an adjoining bedroom. A few times I temporarily had a different living room because of some alterations and

[58] "Amongst the fossils", [English in the original] was Flechsig's soul's favourite expression for "among the fleeting-improvised-men", following its tendency when referring to supernatural matters, to replace the basic language by some modern-sounding and therefore almost ridiculous terms. Thus it also liked to speak of a "principle of light-telegraphy", to indicate the mutual attraction of rays and nerves.

decorations; the bedroom destined for me, however—as I will mention again later—I did not use for about two years but slept in padded cells, particularly number 97 of the round wing on the ground floor. In contrast to the fairly elegantly furnished Asylum of Dr. Pierson, the rooms struck me as rather poor at first. I also wish to mention that for about a year I did *not* have the view from my windows which now offers itself freely to me over the whole
p. 119 Elbe Valley. There were some dense chestnut trees, since felled, which at the time obstructed the view almost completely, so that even by looking out of the windows I could not learn anything of what went on in the outside world.

I can divide the time of my stay at Sonnenstein into two periods, of which the first on the whole still retained that serious, holy and sometimes awesome quality which characterized my life in the latter part of my stay in Flechsig's Asylum and in Dr. Pierson's Asylum; in contradistinction the second period merged gradually more and more into ordinary (not to say vulgar) channels. The first period lasted about a year; the second period continues, modified of late only by becoming less vulgar in some respects. In the first period the miracles were still terrifying and threatening in their bodily and mental effects, so that for a long time I was most seriously concerned for my life, my manliness and later my reason; in the second period—naturally very gradually and not without some set backs—the miracles became increasingly harmless, not to say senseless and childish, although to some extent still repugnant.

In the first period I was still convinced that I was dealing not with real human beings but "fleeting-improvised-men".[59] I still cannot see that this was an error on my part; from what I experienced at the time and still experience daily I must rather leave open the possibility that I was right; in other words the so-called "play-with-human-beings" has only gradually changed
p. 120 to that state in which, *now regarded from outside*, it would appear that mankind had not changed. In order to make this idea, which is hard to understand and not even completely clear to me, somewhat comprehensible, I must first give an account of the conditions of my external environment during the first years of my stay in this Asylum. Of the doctors of the Asylum, I got to know the Superintendent of the Asylum, Dr. Weber, and his assistant Dr. R., at first only in person and not by name, on the very first day during a physical examination in the bathroom (on the ground floor) when a stethoscope was used; I only learnt

[59] For this reason I kept almost total silence.

their names by chance at the end of a year or more. I have since received daily visits from these gentlemen; apart from them I only occasionally saw the senior attendant R. and a few attendants (M., Th.) and Sch. who has since left. M. was the attendant particularly charged with my care.

Other patients did not seem to exist in the Asylum at the time; at least on the corridor which I inhabited where there were nine rooms I did not notice any; only after some time had elapsed did I notice one patient addressed as Prince J . . . . sky and a second as Mr. B., the latter particularly through his playing the violin. Even during my daily walks in the garden of the Asylum with two or three attendants (the above-mentioned) I was *always alone* during the first months; at that time there was nothing to be seen of the large number of other patients of whom I now see up to 80 and 100 with me in the garden. The voices called the attendants "rascals" (compare footnote 56); I must assume that they had the properties of "fleeting-improvised-men" (and therefore were really souls), because they kept up nerve-contact with me in which I frequently heard from them expressions belonging to the basic p. 121 language; I heard phrases, particularly from the attendant Sch., which in the basic language serve to express astonishment—"Good Heavens" and "Hail and Thunder"—(not aloud but in the nerve-language) while he personally was in another room. At times M. and Sch. unloaded into my body a part of their bodies in the form of a foul mass in order "to remove themselves"; M. repeatedly placed himself into my arm as a so-called "large nerve" (a jelly-like mass about the size of a cherry) through which in a certain sense he participated in my thinking and my sensations like the other rays or nerves. The "rascals", in their capacity as souls, were said to have the gift of miracles; at certain special events there was talk of "rascals' miracles", through which these were said to have come about.

My wife visited me at Sonnenstein at longish intervals—probably of a few months. I was petrified when I saw her the first time entering my room on such a visit; I had long believed she was no more among the living. This belief was based on very definite evidence—as also in the case of other human beings—so that my wife's reappearance remains an unsolved riddle to this day. I repeatedly had the nerves belonging to my wife's soul in my body or felt them approaching my body from outside—here again the certainty of my memory leaves no room for doubt about the objective reality of the event. These soul parts were filled with

the devoted love which my wife has always shown me; they
p. 122 were the only souls who showed willingness to renounce their own further existence and find their end in my body, expressing it in the basic language as "let me"[60].

When my wife visited me in person at Sonnenstein I believed for a long time that she was only "fleetingly-improvised" for the occasion; and that she would therefore dissolve, perhaps even on the stairs or directly after leaving the Asylum. It was said that her nerves would be "encapsulated" again after every visit. On one of her visits—probably on my birthday in 1894—my wife brought me a poem, which I reproduce here word for word because it made such a deep impression on me at the time. It went as follows:

> Ere true peace can embrace you—
> God's still and silent peace—
> The peace life never giveth
> Nor worldy joys beneath,
> It needs God's arm must strike
> A blow and wound you deep,
> So that you cry: Have mercy,
> God, have mercy on my days;
> It needs a cry must ring,
> Ring from your soul
> And darkness be within you
> As 'fore the world's first day.
> It needs that crushing pain
> Must wholly vanquish you,
> And not a lonely tear be left
> In your poor wretched soul.
> And when you've done with weeping
> And weary art, so weary,
> Then comes to you a faithful guest
> God's still and silent peace.

This poem, by an unknown author, made such a singular impression on me because the phrase "God's peace" which
p. 123 recurs in it, is *the expression used in the basic language for sleep produced by rays* which I heard innumerable times before and since. At the time I could hardly believe that this was mere coincidence.

[60] This expression could be rendered, grammatically complete, in the following words: "Let me—you rays that are trying to pull me back—do let me follow the power of attraction of my husband's nerves: I am prepared to dissolve in my husband's body".

During the first weeks of my stay at Sonnenstein (in early July 1894), certain changes occurred both in my longstanding nerve communication with rays, and closely related with it in the heavenly conditions; these seem to have been of fundamental importance for the whole period of time which has since passed. Again it is extremely difficult to describe these changes in words because matters are dealt with which lack all analogies in human experience and which I appreciated directly only in part with my mind's eye,[61] in part only by their effects, so that I may have formed but an approximate picture. In the previous chapter it was related that the number of "tested" souls and soul parts present in the p. 124
sky had increased markedly through soul-division. Among these souls Flechsig's, which had for a time retained a fair proportion of its human intelligence in virtue of the size of its two main forms (as "superior Flechsig" and as "middle Flechsig"), was still prominent; in the course of years, however, it progressively lost its intelligence so that now hardly a trace of awareness of its own identity remains. For my part I was always led by the desire to draw these souls and soul parts to myself and so ultimately to cause their dissolution; I started from the perfectly sound supposition that when all "tested" or impure souls had been eliminated from their position of so-called middle instances between myself and God's omnipotence, a solution of the conflict in consonance with the Order of the World would follow automatically; either a cure by a complete calming of my nerves through sleep, or—a possibility I later considered—unmanning, in consonance with the Order of the World, with the purpose of creating new human beings. These "tested" souls, however, were possessed only by the opposite endeavour, namely to assert themselves in their usurped heavenly position which gave them the gift of miracles; whenever they came closer they tried to withdraw again by pushing other souls or soul parts in turn into the foreground.

[61] I use here the expression "seeing with the mind's eye", which I used before (Chapter VIII, p. 110), because I cannot find a more suitable one in our human language. We are used to thinking all impressions we receive from the outer world are mediated through the five senses, particularly that all light and sound sensations are mediated through eye and ear. This may be correct in normal circumstances. However, in the case of a human being who like myself has entered into contact with rays and whose head is in consequence so to speak illuminated by rays, this is not all. I receive light and sound sensations which are projected direct on to my *inner* nervous system by the rays; for their reception the external organs of seeing and hearing are not necessary. I see such events even with eyes closed and where sound is concerned would hear them as in the case of the "voices", even if it were possible to seal my ears hermetically against all other sounds.

One night—perhaps the fourth or fifth after my arrival at Sonnenstein—I succeeded with immense mental effort in temporarily drawing down to myself all impure ("tested") souls; it would only have required a thorough "covering with rays" for my recovery through one nerve-restoring sleep and with it the disappearance of the impure souls. (Unfortunately one could not decide to adopt this course for the reason mentioned previously).
p. 125 In consequence Flechsig's soul took special measures to exclude the recurrence of such a danger to its existence and to that of other impure souls. It resorted to *mechanical fastening* as an expedient; a technique of which I was only able to get a rough idea. This mechanical fastening first occurred in a looser form called "tying-to-rays", where the word "rays" seems to have been used in a special sense which I did not fully understand. I can only describe the picture I saw with my mind's eye. According to this the souls hung on a kind of bundle of rods (like the fasces of the Roman Lictors), but in such a manner that the rods spread out below like a cone, while the nerves of the souls were tied fast around the upper points. When this looser form of fastening seemed not to afford sufficient defence against my power of attraction and the danger of dissolving in my body, a more resistant form was chosen which was called "tying-to-celestial-bodies". As the expression denotes, a tying to some distant stars occurred which from then on excluded the possibility of a complete dissolution in my body in consequence of my power of attraction; on the contrary withdrawal was safeguarded through the mechanical fastening so established. When the "middle Flechsig" used this form of fastening for the first time, it was felt in God's realms that behaviour so contrary to the Order of the World could not be tolerated. The "middle Flechsig" was therefore forced to untie himself again. But when the experiment was later repeated there was no longer sufficient energy for such measures; the tying was permitted, in which not only all other Flechsig soul parts participated, but
p. 126 also the souls in their train, particularly that of v. W. and finally God's omnipotence itself. In this way "tying-to-celestial-bodies" became a permanent institution continuing to the present day and led to further consequences, particularly the "writing-down-system", now to be described. I realize that such a conception, according to which one must think of my body on our earth as connected to other stars by stretched out nerves, is almost incomprehensible to other people considering the immense distances involved; for me however as a result of my daily experiences

over the last six years there can be no doubt as to the objective reality of this relation.

The mentioned writing-down-system is extraordinarily difficult to explain to other people even vaguely. That it exists is overwhelmingly proved to me day after day; yet it belongs even for me to the realm of the unfathomable because the objective it pursues must be recognized by all who know human nature as something in itself unattainable. It is obviously a stop-gap measure and it is difficult to decide whether it arises from a wrong (that is contrary to the Order of the World) intent or from faulty reasoning.

Books or other notes are kept in which for years have been *written-down* all my thoughts, all my phrases, all my necessaries, all the articles in my possession or around me, all persons with whom I come into contact, etc. I cannot say with certainty who does the writing down. As I cannot imagine God's omnipotence lacks all intelligence, I presume that the writing down is done by creatures given human shape on distant celestial bodies after the p. 127
manner of the fleeting-improvised-men, but lacking all intelligence; their hands are led automatically, as it were, by passing rays for the purpose of making them write down, so that later rays can again look at what has been written.

To illuminate the purpose of this whole system I must enlarge further. All the attacks made over the years, on my life, my bodily integrity, my manliness and my reason, were and still are based on the same idea: to withdraw again as far as possible from the power of attraction of my over-excited nerves, which far surpasses anything that has ever existed before. To that end one at first considered my *unmanning*, apparently in recognition of the fundamental tendency of the Order of the World (see Chapter V). This was not unmanning aimed at renewing mankind in consonance with World Order, but only an intended insult, for in a peculiar way it was imagined, or perhaps wishfully thought, that an unmanned body would lose its power of attraction for the rays. Years after my arrival at Sonnenstein, the idea of unmanning still appeared, if I may so express myself, in the minds of the souls. Small parts of Flechsig's soul which were distant, and therefore not in contact with my nerves for quite some time, used repeatedly to exclaim as if astonished: " Is he not unmanned yet? " God's rays frequently mocked me about a supposedly imminent unmanning as " Miss Schreber " [in English in the original]; an expression used frequently and repeated *ad nauseam*

p. 128 was: " You are to be *represented* as given to voluptuous excesses "[62],
etc. I myself felt the danger of unmanning for a long time as
a threatening ignominy, especially while there was the possibility
of my body being sexually abused by other people.

For over a year therefore the female nerves, or nerves of
voluptuousness, which had penetrated my body in great masses,
could not gain any influence on my behaviour or on my way of
thinking. I suppressed every feminine impulse by exerting my
sense of manly honour and also by the holiness of my religious
p. 129 ideas, which occupied me almost exclusively; indeed I really
became aware of the presence of female nerves only when they
were artificially set in vibration by rays on certain occasions so as to
produce a sensation of timidity and to " respresent " me as a human
being trembling with feminine anxiety. On the other hand my
will power could not prevent the occurrence, particularly when
lying in bed, of a sensation of voluptuousness which as so-called
" soul-voluptuousness " exerted an increased power of attraction
on the rays; this expression used by the souls meant a voluptuousness
sufficient for souls but felt by human beings only as general
bodily well-being without real sexual excitement. (Compare
Chapter VII towards the end.)

With this phenomenon becoming increasingly manifest in the course of time, God might have become aware that unmanning was not a way of "*forsaking* " me, that is of freeing Himself again from the power of attraction of my nerves. From this the idea arose to " retain me on the masculine side ", but—again under basically false pretences—not in order to restore my health, but to destroy my reason or to make me demented. Again one paid no attention to the fact that the nerves, even of a demented human

[62] The notion of " representing ", that is to say of giving to a thing or a person a semblance different from its real nature (expressed in human terms " of falsifying ") played and still plays a great role generally in the ideas of souls. In this vein it was said innumerable times on later occasions: You are to be represented as a scoffer of God, or as somebody who has committed soul-murder (compare above Chapter II, p. 23), etc. I think this relates to God's having as a rule only an outward impression of the living human being and to rays, which had come in nerve-contact with a human being, having at every " sight " (twinkle of an eye) *only a single* (momentary) impression. Only in this way can I comprehend the total inability to understand living man as an organism, of which I will later bring more striking proof. One may therefore have tried to persuade oneself—in the calamity in which God's omnipotence found itself through the existence of Flechsig's " tested " soul—that if one obtained an *impression* of a human being different from his real nature, it would then also be possible to *treat* him according to this impression. The whole thing amounts therefore to a *self*-deception quite useless in practice; for a human being naturally has always in his actual behaviour, and particularly in the (human) language, the means of establishing his true nature against intended " representing ".

being, would in a state of highly pathological excitement retain their power of attraction—provided, of course, that they were still generally capable of sensation as of pain, voluptuousness, hunger, cold, etc. Incessantly therefore, day after day and hour after hour, poison of corpses and other putrid matter which the rays carried was heaped upon my body, in the belief that it would be possible in this way to suffocate me eventually and in particular to rob me of my reason. In the next chapter I will relate what temporary damage was thus wrought on my body in a most threatening manner.

I have reason to assume that the poison of corpses or the putrid matter was taken from the same celestial bodies to which the p. 130
rays had been tied, and where they were packed as it were with it or soaked it up in passing. Some of the rays had been given the shape of miracled birds about which I shall have more to say later. It became apparent that the tested souls which were still in heaven, and what had remained of the erstwhile forecourts of heaven, which one had kept in reserve in order to be able to take refuge behind them, had in the course of time totally lost their intelligence, that is to say they had no thoughts of their own left. On the other hand it seems to lie in the nature of rays that they must *speak* as soon as they are in motion; the relevant law was expressed in the phrase "do not forget that rays must speak", and this was spoken into my nerves innumerable times, particularly early on. But in fact for years, lacking own thoughts, they have spoken of nothing but their own miracles, falsely attributing fear of them to my nerves (for instance, "If only my fingers were not paralysed", or "If only miracles would not affect my knee-cap"); further, everything I was about to do was cursed (for instance, "If only the cursed piano-playing would cease", as soon as I sit down at the piano, or even "If only the cursed cleaning of nails would cease", as soon as I start cleaning my nails). Over and above this one has the boundless impudence—I can use no other expression—to demand that I should express this falsified nonsense in spoken words as if it were my own thoughts, in this fashion: "If only the cursed piano-playing would cease" was followed by the question: "Why don't you say it (aloud)?", and this again was followed by the falsified answer: "Because I am stupid, perhaps", p. 131
or again "Because I am frightened of Mr. M." (compare footnote 26, Chapter V). Naturally there are now also pauses in which there is nothing to report of miracles directed against my person, nor any definite "thought of resolution" to undertake this or

that occupation which the rays, *being able to read my thoughts*, can recognize; in other words, when I indulge in thinking nothing, particularly at night when I sleep or in daytime when I temporarily rest or walk about in the garden without thinking, etc. The writing-down-material, mainly *my* previous thoughts besides a few constantly recurring additions of more or less senseless and partly offensive phrases, vulgar terms of abuse, etc., serves to fill in these pauses (that is to say to give the rays something to talk about even during these pauses). I will perhaps append an anthology of these phrases to the present essay in order to give the reader at least some inkling of the nonsense my nerves have for years had to put up with.

The offensive phrases and abusive words serve the particular purpose of inciting me to talk aloud and so to make sleep impossible at the proper times; for the whole policy of souls culminates in the prevention of sleep and soul-voluptuousness; but the aim of the whole policy remains totally obscure. The writing-down also serves as another peculiar trick which again is based on a total misunderstanding of human thinking. It was believed that my store of thoughts could be exhausted by being written-down, so that eventually the time would come when new ideas could no longer appear in me; this of course is quite absurd, because human thinking is inexhaustible; for instance reading a book or a news-
p. 132 paper always stimulates new thoughts. This was the trick: as soon as an idea I had had before and which was (already) written-down, recurred—such a recurrence is of course quite unavoidable in the case of many thoughts, for instance the thought in the morning "Now I will wash" or when playing the piano the thought "This is a beautiful passage", etc.—as soon as such a budding thought was spotted in me, the approaching rays were sent down with the phrase "We have already got this", *scil.* written-down; in a manner hard to describe the rays were thereby made unreceptive to the power of attraction of such a thought.

I must deny myself expounding the writing-down-system and its consequences further; it would in any case be impossible to make this fully clear to anyone who has not had the same experience on his own nerves. I can only give the assurance that the writing-down-system and particularly the intrusion of "We have already got this" when any of my earlier thoughts recurred, became a mental torture, from which I suffered severely for years and to which I am only slowly getting a little accustomed; because of it, I had to endure trials of patience as they have probably never before had to be borne by a human being[63], made all the worse by the difficulties of my outward circumstances (restriction of freedom, etc.).

I have only to add that in the above description I have anticipated p. 133
somewhat in time for the sake of coherence; in actual fact the development described belongs in part to a much later period, for p. 134
instance there was no question of playing the piano, which I mentioned above, for almost a year after my arrival at Sonnenstein.

X p. 135

During the first weeks of my stay at Sonnenstein (in July or August 1894), I am convinced certain important changes took place with the sun. As before when discussing supernatural

[63] There had been times when I could not help myself but speak aloud or make some noise, in order to drown the senseless and shameless twaddle of the voices, and so procure temporary rest for my nerves. This might have appeared as raving madness to the physicians who did not know the true reason, and so might have caused the corresponding treatment which indeed was meted out to me for years, in any case at night-time. That the expression "*mental torture*" is no exaggeration can be gauged from the fact that during the time I slept in the cell (1896–1898), I spent several hours of almost every night outside the bed, pounding with my fists against the closed shutters or, when the shutters had been removed, standing next to the open window clad only in a shirt at a temperature in winter of minus 8 to minus 10 degrees R., shivering with cold (the more so as the natural frost was increased by miracled frost), or groping in the totally darkened cell and by miracles being made to hit my head against the low ceiling; yet all this I found more bearable than to remain in bed, which I simply could not endure when sleep could not be procured.

I must be prepared for the question, why did I not inform my physicians of all these things early on by lodging a complaint? I can only answer by asking a question in turn: would one have given my description of these supernatural events the slightest credence? Even now I would count it a great triumph for my dialectical dexterity if through the present essay, which seems to be growing to the size of a scientific work, I should achieve only *the one* result, to make the physicians shake their heads in doubt as to whether after all there was some truth in my so-called delusions and hallucinations. Had I merely attempted a verbal discussion, I could hardly have counted on sufficient patience to listen to a longish disquisition from me; still less would one have found it worth while to think about the supposed nonsense. Added to this I thought during my early stay in this Asylum that the physicians themselves were only fleeting-improvised-men and that their deliberations were influenced by the rays hostile to me—a notion, the latter part of which in any case, I must still maintain as correct, however little the physicians, in the nature of the matter, will realize it themselves. Besides, the hostile disposition of the rays (that is of God) ceases as soon as they are reassured that they can spend themselves in my body with soul-voluptuousness, or if I am in a position to give immediate proof of the indestructibility of my reason, which amounts to showing them that the policy which aims at its destruction is doomed to failure. More about this later.

matters, I have to confine myself to relating impressions which I received and can only conjecture in how far these changes were objective events. I recollect that for a longish period there appeared to be a *smaller* sun. This sun, as mentioned at the end of Chapter VIII, was first led by Flechsig's soul but later by a soul whose nerves I identified as those of the Director of the present Ayslum, Dr. Weber. While writing these lines I am fully aware that other people can only think this is sheer nonsense, as Dr. Weber is still among the living, a fact I myself have occasion to verify daily. Yet the impressions I received seem to me so certain that I must assume that some time in the past Dr. Weber departed from this life and ascended with his nerves to Blessedness, but then returned to life among mankind; this notion may be unfathomable for
p. 136 human beings and a possibility only to be explained in a supernatural manner[63A]. After the power of its rays had been exhausted this smaller sun was then probably replaced by another sun. For several days and nights I had at that time the most wonderful and magnificent impressions as already mentioned in footnote 11, Chapter I; in my opinion this was the time when the anterior realms of God had been exhausted and the posterior realms of God appeared on the scene for the first time.

I believe I may say that at that time and at that time *only*, I saw God's omnipotence in its complete purity. During the night—and as far as I can remember in one *single* night—the lower God (Ariman) appeared. The radiant picture of his rays became visible to my inner eye (compare footnote 61), while I was lying in bed not sleeping but awake—that is to say he was reflected on my inner nervous system. Simultaneously I heard his voice; but it was not a soft whisper—as the talk of the voices always was before and after that time—it resounded in a mighty bass as if directly in front of my bedroom windows. The impression was intense, so that anybody not hardened to terrifying miraculous impressions as I was, would have been shaken to the core. Also *what* was spoken did not sound friendly by any means: everything seemed calculated to instil fright and terror into me and the word " wretch " was frequently heard—an expression quite common in the basic language to denote a human being destined to be destroyed by God and to feel God's power and wrath. Yet everything that was spoken was *genuine*, not phrases learnt by rote as they later were, but the immediate expression of true feeling.

[63A] With regard to this and some other points, compare the reservations in the Preface.

For this reason my impression was not one of alarm and fear, p. 137
but largely one of admiration for the magnificent and the sublime; the effect on my nerves was therefore beneficial despite the insults contained in some of the *words*; when the "tested" souls which had for a time kept shyly in the background dared to appear again, I could not but express my feelings repeatedly in words such as "Oh how pure!"—towards the majesty of the divine rays—and "Oh how vulgar!"—towards the tested souls. Further, the divine rays read my thoughts correctly, without falsifying them, as has been done without exception since; they even gave them verbal expression in a rhythm corresponding to the natural movement of human nerves[64], so that despite all the frightening side effects, the total impression I received was a calming one and eventually I fell asleep.

On the following day and perhaps on one or two more days (in fact in day-time while I was in the garden) I saw the upper God (Ormuzd), this time not with my mind's eye but with my p. 138
bodily eye. It was the sun, although not the sun in her usual appearance as known to every human being, but surrounded by a silver sea of rays which covered a 6th or 8th part of the sky, as mentioned in footnote 19, Chapter II. Figures of course do not matter very much; but to guard against any danger of exaggeration I concede that from my recollection it might as well have been only a 10th or the 12th part of the sky. However that may be, the sight was of such overwhelming splendour and magnificence that I did not dare look at it continually, but tried to avert my gaze from the phenomenon. One of the many things incomprehensible to me is that other human beings should have existed at that time apart from myself, and that the attendant M., who alone accompanied me at the time, remained apparently totally indifferent to this phenomenon. But his indifference did not really astonish me, because I considered him a fleeting-improvised-man, who of course led a dream-life and so could not be expected to have any understanding for those impressions which must inspire a thinking human being with the highest interest. But I am absolutely at

[64] The vibrations of human nerves follow a certain regular cadence, which I feel is best described by the expression "rhythm" used above. But I cannot decide whether this is the same phenomenon which Kraepelin calls "the ticking of the carotid pulse" at the end of Chapter VI of his work mentioned before (6th Edition), volume I, page 117, as I am not acquainted with the meaning of that expression. Words of four or perhaps six syllables accord most easily with this cadence. For this reason the phrases *learnt by rote* used in the writing-down-material, which aimed at withdrawing from my nerves, chose and still choose preferably words in discord with this natural cadence, as for instance my own title "Senatspräsident".

a loss to make sense of the fact that such a phenomenal impression should have passed him by (if he was a real human being) and the many thousands of other people in other places who must have had the same impression at the time. Of course other people will be ready to counter with the slogan that I suffered from a mere "hallucination". But the certainty of my recollection makes this for me subjectively quite out of the question, the more so as the phenomenon was repeated on several consecutive days and lasted for several hours on each single day; nor do I believe that my memory fails me when I add that that more radiant sun
p. 139 spoke to me in the same way as the sun did before and still does without interruption.

After a few days the miraculous phenomena of which I have spoken were over; the sun assumed the shape which she has since then retained without interruption[65]; the talk of the voices also turned again into a low whisper. I believe the reason for this change lies in the fact that at that time even God's omnipotence was induced to follow the example of Flechsig's soul and attempted "tying-to-celestial-bodies". If the influx of God's pure rays had lasted unhindered, as in the days described above and the nights following, I am certain that in a short time my recovery would have had to follow, or perhaps even that I would have been unmanned and simultaneously impregnated. But as one wanted neither the one nor the other, but always started from the mistaken notion that it would soon be possible to free oneself from the power of attraction of my nerves by "forsaking" me, tying-to-celestial-bodies was started to prevent pure rays reaching my body. How little this policy was permanently successful will be shown later[66].

[65] By the way, even today the sun looks different to me than before my illness. Her rays pale before me if, turned towards her, I speak with a loud voice. I can look into the sun unperturbed and am dazzled only very little, whereas in days of health, I, like other people, would have found it impossible to look into the sun for minutes on end.

[66] In the above description of the appearance of the posterior realms of God in their pure form I have followed exactly the ideas I had formed at the time (in July or August 1894) from the impressions I received, and which I retained throughout the years. Thinking it over again today, it seems that I made a mistake in believing that the phenomena during the night were only those of the lower God (Ariman) and the phenomena in daytime *only* those of the higher God (Ormuzd). This error is explained by the fact that I did not then recognize the signs of distinction which I *now* know between the rays of Ariman and the voices of Ariman, and the rays of Ormuzd and the voices of Ormuzd from years of further uninterrupted contact: the first name I heard was "Ariman" which led me to believe that the whole influx of rays during the night described above started from the lower God Ariman. But as in the course of the years that have since passed there has *never* been a time without both the lower God and the upper God appearing alternately at short

My *outward life* was extremely *monotonous* during that time— p. 140
the first months of my stay at Sonnenstein. Apart from daily morning and afternoon walks in the garden, I mainly sat *motionless*
the whole day on a chair at my table, did not even move towards p. 141
the window, where by the way nothing was to be seen except green trees (compare above); even in the garden I preferred to remain seated always in the same spot, and was only occasionally urged by the attendants to walk about, really against my will. Naturally opportunities for occupation were almost completely lacking even had I had the inclination; during that period everything was kept locked in both my rooms and the keys removed; I had access only to one single drawer containing a few brushes and similar things. I did not possess writing material; all my necessaries (articles of clothing, watch, purse, knife, scissors, etc.) were taken from me, there were only about 4 to 5 books in my room which I might have read had I been so inclined. All the same the main reason for my immobility was not so much the actual lack of means of occupation but that I considered absolute passivity almost a a religious duty.

Although this idea did not originate spontaneously in me but was induced by the voices that talked to me, I kept it up myself for a time until I realized that it was purposeless. That rays could ever expect me to remain totally immobile ("not the slightest movement" was an often-repeated slogan), must again be connected I am convinced, with God not knowing how to treat a living human being, as He was accustomed to dealing only with corpses or at best with human beings lying asleep (dreaming). Thus arose
the almost monstrous demand that I should behave continually as p. 142
if I myself were a corpse, as also a number of other more or less absurd ideas, which were all contrary to human nature. Every

---

intervals, I must assume it was so from the very first appearance of the posterior realms of God; so that both the lower and the upper God alternately produced the phenomena of the night and the following day.

I want to add that the lower God (Ariman) and the upper God (Ormuzd) must be considered as two distinct beings in spite of God's omnipotence, which in certain respects exists as a unity, and that each of them, *also in their mutual relationship*, has his own particular egoism and own instinct of self-preservation and that they therefore tend to push one another forward alternately. I have learnt to recognize this especially in their respective writing-down-material which I will give in some detail later (compare also footnote 37). Naturally this clash of otherwise harmonious interests could only come about because the conditions in consonance with the Order of the World had been disturbed in their purity by the intrusion of strange, impure elements (the "tested souls"); this allowed the power of attraction of a single person's nerves to become so strong as to be contrary to the Order of the World and so constitute a real danger for the realms of God.

noise created by miracle around me—and this recurs continually at short intervals, either by somebody speaking or making himself otherwise conspicuous, by cracking of walls, creaking of floors, etc.—is in a peculiar confusion of terms called an " interference " annoying to me. One falsely produces in me the phrase " if only the cursed interference would stop ", which is reiterated innumerable times every day, by producing vibrations in my nerves which correspond to these words; whereas in reality these noises are felt as frightening *by the rays*, since they produce the so-called " listening-in-thought ". Further—in conditions in consonance with the Order of the World—it would never occur to a human being to consider the talk of his fellow men, for instance, as an unpleasant interference[67].

I believe I can explain how the wholly absurd notion arose by recalling the usual phenomena which accompany nerve-contact made with a sleeping human being (in his dreams). Through such nerve-contact a temporary connection was effected between divine rays and the nerves of that person; of course it was calculated to last only a short time, perhaps for the purpose of imparting information about matters concerning the beyond (compare Chapture I), or to stimulate poetic imagination, etc. To succumb
p. 143 permanently to the power of attraction of such nerves would endanger God Himself; therefore one had to attempt to get away again when the purpose was achieved; one only had to produce little noises by miracle (the so-called " interferences ") through which the attention of the sleeping, perhaps just waking, human being was diverted, and this short period of diverted attention sufficed the rays in the case of nerves not as highly excited as mine, to give up the nerve-contact and enable them to withdraw from the person. No really serious danger could arise for God while it was easy for rays to withdraw, as from only moderately excited nerves. These circumstances were then taken as pertaining equally to me without making allowance that my relation to divine rays had long ago become indissoluble owing to the enormously increased power of attraction of my nerves.

I considered the immobility demanded from me a duty incumbent on me both in the interests of self-preservation and of God, so as to

[67] Some unpleasantness however is connected with this since, as mentioned in Chapter VII, I feel a certain painful sensation with every word spoken around me (in consequence of the respective human nerves being stimulated by miracle) due to rays (which are fixed to celestial bodies) attempting to withdraw from me, causing a very unpleasant tearing in my head.

liberate Him from the embarrassment in which He found Himself owing to the " tested souls ". I had formed the opinion—probably not altogether unfounded—that more rays would be lost if I myself moved to and fro (equally when a draught went through the room); as I was then still filled with holy awe towards divine rays because of their high purposes, and being also uncertain as to whether eternity really existed or whether the store of rays might suddenly be exhausted, I considered it my task to prevent any squandering of rays as far as it was in my power. I had also formed the view, p. 144
influenced by the opinions of the voices continually talking to me in this sense, that a drawing down of " tested souls ", so that they should spend themselves totally in my body and thus allow the restoration of God's sole power in the sky, would be much facilitated if I kept my body immobile. I therefore made the almost incredible sacrifice of desisting from every movement and of course from every occupation for several weeks and months, the conversation of voices excepted; this went so far that not even at night did I dare change my position in bed, because the spending of tested souls was to be expected mostly during sleep. I made this sacrifice, although I had already then received some taste of the " half and half " policy which God's omnipotence pursued towards me, but I could not get myself to believe that God harboured really evil intent towards me.

No change in these conditions occurred until the end of 1894 or early 1895. It coincided with another miraculous phenomenon, the " *cursed creation of a false feeling* "; this was the name given to it by the voices who recognized the tort intended by it. The constant endeavour of rays to withdraw from me (to " forsake " me) was checked only by the holiness of my purpose which was bound to attract all pure souls or rays, and by my deep and sincere concern about my relation to God and my own situation in life. One started therefore to falsify my own frame of mind through miracles, in order to create the impression of a frivolous human being given only to the pleasures of the moment (to " represent " me as such, compare footnote 62). Such an influence by miracles p. 145
on one's mood is *possible* as I have learned by experience, but I am unable to say more as to how it comes about; in order to give the reader an approximate idea I can only use a comparison, and point to the use of morphine which has the effect of producing a relatively serene, in any case indifferent mood, in a person who is harassed by bodily pain or in the throes of a depression.

At the beginning I resisted the influence of the " creation of a false feeling" (the mood—falsifying—miracle); but as time went by I found it easier to allow its influence, because I noticed that subjectively I really felt less unhappy and because I had to admit, that with all holiness of mind and with all my self-sacrificing endeavours to assist God in His fight against the "tested souls", I had not really achieved very much. I became more indifferent to my own situation, remembered Horace's "*Carpe diem*", attempted to brush aside cares for the future, simply to live for the day and accept what life still had to offer. For instance this led me to resume smoking cigars at the turn of 1894–95, which I had totally given up for years. On the other hand the rays did not achieve their purpose with the "creation-of-a-false-feeling". The power of attraction of my over-excited nerves remained undiminished in spite of the changed mood, the only difference being that I did not feel as unhappy as before. Here also *as in almost all miracles which are contrary to the Order of the World*, it seems the poet's word of the power "which always wills the evil and yet creates the good" applies.

p. 146 It goes almost without saying that my behaviour as described above could not be correctly judged by my environment, least of all by my physicians and attendants, assuming always that they were then real human beings. As I had shown no interest in anything nor displayed any intellectual needs, they could hardly see in me anything but a stuporose dullard. And yet the real situation towered sky-high above this appearance: I lived in the belief—and it is still my conviction that this is the truth—that I had to solve one of the most intricate problems ever set for man and that I had to fight a sacred battle for the greatest good of mankind. Unfortunately my deceiving appearance to the contrary brought with it innumerable indignities in the way I was treated; for years I suffered from them severely, and it seemed that one had altogether forgotten my standing and the high official position I had occupied in life. The attendant M. repeatedly threw me back into the bath when I wanted to leave it after a time, or in the morning when it was time to get up and I wanted to, threw me back into bed for reasons unknown to me; or in day-time when I was about to doze sitting at the table, he wakened me out of my sleep by pulling my beard, or he combed my hair with a fine comb while I was in the bath—and this at a time when flights of rays ploughed through my skull (compare the next chapter). At meal-times he used to tie a napkin round my neck as if I were a little child. Cigars were given me one at a time at certain hours

of the day; only several years afterwards did I succeed in obtaining all the cigars for the day in the morning; later still a box of a p. 147
hundred was put at my disposal as reserve. From another attendant I once had to suffer the indignity of having my ears boxed. Sometimes I opposed such indignities with actual resistance, particularly when one wanted to remove the washbasin for the night from my bedroom, which was locked from the outside; or when one tried to move me from my own bedroom to sleep in the cells fitted out for raving madmen. Later on I desisted from all opposition because it led to senseless scenes of violence; I kept silent and suffered.

Naturally nothing is further from my mind than to wish to denounce the attendant M. or any other attendant to his superiors by relating the indignities I had to suffer. I condone the excesses which M. was guilty of in view of his low education; it is also true that in later years he served me satisfactorily on the whole, although he continued to give himself airs. But I could not avoid mentioning these little traits if I wanted to demonstrate the measure of ignominy which I had to endure for years and the deep wounding of my sense of honour which at all times was fully alive.

In order to complete the picture of my situation during the early part of my stay at Sonnenstein it is necessary to give an account of the miracles which were enacted against me, and I will do this in the following chapter.

XI p. 148

From the first beginnings of my contact with God up to the present day my body has continuously been the object of divine miracles. If I wanted to describe all these miracles in detail I could fill a whole book with them alone. I may say that hardly a single limb or organ in my body escaped being temporarily damaged by miracles, nor a single muscle being pulled by miracles, either moving or paralysing it according to the respective purpose. Even now the miracles which I experience hourly are still of a nature as to frighten every other human being to death; only by getting used to them through the years have I been able to disregard most of what happens as trivialities. But in the first year of my stay at Sonnenstein the miracles were of such a threatening nature that I thought I had to fear almost incessantly for my life, my health or my reason.

In itself a state of affairs must be considered contrary to the Order of the World in which the rays serve mainly to inflict damage on the body of a single human being or to play tricks with the objects
p. 149 with which he is occupied—such harmless miracles have become particularly frequent latterly. For rays have the task of creating not just of destroying or playing childish pranks. Hence all miracles directed against me fail *in the long run* in their purpose; what has been destroyed or damaged by impure rays must always later be built up or mended again by pure rays (compare above Chapter VII, footnote 48). But this does not exclude that *temporarily* most serious damage is caused and very painful conditions arise giving the impression of extreme danger.

Most nearly in consonance with the Order of the World were those miracles which were somehow connected with a process of unmanning to be carried out on my body. To them belonged especially the various changes in my *sex organ*: several times (particularly in bed) there were marked indications of an actual retraction of the male organ; frequently however, particularly when mainly impure rays were involved, of a softening approaching almost complete dissolution; further the removal by miracles of single *hairs* from my *beard* and particularly my *moustache*; finally a *change in my whole stature* (diminution of body size)—probably due to a contraction of the vertebrae and possibly of my thigh bones. The last-mentioned miracle which emanated from the lower God (Ariman), was always accompanied by him with the announcement "I wonder whether to make you somewhat smaller"; I myself had the impression that my body had become smaller by about 6–8 cms., that is to say approximating the size of the female body.

The miracles enacted against the organs of the thoracic and abdominal cavities were very multifarious. I know least about
p. 150 those concerning the *heart*; I only remember that I once had a different heart[68]—still during my stay in the University Clinic of Leipzig. On the other hand my *lungs* were for a long time the object of violent and very threatening attacks. By nature my

[68] This, as indeed the whole report about the miracles enacted on my body, will naturally sound extremely strange to all other human beings, and one may be inclined to see in it only the product of a pathologically vivid imagination. In reply I can only give the assurance that hardly any memory from my life is more certain than the miracles recounted in this chapter. What can be more definite for a human being than what he has lived through and felt on his own body? Small mistakes in naming the organs involved may have occurred as my anatomical knowledge is naturally only that of a layman; but generally I think I have achieved accuracy even in that.

lungs and chest are very healthy; but my lungs were so affected by miracles that for a time I seriously believed I had to fear a fatal outcome in consequence of pulmonary phthisis. A " lung worm " was frequently produced in me by miracles; I cannot say whether it was an animal-like being or a soul-like creature; I can only say that its appearance was connected with a biting pain in the lungs similar to the pains I imagine occur in inflammation of the lungs. The lobes of my lungs were at times almost completely absorbed, I cannot say whether as the result of the activity of the lung worm alone or also because of miracles of a different kind; I had the definite feeling that my diaphragm was raised high in my chest to almost directly under my larynx and that there remained only a small remnant of lung in between with which I could hardly breathe. There were days when during my walks in the garden I had to reconquer my lungs anew with every breath. For the p. 151
part which is so miraculous is that the rays cannot but furnish a suffering body with whatever is most essential for its preservation, because to create is their essence and nature.

At about the same time some of my *ribs* were sometimes temporarily smashed, always with the result that what had been destroyed was re-formed after a time. One of the most horrifying miracles was the so-called *compression-of-the-chest-miracle*, which I endured at least several dozen times; it consisted in the whole chest wall being compressed, so that the state of oppression caused by the lack of breath was transmitted to my whole body. The compression-of-the-chest-miracle recurred several times in later years; but like the other miracles described here, it belongs mainly to the second half of the year 1894 and perhaps the first half of the year 1895.

Concerning the *stomach:* already during my stay in Flechsig's Asylum the Viennese nerve specialist named in Chapter V miraculously produced in place of my healthy natural stomach a very inferior so-called " Jew's stomach ". Later for a time the miracles were in preference directed against my stomach, partly because the souls begrudged me the sensual pleasure connected with the taking of food, partly because they considered themselves superior to human beings who require earthly nourishments; they therefore tended to look down on all eating and drinking with some disdain[69]. I existed frequently without a stomach; I expressly p. 152

[69] It was the same feeling which, for instance, made the Commandatore in Don Giovanni when he appears to the latter as a departed spirit, refuse the proffered meal with the words: " Know that I abhor all earthly food," etc.

told the attendant M., as he may remember, that I could not eat because I had no stomach. Sometimes immediately before meals a stomach was so to speak produced *ad hoc* by miracles. This was done particularly by von W.'s soul, which in at least some of its forms sometimes showed a friendly spirit towards me. Naturally this never lasted long; the stomach which had been produced by miracles, in any case only an inferior stomach, was usually removed again miraculously by v. W.'s soul during the meal " because of a change of mind "; great changeability is a marked feature of the soul-character, absolutely divine rays perhaps excluded. Food and drink taken simply poured into the abdominal cavity and into the thighs, a process which however unbelievable it may sound, was beyond all doubt for me as I distinctly remember the sensation.

In the case of any other human being this would have resulted in natural pus formation with an inevitably fatal outcome; but the food pulp could not damage my body because all impure matter in it was soaked up again by the rays. Later, I therefore repeatedly went ahead with eating unperturbed, without having a stomach; all in all I gradually got used to regarding everything which happened in my body with complete equanimity. Even now I am convinced that I am immune to all natural disease influences; disease germs only arise in me through rays and are removed again in the same way by rays. Indeed I doubt very much whether I am at all mortal as long as the communication with rays lasts; for instance, I think I could take the strongest poison without particular danger to my life and my health.[70]
p. 153 After all what can poisons do but destroy some important organs or have a destructive effect on the blood? Both have happened to me innumerable times through rays without any permanent ill effect.[71]

Of other internal organs I will only mention the *gullet* and the *intestines*[72], which were torn or vanished repeatedly, further the

[70] I need hardly say that this is purely hypothetical speculation, and that I have not the least intention of actually carrying out such experiments on my body which, if nothing else, would certainly cause me severe pain.

[71] The correctness of my assertion that I have so to speak become invulnerable, is evidenced by the fact that while I was well I used to suffer several times every winter from a heavy cold which lasted a number of days; during the 6 years of my stay here I have hardly ever had a real cold at all. Should a catarrhal inflammation of the mucous membrane of the nose—which is the essence of a cold—tend to develop, rays would immediately shoot to the diseased part of my body in such numbers that the cold would be stifled in its very beginnings.

[72] Dangerous *obstruction of my gut* was also repeatedly produced by miracles, which was however mostly resolved again, usually after a short time.

pharynx, which I partly ate up several times, finally the *seminal cord*, against which very painful miracles were directed, with the particular purpose of suppressing the sensation of voluptuousness arising in my body. I must further mention a miracle which affected my whole abdomen, the so-called *putrifaction of the abdomen*. This miracle originated regularly from von W.'s soul in one of its most impure shapes—in contrast to other parts of von W.'s soul—hence the name "abdominal putrifaction of von W.". It threw the putrid matter which caused the abdominal putrifaction into my belly with such ruthlessness, that more than once I believed I would have to rot alive, and the rotten smell escaped from my p. 154
mouth in a most disgusting manner. Von W.'s soul assumed that the abdominal putrification would be removed again by God's rays; this happened through rays of a particular kind adapted to this purpose, which pushed their way into my intestines like a wedge and absorbed their putrid content. God's rays appeared to act from the instinctive knowledge that it would be most distasteful for them to have to allow themselves to be attracted by a rotting body. This notion was expressed repeatedly in the slogan, that if I were to be forsaken, I should be forsaken with "a pure body"; but naturally this notion too suffered from the usual obscurity, as apparently one was not at all clear how the nerves of a "forsaken" body would lose their power of attraction. Those miracles always appeared most threatening to me which were in one way or another directed against my reason. These concerned firstly my *head*; secondly during a certain period—of probably several weeks round the autumn of 1894—also the *spinal cord*, which next to the head was considered as the seat of reason. One therefore attempted to pump the spinal cord out, which was done by so-called "little men" placed in my feet. Later I will have more to say about these "little men", which have some similarity to the phenomenon of the same name which I discussed in Chapter VI; as a rule there were two of them a "little Flechsig" and a "little von W.", whose voices I could also hear in my feet. The effect of the pumping out was that the spinal cord left my mouth in considerable quantity in the form of little clouds, particularly when I was walking in the garden. One can imagine the apprehension with which such events filled me, as I did not then know whether or not any part of my reason would thus in fact p. 155
vanish into the air. The miracles directed against my *head and the nerves of my head* happened in manifold ways. One attempted to pull the nerves out of my head, for a time even (during the nights)

to transplant them into the head of M. who slept in the next room. These attempts caused (besides the fear of an actual loss of my nerves) an unpleasant tension in my head. However the pulling out succeeded only moderately, the staying power of my nerves proved the greater force and the half pulled-out nerves always returned to my head after a short time. Serious devastation was caused in my head by the so-called " flights of rays ", a phenomenon difficult to describe, the effect of which was that my skull was repeatedly sawn asunder in various directions. I frequently had —and still have regularly daily—the sensation that my whole skull had temporarily thinned; in my opinion this was brought about through the bony material of my skull being partly pulverised by the destructive action of the rays; but it is restored again by pure rays particularly during sleep. One can form some picture of the disagreeable sensations these happenings cause if one considers that these are the rays of a whole world—somehow mechanically fastened at their point of issue—which travel around one single head and attempt to tear it asunder and pull it apart in a fashion comparable to quartering.

Further, in the time I am discussing attempts were repeatedly made to cover my nerves with some noxious matter; it appeared
p. 156 as if the natural capacity of nerves to vibrate were thereby really impaired, so that even I myself had at times the impression of becoming temporarily stupid. One of the agents concerned was called " poison of intoxication "; I cannot say what its chemical nature was. From time to time also the liquids of the food I had taken were by miracle placed on the nerves of my head, so that these were covered with a sort of paste, and the capacity to think temporarily impaired; I remember distinctly that this happened once with coffee.

All my *muscles* were (and still are) the object of miracles for the purpose of preventing all movements and every occupation I am about to undertake. For instance attempts are made to paralyse my fingers when I play the piano or write, and to cause some damage to my knee-cap to make marching impossible when I walk about in the garden or in the corridor. Lately the effect has mostly been only to make such occupations difficult or cause only moderate pain on walking.

My *eyes* and the *muscles of the lids* which serve to open and close them were an almost uninterrupted target for miracles. The eyes were always of particular importance, because rays lose the destructive power with which they are equipped after a relatively

short time as soon as they *see something*, and then enter my body without causing damage. The object seen can be either visual (eye) impressions, which are communicated to the rays when my eyes are open, or images which I can cause at will on my inner nervous system by imagination, so that they become visible to the rays. I shall return to these events, which in the soul-language are called the "*picturing*" of human beings, in another context. Here I will only mention that attempts were made early on and p. 157
kept up throughout the past years, to close my eyes against my will, so as to rob me of visual impressions and thus preserve the rays' destructive power. This phenomenon can be observed on me at almost every moment; whoever watches carefully will observe that my eyelids suddenly droop or close even while I am talking to other people; this never occurs in human beings under natural conditions. In order to keep my eyes open nevertheless, a great effort of will is needed; but as I am not always particularly interested in keeping my eyes open I allow them to be closed temporarily at times.

During my first months here the miracles on my eyes were performed by "little men", very similar to those I mentioned when describing the miracle directed against my spinal cord. These "little men" were one of the most remarkable and even to me most mysterious phenomena; but I have no doubt whatever in the objective reality of these happenings, as I saw these "little men" innumerable times with my mind's eye[73] and heard their voices. The remarkable thing about it was that souls or their single nerves could in certain conditions and for particular purposes assume the p. 158
form of tiny human shapes (as mentioned earlier only of a few millimetres in size), and as such made mischief on all parts of my body, both inside and on the surface. Those occupied with the opening and closing of the eyes stood above the eyes in the eyebrows and there pulled the eyelids up or down as they pleased with fine filaments like cobwebs. Here too those concerned were usually a "little Flechsig" and a "little v. W." and sometimes in addition another "little man", who had originated from Daniel Fürchtegott Flechsig's soul which still existed at that time. Whenever I showed signs of being unwilling to allow my eyelids to be pulled up and down and actually opposed it, the "little men" became annoyed and expressed this by calling me "wretch"; if I wiped

[73] Of course one can *not* see with the *bodily* eye what goes on inside one's own body, nor on certain parts of its surface, for instance on the top of the head or on the back, but—as in my case—one can see it *with one's mind's eye*, as the necessary illumination of the inner nervous system is provided by rays.

them off my eyes with a sponge, it was considered by the rays as a sort of crime against God's gift of miracles. By the way, wiping them away had only a very temporary effect, because the "little men" were each time set down afresh. Other "little men" were assembled almost continuously on my head in great number. They were called "little devils". They literally walked around on my head, curiously nosing about to see whether any new destruction had been caused on my head by miracles. In a way they even partook of my meals, helping themselves to a part, though naturally only a tiny part, of the food I ate; it made them appear temporarily somewhat swollen, but also less active and less destructive in their intentions. Some of the "little devils" participated in a miracle which was often enacted against my head and of which I will now say a little more. This was perhaps the
p. 159 most abominable of all miracles—next to the compression-of-the chest-miracle; the expression used for it if I remember correctly was "the head-compressing-machine". In consequence of the many flights of rays, etc., there had appeared in my skull a deep cleft or rent roughly along the middle, which probably was not visible from outside but was from inside. The "little devils" stood on both sides of this cleft and compressed my head as though in a vice by turning a kind of screw, causing my head temporarily to assume an elongated almost pear-shaped form. It had an extremely threatening effect, particularly as it was accompanied by severe pain. The screws were loosened temporarily but only very gradually, so that the compressed state usually continued for some time. The "little devils" responsible mostly derived from v. W.'s soul. These "little men" and "little devils" disappeared after a few months never to appear again. The moment of their departure coincided approximately with the appearance of the posterior realms of God. It is true that miracles are still responsible for opening and closing my eyelids in the manner described, but for almost six years now it has no longer been done by the "little men" but directly by rays which set the muscles concerned in motion. In order to prevent my closing or opening my eyes at will the thin layer of muscle situated in and above the eyelids and serving their movement has several times been removed by miracle. But again the effect was only temporary: the muscle tissue so lost was always restored again—for reasons often mentioned before.

p. 160 Manifold miracles were also directed against my *skeleton*, apart from those against my ribs and skull mentioned earlier. In the foot bones particularly in the region of the heel, *caries* was often caused by miracle, causing me considerable pain; luckily, however, the severest pains did not last long. A similar miracle was the so-called *coccyx miracle*. This was an extremely painful, caries-like state of the lowest vertebrae. Its purpose was to make sitting and even lying down impossible. Altogether I was not allowed to remain for long in one and the same position or at the same occupation: when I was walking one attempted to force me to lie down, and when I was lying down one wanted to chase me off my bed. Rays did not seem to appreciate at all that a human being who actually exists *must be somewhere*. Because of the irresistible attraction of my nerves I had become an embarrassing human being for the rays (for God), in whatever position or circumstance I might be or whatever occupation I undertook. One did not want to admit that what had happened was not my fault, but one always tended to reverse the blame by way of "representing"[74].

I believe I have given an almost complete description in this chapter of those miracles which I was led to consider the *essential* ones, because of their threatening character. In the course of this essay I will frequently have to mention many other miracles of a less dangerous kind (partly on my body, partly on the objects p. 161
around me); some of them had already appeared side by side with the miracles described above, some only started later.

XII

p. 162

As mentioned in Chapter IX the talk of the voices had already become mostly an empty babel of ever recurring monotonous phrases in tiresome repetition; on top of this they were rendered grammatically incomplete by the omission of words and even syllables. However, the description of a certain number of phrases used is of interest, because of the sidelight thrown on the souls' whole way of thinking, their idea of human life and of human thinking. Among these phrases are those in which I was called

[74] I for one am sufficiently just not to speak of moral guilt in the ordinary sense on the part of God (compare what has been said at the end of Chapter V, also at the end of the second series of Postscripts). The concept of guilt or sin is a human concept, which in its essence cannot be used towards souls whose nature differs from the human. After all one cannot expect of souls the *human* virtues of perseverance, self-sacrifice, etc.

a "*Prince of Hell*"—roughly since the time of my stay in Pierson's Asylum. It was said innumerable times for instance, that "God's omnipotence has decided, that the Prince of Hell is going to be burned alive", "The Prince of Hell is responsible for the loss of rays", "We announce victory over the beaten Prince of Hell", but then again by some of the voices: "Not Schreber, but Flechsig is the true 'Prince of Hell,'" etc.

Anybody who knew me in my former life and had the opportunity of observing my cool and sober nature, will readily believe that
p. 163 I myself could never have ventured on so fantastic a term as that of "Prince of Hell", still less as it was in such queer contrast to the poverty of my outward life situation, to the many limitations of freedom to which I was subjected, etc. There was certainly nothing in the appearance of my surroundings which was remindful of either Hell or of a princely setting. In my opinion the expression "Prince of Hell", which was only erroneously applied to me, was originally based on an abstraction.

The realms of God may always have known that the Order of the World however great and magnificent, was yet not without its Achilles' heel, inasmuch as the human nerves' power of attracting God's nerves constituted some danger for the realms of God. These dangers were likely to become more acute when somewhere on earth or on any other star nervousness or moral depravity gained the upper hand. In order to form a clearer picture of these dangers the souls had apparently adopted a kind of personification, similar to the way in which nations in their infancy try to understand the idea of God better by means of graven images of false gods. The phrase "Prince of Hell" was probably meant to convey the uncanny power inimical to God that could develop from moral decay among mankind or a general spread of nervous over-excitement in consequence of over-civilization. As my nerves' power of attraction became more and more irresistible, the "Prince of Hell" appeared suddenly to have become reality in my person. An enemy was therefore seen in me who had to be destroyed by all the might of divine power; one refused to recognize that on the contrary I was the best friend to *pure* rays from whom alone
p. 164 I could expect my recovery or other satisfactory solution of the conflict. One was apparently more inclined to share one's own power with impure ("tested" souls)—God's real enemies—than to put up with the idea of being dependent on a single human being whom one would otherwise have looked down upon in the proud awareness of distant power.

Phrases of another group having certain factual significance were those in which one talked of the "*soul-conception*". Fundamentally this contained significant and valuable ideas. In its original meaning soul-conception is I think *a somewhat idealized version which souls had formed of human life and thought.* One must remember that souls were the departed spirits of erstwhile human beings. As such they had a lively interest not only in their own human past but also in the fortunes of their still living relatives and friends and in everything that happened to mankind; they could gain such knowledge either through nerve-contact or outward impressions by actually seeing (compare Chapter I). They were able to express in more or less distinct words some rules of conduct and attitude to life. I will quote a few of these sentences as examples. "Do not think about certain parts of your body" was a rule of conduct apparently expressing the idea that man in his normal healthy state has no reason to think of particular parts of his body, unless reminded of them by pain. "Not at the first demand", was another phrase, indicating that a sensible human being would not allow himself to be led into one or other action by a momentary impulse. "A job started must be finished" was the formula p. 165
expressing that man should pursue to its ultimate goal what he starts, without being distracted by adverse influences, etc.

In man's thought processes one distinguished the "thought of decision"—man's exertion of will to do a certain thing—"wishful thoughts", "thoughts of hope" and "thoughts of fear". The "thinking-it-over-thought" denoted something perhaps also known to psychologists: it often leads a person to turn his will power in the opposite direction or at least change it from that which at first he may have felt inclined to follow, but which on further consideration *automatically causes doubts.* "The-human-thought-of-recollection" was used to indicate man's automatic need to imprint on his mind by repetition an important thought which had occurred to him. How deeply ingrained the "human-thought-of-recollection" is in the nature of the human processes of thought and feeling, can be seen from very characteristic instances when in poems rhymes (refrains) recur, or when in musical compositions a certain sequence of notes expressing the embodiment of beauty occurs not only once but is repeated again and again. A very prominent part was played in the "soul-conception" by ideas about the relation between the two sexes and their respective mode of occupation, their tastes, etc. For instance beds, hand-mirrors and rakes were considered feminine,

basket-chairs and spades masculine; of games, chess as masculine,
p. 166 draughts as feminine, etc.

Souls knew very well that a man lies on his side in bed, a woman on her back (as the "succumbing part", considered from the point of view of sexual intercourse). I myself, who in earlier life never gave it a thought, have only learned this from the souls. From what I read in for instance my father's MEDICAL INDOOR GYMNASTICS (23rd Edition, p. 102), physicians themselves do not seem to be informed about it. Further, the souls knew that male voluptuousness is stimulated by the sight of female nudes, but on the contrary female voluptuousness to a very much lesser extent if at all by the sight of male nudes, while female nudes stimulate *both* sexes equally. For instance the sight of a nude male body perhaps at a swimming exhibition, will leave the female public cold (for this reason their admission is rightly not considered immoral to the same extent as the presence of men at a female swimming exhibition), whereas a ballet will produce some sexual stimulation in *both* sexes. I do not know whether these phenomena are generally known and considered correct. My own observations and the behaviour of my own nerves of voluptuousness leave me in no doubt that the soul-conception is correct in this respect. I am of course fully aware that the reaction of my own (female) nerves of voluptuousness does not in itself constitute proof for the very reason that it is exceptional for female nerves to be present in a male body as in my case.

A distinction between masculine and feminine with respect to articles of clothing (the "armamentarium" as it was called in the basic language) is almost self-evident; boots appeared to the souls an especial symbol characteristic of manliness. To the souls "to
p. 167 take off boots" meant much the same as unmanning.

These short remarks may suffice to give an approximate idea of the original meaning of the expression "soul-conception". What I know about it I owe partly to definite information—during the early part of my illness—and partly to impressions received in my contact with souls. I have thus gained insight into the nature of human thought processes and human feelings for which many a psychologist might envy me.

The phrases about "soul-conception" received a quite different meaning later. They degenerated into mere flourishes with which one tried to satisfy the need for speech, while totally lacking in own thoughts (compare Chapter IX). "Do not forget that you are bound to the soul-conception" and "Now then, that is too much according to the soul-conception", became constantly recurring empty phrases, by the endless repetition of which I was tortured for years almost beyond endurance and still am. The latter phrase especially was the souls' almost constant retort when they could not think of what to say further to a new thought of mine, and it also shows by its poor stylistic form the degeneracy which had set in. In contrast the genuine basic language, that is the expression of the souls' true feelings before the time the mechanically repeated phrases commenced, excelled in form also by its dignity and simplicity.

Certain other phrases with quite important meanings can only be mentioned in the next chapter because of their context.

My *outward living conditions* have in some respects at least become p. 168
more bearable since about the first half of the year 1895, as mentioned at the end of Chapter X. Most important was that I started to occupy myself in different ways. It is true I still declined to write to my relatives, in particular to my wife, although the attendant M. tried to persuade me. I did not then believe in the existence of a real mankind outside the Asylum, but thought that all the human shapes I saw, in particular my wife when she visited me, were "fleeting and improvised" for only a limited time, so that to write letters as was suggested to me would have been a sheer farce in which I was not prepared to take part. Since then however there have been opportunities to play chess (with other patients or with attendants) and to play the piano. Having once or twice played the piano in the common-room or library of the Asylum during my wife's visits, a small piano was put into my room in the Spring of 1895 for my regular use. The feelings aroused in me when I resumed this occupation which in days of health I had enjoyed, I can best describe with a quotation from Tannhäuser:

> "Total forgetting descended between today and yesterday. All my memories vanished rapidly and I could only remember *that I had lost all hope of ever greeting you again or ever raising my eyes to you.*"

The only time I played the piano in Flechsig's Asylum was on my wife's urgent persuasion; it was the aria from Handel's Messiah "I know that my Redeemer Liveth" from a score which happened to be at hand. My state was such that I played in the certain conviction of it being the last time in my life that my p. 169

fingers would touch the keys of a piano. Having resumed chess and piano playing in the Asylum, they became my two main occupations during the whole five years which have since passed. Playing the piano in particular was and still is of immense value to me; I must confess that I find it difficult to imagine how I could have borne the compulsive thinking and all that goes with it during these five years had I not been able to play the piano. During piano playing the nonsenscial twaddle of the voices which talk to me is drowned.[74] Next to physical exercises it is one of the most efficient forms of the so-called not-thinking-of-anything-thought; but again one wanted to deprive me of it by introducing the " musical-not-thinking-of-anything-thought " as it was called in the soul-language. The rays always at least have a visual impression from my hands and from my reading the score, and every attempt at " representing " me by the " creation of a false feeling " and suchlike is doomed to end in failure because of the real feeling one can put into piano playing. Piano playing therefore was and still is one of the main objects of curses.

The difficulties which were put in my way defy description. My fingers are paralysed, the direction of my gaze is changed in order to prevent my finding the correct keys, my fingers are diverted on to wrong keys, the tempo is quickened by making the muscles of my fingers move prematurely; all these were and still are daily occurrences. Even the piano itself was frequently the object of miracles and strings were broken (luckily much more
p. 170 rarely in recent years). In 1897 alone the bill for broken piano strings amounted to no less than 86 Marks.

This is one of the few instances which I believe furnishes sufficient proof to convince other people of the reality of the miracles which I maintain happen. Superficial judgment might lead some to assume that I myself have caused the piano strings to snap by senseless banging on the piano; this was for instance my wife's repeatedly stated opinion, possibly having heard it from the physicians. In reply I maintain—and I am convinced that every expert will support me in this—that it is *altogether impossible* to snap the strings of a piano merely by banging on the keys, however violently. The small hammers linked with the keys only lightly touch the strings, and could never strike them sufficiently hard to

[74] As one cannot play the piano continually, musical clocks serve the same purpose, and (for the garden) mouth organs, which I recently (spring 1900) asked my relatives to get for me.

break them. Let anyone try to hit the keys as hard as he likes, even with a hammer or a log of wood; the keyboard may perhaps be broken to pieces but he will never be able to break a string. Strings have broken much less frequently in recent years—it still happens occasionally—because the rays' (God's) intent towards me has become less unfriendly (more about this later) owing to my constantly increasing soul-voluptuousness; the rays were also forced by still more unpleasant conditions (even for them) in particular by the so-called " bellowing ", to consider piano playing the most congenial pasttime for all concerned.

I must mention another miraculous event in this connection,
although it really belongs to an earlier time, which is one of the p. 171
most mysterious things even I ever experienced who, after all, has seen so much of miraculous things. I remember that on a certain day while I still kept immobile (that is in the summer or autumn of 1894) the attempt was made on one occasion to place a whole grand piano (Blüthner) in my room by miracle; it seems to have been one of v. W.s' miracles. I am fully aware how absurd this sounds and I must therefore ask myself whether it could not have been a hallucination. But certain circumstances make it extremely difficult for me to think so. I remember clearly that it took place in broad daylight while I was sitting in a chair or on the sofa; in front of me I distinctly saw the polished brown surface of a grand piano in the making (hardly a few paces away). Unfortunately I disregarded the miracle at the time; I wanted nothing whatever to do with any kind of miracle; they all filled me with disgust, particularly as I had made absolute passivity my duty. Later I sometimes regretted that I did not encourage the miracle (" pacify it " was the expression in the basic language) to find out whether it could really be completed. Almost without exception all miracles were and are doomed to failure or rendered much more difficult if I oppose them resolutely with my will. And so I must leave undecided what objective background the reported event had: if it really was a hallucination it must have been of a most extraordinary kind in view of the immediate proximity of the object supposedly seen.

Miracles of heat and cold were and still are daily enacted against me during walks in the garden and when I am indoors, always
with the purpose of preventing the natural feeling of bodily well- p. 172
being which is caused by the soul-voluptuousness; for instance miracles make my feet cold and my face hot. I think the physiological mechanism is that during the cold-miracle the blood is

forced out of the extremities, so causing a subjective feeling of cold, and that conversely during the heat-miracle the blood is forced towards my face and head, in which of course coolness is the condition corresponding to a general sense of well-being. From youth accustomed to enduring both heat and cold, these miracles troubled me little, except when miracles made my feet cold while lying in bed, as happened often. Conversely I myself have often been forced to seek heat and cold. This was particularly necessary during the first years of my stay here, when soul-voluptuousness had not yet reached its present degree, in order to divert the rays towards the chilly parts particularly to the hands and feet, and so protect the head from the injurious influences intended. I frequently clung to the icy trees with my hands for many minutes during the winter or held balls of snow until my hands were almost paralysed. For some time (probably in the spring or autumn of 1895) I put my feet through the iron bars of the open window at night in order to expose them to the cold rain. As long as I did this the rays could not reach my head, which of course was of foremost importance to me, and I felt therefore perfectly well apart from frozen feet.[75] I have reason
p. 173 to assume that this behaviour of mine somehow came to the notice of my physicians and caused them to adopt a measure which provoked my severest displeasure. For a few days I was moved from my usual rooms and on my return I found that heavy wooden shutters had been fixed before my bedroom window, which were locked at night so that my bedroom was in total darkness and even the first light of day in the morning could hardly penetrate. Naturally the physicians probably had no idea of how deeply this measure affected me in my extremely hard struggle in defending myself against the attempts directed at destroying my reason. But it is understandable that it filled me with a deep and long-lasting sense of bitterness. Light, necessary for every human occupation, had become almost more essential for me than my daily bread in my allotted task of at all times convincing God, Who does not know the living human being, of my undiminished powers of reason. Therefore depriving me of artificial light and prolonging the time of natural darkness made my position immeasurably more difficult. I will not dispute with the physicians

[75] For this reason the effect of the one cold shower I was allowed to take in the bathroom was almost miraculous. All at once I felt perfectly well and free from all the threatening manifestations of miracles by which my head and other parts of my body had been visited—although only for a short time.

whether the measure they imposed was necessary from a purely human point of view to protect my health from the consequences of harmful actions. But here too I cannot help remarking that the means did not seem to fit the end. What could possibly have happened to me other than contracting a cold? The iron bars p. 174
gave sufficient protection against the danger of falling out of the window, and as regards the danger of contracting a cold, one might well have waited to see whether human beings' natural need for warmth would not have prevented me from keeping the windows open too long. But these neither were nor are the decisive factors. For me the main point was that I could only see the physicians as tools in whose nerves decisions were aroused by divine rays aimed at furthering the plans directed at destroying my reason; naturally without the physicians themselves becoming subjectively conscious of this but thinking that they were acting simply from human deliberations. I must still maintain this opinion because behind every word which the physicians and other people speak to me I notice the divine influence as revealed to me by the writing-down-material I know so well, which I will perhaps try to explain further later on. In writing these lines I do not mean to recriminate about the past. I harbour no ill-will against any human being for what happened in times gone by; happily it has mostly been overcome. But I thought it necessary to discuss the affair about the window shutters in greater detail to explain the deep mistrust of the physicians which filled me for years, and of which they possibly noticed some signs in my behaviour.

These shutters (the only ones in the whole wing of the Asylum I inhabited) still exist, but have not been closed for a long time. p. 175
Usually such shutters are found only in the cells equipped for raving madmen on the ground floor and first floor of the *round wing* of the Asylum. For two years (1896–1898) I slept in several of these cells as I will relate later, in which time the adverseness of my circumstances was if possible increased by the darkness.

XIII p. 176

The month of November 1895 marks an important time in the history of my life and in particular in my own ideas of the possible shaping of my future. I remember the period distinctly; it coincided with a number of beautiful autumn days when there was a heavy morning mist on the Elbe. During that time the signs of a transformation into a woman became so marked on my body, that I could no longer ignore the imminent goal at which the whole development was aiming. In the immediately preceding nights my male sexual organ might actually have been retracted had I not resolutely set my will against it, still following the stirring of my sense of manly honour; so near completion was the miracle. Soul-voluptuousness had become so strong that I myself received the impression of a female body, first on my arms and hands, later on my legs, bosom, buttocks and other parts of my body. I will discuss details in the next chapter.

Several days' observations of these events sufficed to change the
p. 177 direction of my will completely. Until then I still considered it possible that, should my life not have fallen victim to one of the innumerable menacing miracles before, it would eventually be necessary for me to end it by suicide; apart from suicide the only possibility appeared to be some other horrible end for me, of a kind unknown among human beings. But now I could see beyond doubt that the Order of the World imperiously demanded my unmanning, whether I personally liked it or not, and that therefore it was *common sense* that nothing was left to me but reconcile myself to the thought of being transformed into a woman. Nothing of course could be envisaged as a further consequence of unmanning but fertilization by divine rays for the purpose of creating new human beings. My change of will was facilitated by my not believing at that time that apart from myself a real mankind existed; on the contrary I thought all the human shapes I saw were only "fleeting and improvised", so that there could be no question of any ignominy being attached to unmanning. It is true however that those rays which were intent on "forsaking" me and which for that purpose wanted to destroy my reason, did not fail to make a hypocritical appeal to my sense of manly honour; some of the phrases, since repeated innumerable times whenever soul-voluptuousness appeared, were: "Are you not ashamed in front of your wife?", or still more vulgarly: "Fancy a person who was a *Senatspräsident* allowing himself to be f . . . . d." But however repellent these voices, however often I had occasion to air my just indignation in one way or another during the thousand-fold repetition of these phrases, I did not allow myself to be diverted from that behaviour which I had come to recognize
p. 178 as essential and curative for all parties—myself and the rays.

Since then I have wholeheartedly inscribed the cultivation of femininity on my banner, and I will continue to do so as far as consideration of my environment allows, whatever other people who are ignorant of the supernatural reasons may think of me. I would like to meet the man who, faced with the choice of either becoming a demented human being in male habitus or a spirited woman, would not prefer the latter. Such and *only such* is the issue for me. The pursuit of my previous profession, which I loved wholeheartedly, every other aim of manly ambition, and every other use of my intellectual powers in the service of mankind, are now all closed to me through the way circumstances have developed; even communication with my wife and relatives is denied me apart from occasional visits or exchange of letters.[75B] I must follow a healthy egoism, unperturbed by the judgment of other people, which prescribes for me the cultivation of femininity in a manner to be described more fully later. In this way only am I able to make my physical condition bearable during the day and at night—at least in some measure—and obtain the sleep necessary for the recuperation of my nerves; *high-grade voluptuousness eventually passes into sleep*—maybe this is even known to medical science. Conducting myself in this manner I serve at the same time the express interest of the rays, that is God Himself. If I allow God, Who seems to be led by the erroneous assumption that my reason p. 179
can be destroyed and Who at present pursues aims which are contrary to the Order of the World, to carry on His contrary policy all the time, it only leads to senseless noise in my environment, consisting mostly of madmen, as the experience of years has proved irrefutably. Only later will I be able to say more about this.[76]

At the time when my whole attitude to things changed in the manner just described, an essential change also occurred in celestial conditions—and for the very same reasons. The dissolution in my body of the rays (which are separated from the totality of

75B (Added March 1903.) As will be seen from the content, the present chapter was also written during the time when I was totally isolated behind the walls of Sonnenstein; I would therefore have to change some details although the basic ideas remain correct.

76 I must use particular discretion in contact with my wife, for whom I retain my former love in full. I may at times have failed by being too frank in conversation or in written communications. It is of course impossible for my wife to understand my trends of thought fully; it must be difficult for her to retain her previous love and admiration for me when she hears that I am preoccupied with ideas of possibly being transformed into a woman. I can deplore this, but am unable to change it; even here I must guard against false sentimentality.

God's nerves) due to my power of attraction amounts to the end of their independent existence, like death is to man. It was therefore a matter of course that God should make all attempts to avoid the fate of having to perish in my body with more and more parts of His totality, and indeed one was not very particular in choosing the means of prevention. *But the attraction lost all its terror for these nerves, if and to the extent they met a feeling of soul-voluptuousness in my body* in which they also participated. They
p. 180 then regained in my body a more or less adequate substitute for the lost heavenly Blessedness which itself consisted in enjoyment similar to voluptuousness (compare Chapter I).

The feeling of soul-voluptuousness however, was not always present in my body to the same extent; it reached its full development only when the parts of Flechsig's soul and the other "tested" soul parts lay *in front* and thus all rays were united. However there were also alternate periods in which soul-voluptuousness was either absent or present to a much lesser extent, because the tying-to-celestial-bodies (compare Chapter IX) forced the tested souls to draw back from time to time. This caused a certain periodicity in the appearance of female characteristics on my body of which I will have more to say later. But after the influx of God's rays had been constant for over a year—in November 1895—soul-voluptuousness became so great at times that some rays started to like entering my body. This was noticeable first with the *lower* God (Ariman)—to some extent identical with the sun (see Chapter VII), who being *nearer* partook in soul-voluptuousness much more than the upper God (Ormuzd) who remained at a far greater distance.

Up to the change which took place in November 1895, only the lower God (Ariman) seemed to have a more intimate relationship with Flechsig—perhaps as a human being, perhaps as a "tested soul"—so that this plot, provided it existed as described in Chapter II, did not reach higher than to involve the lower God (Ariman). Up to that time the upper God maintained a more
p. 181 correct, and on the whole more friendly attitude in consonance with the Order of the World towards me. Now this relationship was reversed. The lower God (Ariman) as stated, did not object to losing himself with part of his nerves in my body, because he almost always met soul-voluptuousness there; he severed the close relations which apparently had existed between him and Flechsig's "tested" soul; the latter at that time still possessed of a good deal of its human intelligence, now formed a sort of hostile alliance

against me with the *upper* God. This change in the relation of the parties has persisted mostly unchanged to this day.

The lower God's behaviour towards me has since been generally friendly, that of the upper God much more hostile. This was shown *partly* in the nature of their miracles—in the course of time the miracles of the lower God became more like the relatively harmless tricks mentioned in Chapter II—*partly* in the talk of their respective voices. The voices emanating from the lower God—although also no longer the *genuine* expression of direct momentary feeling, but rather an admixture of phrases learnt by rote—still differ considerably in *form* and *content* from those of the upper God. At least *their content* is not only abusive and full of insulting phrases, but amounts to a kind of neutral nonsense (for instance "David and Solomon", "salad and radishes", "little heaps of flour", etc., are repeated again and again). In their *form* also they are less of a nuisance to me because they fit in better with the natural right of man to think nothing. In time one grows accustomed to letting p. 182
such nonsensical phrases as those mentioned in brackets pass through one's mind as forms of the "not-thinking-of-anything-thought". But the lower God, at least during the first years after the change described in this chapter, had at his disposal also a certain number of phrases which were of actual significance and which showed a quite correct (that is the same as my own) notion of the causes of the conflict, the means of its solution and probable future developments. But as said before, these were not genuine expressions of momentary feeling, but predetermined concoctions of thoughts spoken into my head by senseless voices in tiresome, monotonous repetition (later on mostly by miraculously produced birds). But these phrases were of great interest to me as they permitted me to see that God after all, was not so devoid of all understanding for the necessities arising from the Order of the World as other observations made Him appear. I will therefore record some of these phrases.

In the first place the change in the grouping of the parties which had occurred in consequence of the increase of soul-voluptuousness was signalized by the often-repeated phrase "Two parties have formed". Then there were various ways of expressing the thought that the whole policy God was pursuing against me aimed at destroying my reason had failed. Some phrases were of a general nature without any personal implication, as for instance: "Knowledge and capabilities can in any case never be lost" and "Sleep must come"; further: "All nonsense (that is, the

nonsense of thought reading and falsifying thoughts) cancels
p. 183 itself out", and "Permanent successes are on the side of the human being". Other phrases of the lower God were in part addressed to me personally, in part—spoken through my head as it were—to his colleague, the upper God; the former particularly in the already mentioned phrase: "Don't forget that you are tied to the soul-conception", the latter in phrases such as for instance: "Don't forget that all representing is nonsense", or "Don't forget that the end of the world is a contradiction in itself", or "Well, since you have made the weather dependent on one human being's thoughts", or "Well, you have made any holy occupation impossible (for instance playing the piano or playing chess, through the manifold interfering miracles)". On a very few occasions one even went so far as to make a kind of confession of one's own guilt, for instance: "If only *I* had not put you among the fleeting-improvised-men", or "Well, such are the consequences of the renowned soul-policy", or "What is to become of the whole cursed affair", or "If only the cursed play-with-human-beings would cease". From time to time the confession was *in these words*: "The feeling is lacking", that is the feeling we ought to have for every decent human being, even for the most abominable sinner, considering the means of purification provided in the Order of the World. For a time the aim of the whole development was expressed by the lower God in the phrase—grammatically incomplete as is so often the case in the soul-language: "Hope that voluptuousness reaches a degree", that is to say such a degree that divine rays would lose all *interest* in withdrawing, thus naturally resulting in a solution in consonance with the Order of the World. However, the lower God also had a number of other phrases in readiness which made me shudder, in other words I had to exert all my reason to try to uphold the conviction that
p. 184 he could not possibly succeed. There was talk of "colossal powers" on the part of God's omnipotence and of "hopeless resistance" on my part; it was thought necessary to remind me that the possibility for God to withdraw was boundless with the often-repeated phrase: "Don't forget that eternity is boundless".

Obviously what I have said above about the changed behaviour of the upper and lower God and about the kind of phrases the latter used, contains a tangle of contradictions which cannot be unravelled. Almost insuperable difficulties arise even for me at every attempt to solve these contradictions; a really satisfactory solution would only be possible if one had such complete insight into the nature of God which not even I have attained who have certainly gained deeper insight than all other human beings, because human capacity is limited. I will therefore only venture a few tentative remarks in this connection with all the reservations arising from the insufficiency of the human apparatus for comprehension. Firstly I cannot presume that the upper God's intellectual or moral standard is below that of the lower God. If the latter yet appears to surpass the former in that he recognizes what is possible and respects the Order of the World, I think this can be accounted for by the upper God's *greater distance* from me compared with the lower God's.

The lower and the upper God apparently have in common that they are not able to understand the living human being as an organism *while they are at a distance*; both in particular seem to be caught up in the mistaken notion hardly understandable for a human being, that everything which becomes appreciable to them from the nerves of a human being in my position, mostly only p. 185
in consequence of the falsification of thoughts by the rays, is to be regarded as the manifestation of the human being's own thinking activity; also that cessation of thinking, however temporary, and the resulting state in which definite thoughts formulated in words do not echo from the nerves of a human being in a form appreciable to the rays, implies that this person's mental capacities are extinct, or to use a common though obviously misunderstood[77] human expression, the *advent of dementia*. It appears then that God in both His forms tends to the erroneous idea that the *nerve-language* resulting from the vibrations of the nerves (compare the beginning of Chapter V) is to be regarded as the real language of the human being. Thus, as some excitation of nerves also occurs in a sleeping person when dreaming, one failed to distinguish between the mental activity of a dreaming and that of a fully conscious person using his power of thinking. Naturally I am referring only to *my own* case, that is to say a case in which God entered into continual contact by rays with a single human being, a contact which could no longer be severed and which therefore was contrary to the Order of the World. All these erroneous[78]

[77] Not even in a dement is there complete cessation of mental activity, only a very variable degree of pathological diminution or change of mental activity.

[78] These faulty notions may be accounted for by the fact that while circumstances in consonance with the Order of the World prevail, God deals only with souls which either have already ascended to the forecourts of heaven or are still in the process of purification (compare Chapter I), and besides only occasionally with *sleeping* human beings, who as such (during sleep) naturally also do not make use

ideas which have been mentioned seem only to be given up when God has come closer and then suddenly realizes from my behaviour,
p. 186 my activities and perhaps even from my conversation with other people, etc., that He is still dealing with a human being of completely unimpaired mental powers.

It seems to be impossible for God to draw a lesson for the future from such an experience, perhaps because of some qualities innate in His nature. For these phenomena are repeated in exactly the same way year in year out, day after day, particularly the attempt to withdraw at first sight (in the twinkle of an eye) with every pause in my thinking activity (when the not-thinking-of-anything-thought starts), and the assumption that I have then succumbed to dementia; this is usually expressed in the fatuous phrase "Now he should (*scilicet* think or say) I will resign myself to the fact that I am stupid", followed in senseless monotony like a barrel-organ by all the other tasteless forms of speech "Why do you not say it (aloud)?", or "But then for how much longer" (*scilicet* will your defence against the power of the rays still be successful) etc., etc.; this goes on until I proceed to take up some new occupation which proves my undiminished mental powers. It is an extremely difficult question even for me to explain this inability on the part of God to learn by experience. Perhaps one has to think of it in this way, that the more correct insight is only gained by the most forward nerve endings which are however already condemned to dissolve in my body; those parts at a distance which start the withdrawal action do not partake in this impression or at least not
p. 187 to an extent sufficient for them to change their minds.[79] It therefore seems to me very doubtful whether it makes any practical difference if, as mentioned above, the lower God has included a number of correct ideas in his collection of phrases which he makes the voices which issue from him speak into my head. In any case these thoughts contain nothing new for me, and the upper God receiving only a *formal* acquaintance with them is apparently quite unable to

---

of the loud (human) language. In the relationship of souls among themselves, the *nerve language* arising from the motion or vibration of nerves (therefore only a soft whisper) was in fact the only way of communicating or exchanging ideas.

[79] One might attempt a different explanation in the following manner. One might say—to learn, that is to advance from a lower grade of knowledge to a higher grade, is a human conception only applicable to beings whose knowledge leaves room for improvement. With respect to my own nature, to whose qualities total wisdom belongs as it does to God, the question of learning as such cannot arise. But I must admit that even to me this explanation appears somewhat sophisticated, because total wisdom in absolute completeness does not exist in God and particularly not with respect to His knowledge of living human beings.

assimilate them, that is to change his usual mode of action. As the lower God is informed of the true state of affairs sooner than the upper God, he possibly allowed himself to be led by the idea that rays must speak (compare Chapter IX); this being so, it would be preferable that the content of these spoken words made sense—even if in endless repetition—and not consist of sheer nonsense or frank vulgarities. A long time ago I formulated the idea that God cannot learn by experience, in written notes[80] as follows: "*Every attempt at an educative influence directed outwards must be* p. 188 *given up as hopeless*"; every day which has since passed has confirmed the correctness of this opinion. But here again as on earlier similar occasions I feel I must protect the reader from possible misunderstanding. Religiously minded people who are filled with the concept of God's omnipotence, omniscience and loving kindness must find it incomprehensible that God should here be depicted as so lowly a Being that He can be surpassed both morally and mentally by one single human being. However, I must emphasize that my superiority in both respects is to be understood in *the most relative sense.* I maintain such a superiority *only* as it concerns the condition contrary to the Order of the World originating from permanent and indissoluble nerve-contact with one single human being. In this respect I am both the more reasonable and the better part. Man knows his own nature and in addition I have come to know the soul-character so thoroughly through years of contact with them as no other human being has before. God on the other hand does not know the living human p. 189 being and indeed He had no need to know him, as I have repeatedly stressed before. This is by no means irreconcilable with my acknowledging God's eternal wisdom and goodness in all other respects, particularly in supernatural matters such as the creation and evolution of the world.[81]

[80] These notes are contained in little diaries which I have kept for years; I enter under consecutive numbers and with dates, thoughts about impressions gained, about possible future developments, etc. in the form of little studies. As I consider it probable that my "Memoirs"—the present work—will one day become an important source of information about the structure of an entirely new religious system, the notes in these diaries may form a valuable supplement to my "Memoirs". They will make it possible to recognize how I gradually fought my way to an increasingly correct understanding of supernatural matters. Yet much of it will remain beyond other people's comprehension as I made these notes primarily for the purpose of clarifying these questions for myself, and they lack the detailed explanations which would be necessary for other people.

[81] As tentatively as I expressed myself above about some of God's qualities, as definitely dare I answer other questions though they have always been counted among the thorniest problems since thinking human beings have existed. I refer particularly

I would like to end this chapter by remarking that now at the end of almost five years, things have developed so far that the upper God has taken up the same attitude toward me as the lower God has done since the change of circumstances described in this chapter. The miracles of the upper God are beginning to assume the harmless character which mostly has characterized the miracles of the lower God. As example I will only mention my cigar ash being thrown about on the table or on the piano, my mouth and my hands being soiled with food during meals, etc. It fills me with satisfaction that I predicted this development of things years ago. As proof I will quote the relative entry in my diary (number 17 of 8th March, 1898):

p. 190 "We would like to express the opinion *by way of conjecture*, that *perhaps* even the posterior Ormuzd will lose his interest in disturbing voluptuousness, like the posterior Ariman has lost it in the last two and a half years, so that inner voluptuousness transfigured and ennobled by human imagination would offer greater attraction than outer f.....g when contrary to the Order of the World".

A few explanatory remarks are necessary to understand this quotation. "Posterior" Ariman and "posterior" Ormuzd were the names given (first by the voices and not by me) to the lower God and upper God respectively, when one or the other had got behind by the other pushing into the foreground, which occurred innumerable times daily. "*Inner* voluptuousness" is the soul-voluptuousness which originates in my body. The expression "*outward* f.....g contrary to the Order of the World", refers to my observations that the taking up of putrid matter by pure rays is connected with a kind of voluptuous sensation for them. The choice of the word "f.....g" is not due to my liking for vulgar terms, but having had to listen to the words "f..k" and "f.....g" thousands of times, I have used the term for short in this little note to indicate the behaviour of rays which was contrary to the Order of the World.

---

to the relation of God's omnipotence to human freedom of will, the so-called doctrine of predestination, etc. In consequence of revelations and other impressions I have received, these questions have become almost as clear to me as the sun itself. In view of the deep interest attaching to these questions I will later propound the knowledge I gained, at least in outline.

XIV p. 191

Besides the events described in the previous chapter, certain changes in the heavenly conditions occurred during that time and in the following year or two which, although less important, are touched on here for the sake of completeness. They concern mainly the fate of "tested souls". These as mentioned before had been very numerous for some time in consequence of the partition of souls. A large part of them were occupied almost only in participating in the so-called " circumventory movements ", a manœuvre invented by the main parts of Flechsig's soul; its purpose was to attack the innocently approaching divine rays from behind and so force them to surrender. The picture of this phenomenon is still distinct in my memory; but I must forego describing it in words; nor am I able to say with certainty whether this phenomenon belonged to a time before or after the " tying-to-celestial-bodies ".

So much is certain, that the great number of " tested soul-parts " had eventually become a nuisance to God's omnipotence itself. After I had succeeded in drawing down to myself a considerable part of them, God's omnipotence started a raid among them p. 192
one particular day; the consequence was that from then on Flechsig's soul remained only in one or two shapes and von W.'s soul in one single shape. The latter seems even to have given up the tying voluntarily; from then on it sat for some time—probably a year—mostly in my mouth or eyes, troubling me only little, in fact even providing me with some entertainment, as I could keep up a kind of exchange of ideas with it, in which I however was almost always the giving and von W.'s soul the receiving part. I still remember with some amusement the very funny impression this soul made when finally almost completely without thoughts and limited only to visual impressions, it started to join in searching when I was looking for some object in my environment, that is to say it joined in looking out of my eyes.[82] About the end of 1897 von W.'s soul eventually disappeared altogether unnoticed by me. I had lately become so accustomed to its company that one day, not having thought of it for some time, I suddenly realized that it had vanished; I found myself moved to play the funeral march from Beethoven's "Eroica" on the piano in honour of its departing.

[82] This gave my eyes a peculiar almost glassy expression. The presence of von W.'s soul was felt as a sort of watery mass which covered my eyeballs.

Flechsig's soul is still present as a meagre remnant (tied on to somewhere); but I have good reason to assume that it long ago lost its intelligence, that is to say it is now also totally devoid of thoughts, so that it can hardly even enjoy with satisfaction its own heavenly existence, which it had unlawfully achieved against God's omnipotence—and this once again represents one of the
p. 193 most glowing confirmations of the Order of the World, according to which nothing can maintain itself permanently which contradicts it.

And so the previous " tested souls " vanished from the scene—with one small exception. Thinking of this event I cannot refrain from giving a few details of the very peculiar names which they had up to their disappearance. Even if they are of little interest to readers, it is important for me to remember them and so keep fresh the terrifying and gruesome memories connected with them. The total opposition to God's omnipotence consisting of Flechsig's and v. W.'s soul parts as well as their other party followers (advance guards, etc.) called themselves for some time the " so-what-party ". This hackneyed phrase originated from Flechsig's soul which had the habit of answering all questions about what was to become of this whole " cursed affair " (that the whole affair had gone utterly astray seems to have been known to God's omnipotence) with a mocking and indifferent " so what ". This answer again is most characteristic of the soul-character; souls after all know of no care for the future, but let momentary enjoyment suffice. Translated into the human sphere the " so what " of Flechsig's soul would mean " I do not care a damn for the future, as long as I feel well at the moment ". Therefore when only two parts of Flechsig's soul remained, the more distant one was called " the posterior Flechsig ", and the one that was a little nearer, by the way the one that had always been of weaker intelligence, was called the middle " so-what-party ".

p. 194 Of von W.'s soul parts the " abdominal putrification of von W." has been mentioned earlier; this probably had the most impure nerves and therefore exhibited the most abominable intent towards me, and towards God's omnipotence unabashed impudence. This found expression in certain classical phrases which did not fit in with the movement of my own nerves, nor with the accustomed rhythm of the rays, such as " in a way this is unbearable ", " permit me ", etc. (the latter expression was used when it was to be dislodged from its position). It hung on the opposite wall of my bedroom when I was lying in bed. It was almost equalled in impudence of intent by the so-called " mid-day "—von W.; it had this name because it was said to have charge of meals, particularly mid-day meals. A more decent, almost reasonable, if changeable character, was shown by two other of von W.'s soul's shapes, the " anyhow " von W. and the " O damn " von W., both names used by themselves. The phrase " O damn " in particular was a remnant of the basic language, in which the words " O damn, that is hard to say " were used whenever the souls became aware of a happening inconsistent with the Order of the World, for instance " O damn, it is extremely hard to say that God allows himself to be f..... ".

Particularly dangerous for a time was a really very small part of von W.'s soul which was called " the scourge of von W." because of a miracle practised exclusively by him. He used to move a little scourge about in my skull, and with it caused serious destruction and often fairly severe pain.

During the time of my stay in Dr. Pierson's Asylum (" the Devil's Kitchen ") there was also a shape of von W.'s soul for the formation of which some of my own nerves must have been used, because it was called " the little von W.-Schreber ". This was p. 195
the best intentioned of all; " he " sometimes even achieved (in his miracles) the so-called " golden drop ", a miracle usually practised only by God's omnipotence in which some fluid like balsam was placed on damaged parts of my head and elsewhere—I could feel it distinctly—so that all at once an immediate curative effect was achieved.

My outward life was no longer quite as monotonous during the time after the change described in Chapter XIII as it had been earlier in the period of my immobility; yet there was little variety, as may be expected from living in an Asylum. I still spent the best part of my time playing the piano and chess; the number of printed scores at my disposal had grown considerably through presents from my relatives.

I started to make written notes as I had been provided with some coloured pencils and later with other writing material; my circumstances were so pitiful that even a pencil or a rubber was guarded by me like a real treasure. My note-taking consisted at first only of a few unconnected thoughts or words which I put down; later—beginning with the year 1897—I started to keep regular diaries, in which I entered all my experiences; earlier—but still in 1896—I was limited to meagre entries in a small calendar. But I also started to sketch my future " Memoirs ", which I had already

planned. This sketch is contained in a little brown book, entitled "From my Life"; it has served me as a welcome support of my memory while elaborating the present "Memoirs". Anybody
p. 196 interested in this sketch—which was kept in shorthand—would find there many more items which I have not incorporated into my "Memoirs"; they show the reader that the content of my revelations was immeasurably richer than what I could incorporate in the limited space of the "Memoirs". Finally—since the late autumn of 1897—I have written down certain observations mentioned in footnote 80 and the Little Studies in small note-books *B*, *C* and *I*.

From the start I have had (and I sometimes still have) great difficulties with meals which until Easter of this year (1900) I took by myself in my room. Nobody can imagine how great the difficulties were with which I had to fight; while I was eating, miracles were continually produced inside my mouth; and even the nonsensical questions continued: "Why don't you say it (aloud)?", etc., although speaking aloud is impossible when one has one's mouth full of food. My teeth were constantly in danger; indeed several times during meals some of my teeth were broken by miracle. Frequently during meals a miracle was effected of biting my tongue. The hairs of my moustache were almost regularly miracled into my mouth with the food so that this alone, had no other reason existed, would have made me shave it off in August 1896. To shave my moustache off had become a necessity for me for other reasons, however little I liked myself—in day-time—with a clean-shaven face. Considering the conditions discussed in Chapter XIII it became necessary for me, at least at night-time, to support my imagination of being a female, and a moustache would naturally have been an insurmountable obstacle for this illusion. While I ate alone I had almost regularly to play the piano or to read during meal times, because it was imperative even during meals to furnish the distant God[83] with proof
p. 197 that my mental powers were intact; had I not wanted to do this I would have had to eat my meals standing up or walking about.

[83] After what has been said repeatedly before, for instance in footnote 19, about the *hierarchy* of the realms of God, the reader may have gained some idea of what I wish to express with the term "the *distant* God". One must not think of God as a being limited in space by the confines of a body like a human being, but one has to think of Him as *Many in One or One in Many*. These are not unfounded figments of my brain, but I have definite factual evidence for all these assumptions (that is to say for the expression "a distant God"), for instance at the time when the genuine basic language was current, every anterior leader of rays used to speak of the divine rays or of the representatives of the Divinity in his train as "I Who am distant".

As mentioned earlier—and anticipating a little in time—I passed the nights during the two and a half years from May 1896 to December 1898 not in the room allotted to me, that is in the bedroom adjoining my living room, but in the padded cells for dements on the ground floor and on the first floor of the round wing of the Asylum. The reason for this regulation I cannot understand even today. It is true during the first years of my stay in this Asylum scenes of violence occurred between me and other patients, several times also with the attendants. I have noted all these instances down; all in all there were about ten to twelve such occurrences, the last of which took place on the 5th of March 1898; by the way, in all instances concerning other *patients* I was always the attacked party.

The *deeper* reasons which led to these scenes of violence I will p. 198
discuss later. At any rate I cannot believe that the doctors could have regarded me as a person in general given to maniacal outbursts because of these rare events, as they also had the opportunity of observing that during *day-time* I occupied myself decently, quietly and in accordance with my intellectual standing by playing the piano, playing chess, and later reading books and newspapers. It is possible that every now and then I spoke out aloud at night—which I was forced to do for reasons mentioned in footnote 63; it is therefore possible that other patients sleeping on the same corridor or above me could occasionally have had grounds for complaint. But here too it was not a question of disturbances of the peace which occurred every night, not even most nights, and in any case quite often I have to suffer similarly through other patients, although my bedroom is fairly separate from the other bedrooms.

I must therefore regard it as an extremely strange regulation that I was made to sleep in cells furnished for maniacal patients for *fully two and a half years* with the exception of only a few nights; there was nothing in these cells apart from an iron bedstead, a bedpan and some bedding, and over and above this most of the time they were completely blacked out by heavy wooden shutters. I repeat that I do not wish to raise any complaints about the past; however, I cannot but assume that some degree of *vis inertiae* allowed a state of affairs to persist although it had become unbearable and despite the fact that the reasons which led to such a measure no longer p. 199
actually existed.

I think I can fairly maintain that *nothing similar happened to any other patient in the Asylum;* cases of periodic mania are locked up in cells but are, as far as I know, kept there only for a few weeks.

Therefore, however little I intend lending the subsequent description any personal acrimony, nevertheless an account of how unbearably I suffered during this stay in the cells belongs to the complete picture of the story of my sufferings. My sleep is, as shown before, exclusively dependent on the heavenly constellations; sleep becomes impossible for me as soon as God has withdrawn to too great a distance, which periodically happens for half a day or at least several hours. If I then have to remain awake, the senseless twaddle of voices in my head causes an absolutely unbearable mental martyrdom; added to this are, for over twelve months, more or less severe states of bellowing to be described later, which occur whenever I cannot convince the distant God, who believes I have become demented, that this is not so.

But how was I to do this in sleepless nights in the cell in which I lacked light as well as any objects which could be used for some occupation? It was impossible to remain in bed, and groping around in the darkened cell clad only in a shirt, with bare feet—as even my slippers were taken away—was naturally extremely boring, and in winter-time very cold and further not without danger because miracles directed my head against the low beams
p. 200 of the cell. Necessity is the mother of invention, and so in the course of those years I had recourse to all kinds of measures in order to spend the time in a somewhat bearable way. Sometimes almost for hours on end I tied knots in the four corners of my handkerchief and untied them again, partly in bed and partly while walking around recalled aloud some memories from my life, counted aloud, particularly in French—because questions were also constantly directed at whether I could still speak "foreign languages"; produced parts of my historical and geographical knowledge, for instance repeated all the Russian Governments and French Departments, etc., etc. Naturally I did not like to speak aloud as this meant giving up my sleep, but frequently I could do nothing else. Very painful was the lack of a clock and of matches, because when I woke up at night after some sleep I could not tell the time and did not know what best to do for the rest of the night.

When towards the end of my time in the cells the shutters were no longer closed, I occupied myself with observing the starry sky[84],

[84] This always in the peculiar knowledge not shared by any other human being that it was this starry sky itself from which the miracles emanated which damaged me so multifariously.

and by means of a map of the stars which I had studied during the day I managed to tell the time at night with a fair degree of accuracy, just like the people of old. As long as the shutters were closed I often thundered against them with my fists until my hands were raw; once I succeeded in knocking a shutter down by force which had already been loosened by miracle, with the result that the cross-bar was by miracle made to descend on my head with such force that my head and my chest were covered with blood. p. 201
Conditions have latterly improved a little by my taking a small metal container into the cell with me in which I keep little belongings, a pencil, paper, a so-called *pocket-chess-board* [in English in the original] etc., with which at least during the summer it was possible to occupy myself from daybreak on. I have already said that I suffered these conditions for *two and a half years;* in the last resort only because human beings did not appreciate supernatural matters.

XV p. 202

Some time after the change recounted in Chapter XIII, perhaps at the end of 1895 or the beginning of 1896, I had a number of experiences which led me to a critical examination of my ideas about the "fleeting-improvised-men", "play-with-human-beings", and suchlike, in consequence of which I arrived at a slightly different point of view.

In particular I remember three events which made me hesitate whether what until then I had considered true and correct was really so: firstly taking part in the Christmas festivities of the family of the Director of the Asylum Dr. Weber in the year 1895; secondly receiving a letter from my sister-in-law in Cologne on the Rhine addressed to me and bearing the postmark of Cologne; thirdly a children's procession celebrating the twenty-fifth anniversary of the Peace of Frankfurt—10th of May 1896—which I saw from my window passing along a street of a suburb of Pirna which runs below it. After these and similar events
—soon regular correspondence was added and reading newspapers p. 203
which were subscribed for by my relatives—I could no longer doubt that a real race of human beings in the same number and distribution as before did in fact exist. But this caused

difficulties; how was I to combine this fact with my earlier impressions apparently pointing to the contrary. This difficulty remains even today, and I must confess that I am faced with an unsolved riddle, one which is probably insoluble for human beings.

I have no doubt whatever that my early ideas were not simply " delusions " and " hallucinations " because even now I still receive impressions daily and hourly which make it perfectly clear to me that, in Hamlet's words, *there is something rotten in the state of Denmark*—that is to say in the relationship between God and mankind. But how the present state of things developed historically, whether by sudden changes or gradual transition, and to what extent apart from the manifestations of life caused by the influence of rays (miracles), manifestations of life occur independently and uninfluenced by the rays, remains even for me an obscure point[84B]. I am quite sure that expressions and phrases like " fleeting-improvised-men " and " cursed-play-with-human-beings ", the questions: " What is going to happen to this cursed affair? ", etc., as well as the talk about " new human beings from Schreber's spirit " did not originate in my head, but were spoken into it from outside. This alone would make me assume that the ideas connected with them have some basis in reality corresponding to some historical events. Moreover in the course of the last six years I have unintermittently received impressions—and still receive
p. 204 them daily and hourly—which furnish me with incontestable proof that everything spoken and done by human beings near me is due to the effect of miracles and directly connected with the rays coming nearer and alternately striving to withdraw again.

I have already mentioned in Chapter VII that every word spoken near me or with me, every human action however small which is combined with some noise, for instance opening the door-locks on my corridor, pressing the latch on the door of my room, the entry of an attendant into my room, etc., is accompanied by a sensation of a painful blow directed at my head; the sensation of pain is like a sudden pulling inside my head which calls forth a very unpleasant feeling as soon as God has withdrawn to an excessive distance, and may be combined with the tearing off of part of the bony substance of my skull—at least that is how it feels. As long as I talk aloud—in my room or in the garden—turned towards God, everything around me is deathly quiet and God has no wish to withdraw, as He receives the direct impression

[84B] Compare the Preface.

of the activity of a human being in complete possession of his senses. This creates a feeling in me at times as if I were moving among walking corpses, so completely[85] seem the people (attendants and patients) suddenly to have lost the capacity to say one single word. The same happens as long as my gaze rests on a female being. p. 205
But as soon as I turn my gaze or allow my eyes to be closed by miracles, or as soon as I change from talking aloud to silence without at the same time starting some mental occupation, in other words when I give myself up to thinking nothing, the following phenomena which are interrelated occur almost at once (at first sight):

(1) Noises around me, mostly consisting in violent outbursts among the lunatics who of course form the majority of those around me;

(2) In my own person the advent of the bellowing-miracle when my muscles serving the processes of respiration are set in motion by the lower God (Ariman) in such a way that I am forced to emit bellowing noises, unless I try very hard to suppress them; sometimes this bellowing recurs so frequently and so quickly that it becomes almost unbearable and at night makes it impossible to remain in bed;

(3) The winds arise, however not uninfluenced by the existing state of the weather; but short blasts of wind coinciding with pauses in my thinking are quite unmistakable;

(4) The cries of " help " of those of God's nerves separated from p. 206
the total mass, sound the more woeful the further away God has withdrawn from me, and the greater therefore the distance which those nerves have to travel, obviously in a state of some anxiety.

All these phenomena happen hundreds of times every day; I must have observed them in the course of years tens of thousands if not hundreds of thousands of times with exactly the same

[85] Conditions during meal times, which since Easter of this year (1900) I have taken at the family table of the Director of the Asylum Dr. Weber, are somewhat different; particularly for the reason that a continuous conversation is kept up, interrupted only by short pauses. The manifestations described in the text do not always appear in the same way, in fact they have undergone certain changes in the course of time, particularly in connection with the increased soul-voluptuousness. Some of the manifestations vanish temporarily to make room for others which in earlier years were either not observed at all or only rarely. This refers particularly to the so-called " bellowing ", which I will discuss in more detail later. But the basic reason remains the same, namely God's apparently irresistible temptation to withdraw as soon as soul-voluptuousness is not met in my body, or my speech and my occupation do not provide direct proof of the presence of a human being in complete possession of his mental powers.

regularity. I have repeatedly pointed to the reason. Every time my thinking activity ceases God instantly regards my mental powers as extinct, the desired destruction of my reason[86] (the " dementia ") achieved and the possibility of a withdrawal thus brought about.

And so the withdrawal action is started, and to achieve it an "interference" produced by miracle in the sense given in Chapter X, page 143. This is the noise mentioned in (1) above. Simultaneously and almost immediately the so-called bellowing miracle is produced by the lower God ((2) above). It seems to serve a double purpose, namely to create by " representing " the impression of a person bellowing because he is demented; and also to drown by bellowing the inner voices which the upper God started so that he could withdraw to a greater distance; in this way the lower God, who seems somehow aware of the necessity of allowing himself to be attracted, could count on a union of all rays and on soul-
p. 207 voluptuousness which it causes in my body; in other words he could safeguard himself from entering my body *without soul-voluptuousness.* Withdrawal to a greater distance at once causes (see (3)) the wind to arise (compare Chapter I). Nevertheless the upper God soon becomes aware that the hoped for cessation of the power of attraction of my nerves has once again not been achieved but rather persists undiminished; this causes a state of anxiety in those of God's nerves which first became separated (see (4)) and is expressed with genuine feeling in cries of " help ". It remains a riddle to me that the cries of help are apparently not heard by other human beings[87]: the sound which reaches my own ear—hundreds of times every day—is so definite that it cannot be a hallucination. The genuine " cries of help " are always instantly followed by the phrase which has been learnt by rote: " If only the cursed cries of help would stop ".

That all signs of life of human beings around me, particularly their speech, are caused by miracles (influence of rays), is clearly shown also in the *content* of what is said. I must expand this in order to make it clear. As already remarked on page 130, Chapter IX, when God started the tying-to-celestial bodies (page 125) He spared not only the tested souls which were still about, but also what was left of the erstwhile " forecourts of heaven "—that is to

[86] That this was the aim was previously often acknowledged quite openly in the phrase which I heard emanating from the upper God " We want to destroy your reason ". Of late this phrase has been used less often, because when it is repeated time and again it also amounts to a kind of the not-thinking-of-anything-thought.

[87] Compare the remarks at the end of IV of the Postscripts, First Series.

say the blessed souls of human beings; the purpose was to load them with poison of corpses when the power of attraction of my nerves caused them to come nearer, and send them out in advance as outposts and so slow down the attraction of the genuine rays of God. One probably also believed that at least one could choke me through the mass of poison of corpses which in this manner was daily heaped upon my body, that is to say be able to kill me or p. 208
destroy my reason. These nerves (the remnants of the forecourts of heaven) have appeared for years in the shape of *birds created by miracle*, thereby manifesting a mysterious connection with the innermost nature of divine creation; in so far they are unfathomable even to me. But the fact itself *that the nerves which are inside these birds are remnants* (single nerves) *of souls of human beings who had become blessed* is absolutely certain because of my observations repeated thousands of times every day for years.

I recognize the individual nerves exactly by the tone of their voices from years of hearing them; I know exactly which of the senseless phrases learnt by rote I can expect of each one of them, according to whether they are emitted from the camp of the lower God or from that of the upper God (produced by miracle by the latter or the former). Their property as erstwhile human nerves is evidenced by the fact that *all* the miraculously produced birds *without exception*, whenever they have completely unloaded the poison of corpses which they carry, that is to say when they have reeled off the phrases drummed into them, then express *in human sounds* the *genuine* feeling of well-being in the soul-voluptuousness of my body which they share, with the words " Damned fellow "[88] or " Somehow damned ", *the only words in which they are still capable of giving expression to genuine feeling*. They have not the least understanding of what they have spoken before, i.e. for the p. 209
phrases learnt by rote—to retain this expression which naturally is only to be understood figuratively; they reel them off without knowing the sense of the words; it seems that otherwise their intelligence is no higher than that of natural birds.

I cannot say how their nerves are made to vibrate in such a manner that sounds spoken or more correctly lisped by them sound like human words, of which the phrases learnt by rote are composed: I therefore cannot explain the technicalities of the matter, but I presume that it is a question of supernatural matters which

[88] The words " damned fellow " are here not used in any derogatory sense, in fact just the reverse, as was the rule in the basic language, namely in that of joyous tribute or admiration.

therefore are completely incomprehensible to human beings.[89] But their *effect* is well known to me from years of experience; it consists in the nerves of the miraculously created birds being made *immune* against all sensation which they would otherwise have when entering my body, particularly against soul-voluptuousness or visual impressions, as long as they are occupied with reeling off the phrases drummed into them (learnt by rote), just as if they entered into me blindfolded or with their natural capacity for feeling somehow suspended. This after all is the purpose of the whole business and also the reason for the tempo of these automatic phrases being more and more slowed down in the course of years
p. 210 —in proportion to the increase of soul-voluptuousness: the destructive power of the poison of corpses carried by the entering voices was to be maintained as long as possible. With it, however, a most peculiar phenomenon arose which is of the greatest importance for the extent of the damage the voices or rays concerned cause in my body.

It has already been mentioned that the miraculously created birds do not understand the *meaning* of the words they speak; but apparently they have a natural sensitivity for *similarity of sounds*. Therefore if, while reeling off the automatic phrases, they perceive *either* in the vibrations of my own nerves (my thoughts) *or* in speech of people around me, words which *sound* the same or similar to their own phrases, they apparently experience surprise and in a way fall for the similarity in sound; in other words the surprise makes them forget the rest of their mechanical phrases and they suddenly pass over into *genuine* feeling.

It has already been said that the sounds need not be completely identical; a similarity suffices, as in any case the birds do not understand the *sense* of the words; therefore it matters little to them—in order to give some examples—whether one speaks of

"Santiago" or "Carthago"
"Chinesenthum" or "Jesum Christum"
"Abendroth" or "Athemnoth"
"Ariman" or "Ackermann"

[89] (Written some days later than the above text.) Perhaps it is a similar process to the one (see page 155/156 of Chapter XI) attempted with my own nerves, of which I became aware in the form of transitory dementing or diminution of my powers of thinking. One could imagine that the covering of the nerves of birds with the poison of corpses robs them of their natural capacity to vibrate, that is to say of their natural feeling, and in a way tends to stretch them; the result is that they are only able to perform the long-drawn-out vibrations corresponding to human words which have lately been spoken extremely slowly.

"Briefbeschwerer" or "Herr Prüfer schwört".
etc., etc.[90]

To confuse these talking birds by deliberately throwing in p. 211
similar sounding words became a kind of pastime in the voices' almost unbearably tedious twaddle which afforded me a somewhat queer amusement. However droll this may sound the matter also has its serious side. The upper and lower God who also know that the miraculously created birds fall for similar sounds, use this peculiarity as a trump card against each other. Each wants to hold back and push the other forward; whenever the birds fall for similarity of sound, the attraction of that part is increased from whose camp the voices emanate. Thus the upper God likes to make persons around me say those words which belong to the writing-down-material and to the voices of the lower God and vice versa, while I for my part, aiming at a union of all rays and so at a uniform attraction, always have to counteract these efforts. Here too I could furnish as many examples as there are grains of sand in the sea.

To mention only a few: "electric light" and "railways", as well as—in the connection mentioned on page 184 Chapter XIII—the "colossal powers" and the "hopeless resistance" belong to the writing-down material of the *lower* God. The *upper* God therefore causes a conversation carried on in my presence—also during meals at the Director's table—to turn to "electric railways", everything is found "colossal" and at every opportune or inopportune moment p. 212
one speaks of "hopes" so frequently that it is astounding and excludes all possibility of coincidence. This alone—apart from much else—constitutes absolute proof for me that *the nerves of the human beings who use these words are made to do so through the influence of rays (miracles)*—naturally without their knowing it; in other words it is proof of the reality of the so-called "*play-with-human-beings*" about which the lower God used to speak innumerable times in earlier years. Here too I am conscious of how incredible all this must seem to other human beings; but what I said above is strengthened by hourly and daily experiences, in every place and at every opportunity so overwhelmingly, that it precludes any doubt for me in the objectivity of these circumstances. I may perhaps later go into further details.

90 These examples are taken from the actual writing-down or speech-material; 'Herr Prüfer,' the name of a patient in this Asylum, I used to hear often. I could multiply the examples a hundred or thousandfold but will let the above suffice.

I want to add something about the birds created by miracle; it is queer that the individual nerves or souls which are in them appear in the shape of different *kinds of birds* according to the season of the year. The same nerves are in the spring contained in the bodies of finches or other singing birds, in the summer in those of swallows, and in winter in those of sparrows or crows. I have no doubt about the identity of the souls concerned because I know the tone of their voices well, and I recognize the phrases I regularly hear from them and which have, so to speak, been crammed into them.[92]

p. 213 This naturally leads to the question whether they *can* possibly *have a continual life* or whether they have to be created anew by miracles every day or anyway at longer intervals of time. I can only raise but not answer this question. I observe that the miraculously created birds feed and empty themselves in the manner of natural birds; it would therefore be possible that the miraculously created state is maintained for a time by taking in nourishment; I have also repeatedly observed them building nests in the spring which appears to point to some powers of reproduction. Their language on the other hand makes it certain for me that in other respects they are not completely natural birds. They are very numerous, apparently appear in hundreds, so that I dare not give any definite estimate of their number. From their spoken phrases they can easily be distinguished into two groups, one emanating from the upper and the other from the lower God.

Of the lower God's group one soul in bird's form is usually around me; for years therefore the voices have called it "my little friend". In the spring it usually appears as a woodpecker or blackbird, in the summer as a swallow and in the winter as a sparrow. The joking title "*picus*, the woodpecker", is used by
p. 214 the other voices even when it appears as a blackbird, swallow or sparrow. I know exactly the numerous phrases given it to repeat constantly in the course of the years, and I have often made lists of them as also of those of the other miraculously created birds; they always proved correct. To a large number of the other

[92] The expression "crammed in" which occurred to me only during writing, seems to express the relation even better than the previously used expressions "learnt by rote" and "drummed in". The latter expressions could make one think that the miraculously created birds were aware of the *sense* of the words; but that is not so. Their speech *in respect of the crammed in phrases* is not even as advanced as a parrot's. The parrot repeats words learnt on his own impulse, in other words of his own free will. On the other hand the miraculously created birds *must* reel off the crammed in phrases without any regard to time or circumstance and irrespective of whether they want to or not.

bird-souls I jokingly gave girls' names in order to distinguish them, because all of them can best be compared to little girls in their curiosity, their inclination to voluptuousness, etc. These girls' names were then taken up by God's rays and used for the respective bird-souls concerned. To the miraculously created birds belong all fairly *fast flying* birds, particularly all singing birds, swallows, sparrows, crows, etc.; *of these species of birds I have never once during these years seen a single specimen which did not speak.* On both the occasions when I drove in a carriage this summer (1900)[93] they accompanied me the whole way. On the other hand the pigeons in the court of this Asylum do *not* speak, neither as far as I have observed a canary kept in the servants' quarters, nor the chicken, geese and ducks which I have seen both from my window on the plots of land lying below the Asylum, and on the two mentioned excursions in villages through which I passed; I must therefore presume that these were simply natural birds. The whole phenomenon of the talking birds is so marvellous and like a fairy tale that I would be most interested to observe bird life in other parts of the country; I cannot presume that leafy p. 215
woods further away totally lack a bird population.[93B]

XVI p. 216

In the previous chapters I described the changes in my outward life during the past years and the forms the battle of annihilation assumed which divine rays led against me. I will now add some more about the forms—also vastly changed—of the constant *compulsive thinking*. Compulsive thinking has been defined in Chapter V as having to think continually; this contravenes man's

[93] Up till then, that is to say for almost six years, I had never left the walls of the Asylum.

[93B] (Added March 1903.) The talking of all *free flying birds has persisted without interruption* in the past years in which I frequently changed my residence, and it persists to this day. Besides I would now prefer the expression "talking birds" to "birds created by miracle" which is used in the text. Earlier on I thought I could not explain the talking of the birds other than by assuming that they were *as such* created by miracle, that is to say were created anew each time. After what I have observed meantime I consider it more likely that they were birds produced by natural reproduction, into whose bodies the remnants of the "forecourts of heaven", that is to say erstwhile blessed human souls, had been inserted in some supernatural way or were inserted anew each time. But that these souls (nerves) are actually inside the bodies of these birds (perhaps *in addition* to the nerves which these birds naturally possess and in any case without awareness of their previous identity) remains as before without any doubt for me for reasons developed in the text.

natural right of mental relaxation, of temporary rest from mental activity through thinking nothing, or as the expression goes in the basic language, it disturbs the " basis " of a human being. My nerves are influenced by the rays to vibrate corresponding to certain human words; their choice therefore is not subject to my own will, but is due to an influence exerted on me from without. From the beginning the *system of not-finishing-a-sentence* prevailed, that is to say the vibrations caused in my nerves and the words so produced contain not mainly finished thoughts, but unfinished ideas, or only fragments of ideas, which my nerves have to
p. 217 supplement to make up the sense. It is in the nature of nerves that if unconnected words or started phrases are thrown into them, they automatically attempt to complete them to finished thoughts satisfactory to the human mind.

The system of not-finishing-a-sentence became more and more prevalent in the course of years, the more the souls lacked own thoughts. In particular, for years single conjunctions or adverbs have been spoken into my nerves thousands of times; these ought only to introduce clauses, but it is left to my nerves to complete them in a manner satisfactory to a thinking mind. Thus for years I have heard daily in hundredfold repetition incoherent words spoken into my nerves without any context, such as " Why not? ", " Why, if ", " Why, because I ", " Be it ", " With respect to him " (that is to say that something or other has to be thought or said with respect to myself); further an absolutely senseless " Oh " thrown into my nerves; finally certain fragments of sentences which were earlier on expressed completely; as for instance

1. " Now I shall ",
2. " You were to ",
3. " I shall ",
4. " It will be ",
5. " This of course was ",
6. " Lacking now is ",

etc. In order to give the reader some idea of the original meaning of these incomplete phrases I will add the way they used to be completed, but are now omitted and left to be completed by my nerves. The phrases ought to have been:

p. 218 1. Now I shall resign myself to being stupid;

2. You were to be represented as denying God, as given to voluptuous excesses, etc.;

3. I shall have to think about that first;

4. It will be done now, the joint of pork;

5. This of course was too much from the soul's point of view;

6. Lacking now is only the leading idea, that is—we, the rays, have no thoughts.

The rather tasteless phrase about the joint of pork (number 4) is due to myself having used years ago the figure of speech "done like a joint of pork" in the nerve-language. This phrase was seized on and became a constantly recurring part of the speech-material. The "joint of pork" I was to refer to myself: it was meant to express that I was done, i.e. that my power of resistance against the attacks on my reason by the rays must by now be exhausted.

The purpose of not-finishing-a-sentence is consistent with God's attitude to me throughout: to prevent dissolution in my body which would necessarily result from its attraction. While conditions prevailed which were at least somehow in consonance with the Order of the World, that is before tying-to-rays and tying-to-celestial-bodies was started (compare Chapter IX), a momentary uniform *feeling* was enough to make the freely suspended souls jump down from the sky into my mouth, thus ending their independent existence; an event, as mentioned in Chapter VII, page 83, I actually experienced repeatedly. But mere "intellectual deliberation" had the same effect; whenever expressed in a p. 219
grammatically complete sentence, the rays would be led straight to me, and entering my body (though capable of withdrawing) temporarily increase its soul-voluptuousness. Not-finishing-a-sentence has apparently the effect that the rays are, as it were, held up half way, and could therefore withdraw before having added to soul-voluptuousness in my body; but even this does not permanently prevent the attraction completely; it only slows it down.

It is hard to give a picture of the mental strain the compulsive thinking imposed on me particularly after it had become so much worse, and what mental torture I had to suffer. During the first years my nerves indeed seemed irresistibly compelled to continue[95] each started clause to the satisfaction of the human mind, much as in ordinary human intercourse an answer is regularly given to somebody's question.

I will give an example to illustrate how such a need is inherent

[95] To do this immediately at first sight (in the twinkle of an eye), as the stimulation of nerves demanded, was called "the capacity to answer at first sight".

in the nature of human nerves. Consider the case of parents or
teachers being present during a school examination of their
p. 220 children. If they follow the examination attentively they will
automatically answer every question in their mind, perhaps only
in the form: " I am not at all sure whether the children will know
this ". Of course there is no mental compulsion for parents or
teachers, they have only to divert their attention from the pro-
ceeding examination towards something else in their environment
to spare their nerves this strain. This is the essential difference
between this example and my case. The questions or querying
particles spoken into my nerves compel my mind to work by
setting the corresponding nerves in vibration, in a way that they
cannot possibly escape the impulse to think. I must leave undecided
whether the expression I chose of my nerves being set in corresponding vibrations by the rays, covers the circumstances correctly;
what I directly feel is that the talking voices (lately in particular the
voices of the talking birds) as *inner voices* move like long threads
into my head and there cause a painful feeling of tension through
the poison of corpses which they deposit.

In contradistinction to these inner voices I hear outer voices
particularly spoken by birds, which come to me from outside,
from the birds' throats. However, in both cases my nerves cannot
avoid the sound of the spoken words; the stimulation of my nerves
follows automatically and compels me to think on when I hear
questions or incomplete thoughts. In earlier years my nerves
simply had to think on, to answer questions, to complete broken-
off sentences etc. Only later was I gradually able to accustom
p. 221 my nerves (my " basis ") to ignoring the stimulation which forced
them to think on, by simply repeating the words and phrases and
thus turning them into not-thinking-of-anything-thoughts. I have
done that for a long time now with conjunctions and adverbs which
would need a full clause for their completion. If I hear for instance
" Why, because I ", or " Be it ", I repeat these words for as long
as possible without attempting to complete the sense by trying to
connect them with what I thought before.

I proceed in the same manner when attempts are made with the
words " If only my " to compel my nerves to develop ideas of
fear, not really present in my mind but falsely imputed to me.
I know what can be " expected " to follow—because as a rule the
corresponding miracle happens simultaneously and I feel it on
my body; the intended continuation is sometimes " If only my
voluptuousness were not disturbed ", sometimes " If only my

boots were not removed by miracle", sometimes "If only my nose, my eyes, my knee-cap, my skull, etc., would not be affected by miracles".

Since my nerves have become accustomed to suppress the corresponding stimulation, I no longer elaborate in words the nonsense to which these falsified ideas lead; I am satisfied to keep on repeating the same words "If only my" without adding anything to them. In ordinary conversation of course everybody would simply counter "If only my" with "What do you really mean", or perhaps would use abusive language in self-defence. This is very difficult for me because the rays regularly answer p. 222
"We have had this before" (with the effect mentioned in Chapter IX). It would in any case be unendurable in the long run to submit nerves all day long to the counter question "What do you really mean", or to abusive language.[96]

The infringement of the freedom of human thinking or more correctly thinking nothing, which constitutes the essence of compulsive thinking, became more unbearable in the course of years with p. 223
the slowing down of the talk of the voices. This is connected with the increased soul-voluptuousness of my body and—despite all writing-down—with the great shortage of speech-material at the disposal of the rays with which to bridge the vast distances separating the stars, where they are suspended, from my body.

No one who has not personally experienced these phenomena like I have can have any idea of the extent to which speech has slowed down. To say "But naturally" is spoken B.b.b.u.u.u.t.t.t. n.n.n.a.a.a.t.t.t.u.u.u.r.r.r.a.a.a.l.l.l.y.y.y, or "Why do you not

[96] One can only get an idea of the *enormous infringement of man's most primitive rights* which compulsive thinking constitutes and of how my patience was tested beyond all human conception, when one pictures a human being behaving to another human being in human language in the way that rays behave to me to this day in the nerve-language. Imagine a human being planting himself before another and molesting him all day long with unconnected phrases such as the rays use towards me ("If only my", "This then was only", "You are to", etc.). Can one expect anything else of a person spoken to in this manner but that he would throw the other out of the house with a few fitting words of abuse? I also ought to have the right of being master in my own head against the intrusion of strangers. But this is not possible as regards the rays, because I am not in a position to prevent their influence on my nerves; this rests on God's power of miracles. The human language (spoken aloud) which is the *ultima ratio* for preserving the sanctity of my house cannot always be used, partly out of consideration for my environment, partly because continuous talking aloud would make every sensible occupation impossible; finally because at night it would prevent sleep. Hence one tries to provoke me to talk aloud with the question: "Why do you not say it (aloud)?" or by means of insulting phrases (compare Chapter IX). Of late, having become increasingly clear about these things, I have in fact not refrained from making use of speaking aloud whenever the opportunity arose both in conversation and when I am alone.

then shit?" W.w.w.h.h.h.y.y.y d.d.d.o.o.o. . . . . ; and each requires perhaps thirty to sixty seconds to be completed. This would be bound to cause such nervous impatience in every human being, not like myself more and more inventive in using methods of defence, as to make him jump out of his skin; a faint idea of the nervous unrest caused is perhaps the example of a Judge or teacher always listening to a mentally dull witness or a stuttering scholar, who despite all attempts cannot clearly get out what he is asked or wants to say.

Playing the piano and reading books and newspapers is—as far as the state of my head allows—my main defence, which makes even the most drawn-out voices finally perish; at night when this is not easily done or in day-time when the mind requires a change of occupation, I usually found committing poems to
p. 224 memory a successful remedy. I learnt a great number of poems by heart particularly Schiller's ballads, long sections of Schiller's and Goethe's dramas, as well as arias from operas and humorous poems, amongst others from Max and Moritz, Struwelpeter and Spekter's fables, which I then recite in silence on the quiet verbatim. Their value as poetry naturally does not matter; however insignificant the rhymes, even obscene verses are worth their weight in gold as mental nourishment compared with the terrible nonsense my nerves are otherwise forced to listen to.

Even while reciting poems I have to combat difficulties which at times reduce their effectiveness; miracles aimed at scattering my thoughts act on my nerves and make it impossible to find the continuation of a poem learnt by heart; or when the most persistent inner voices have at last been silenced by the recital of longer poems and I have reached a state of great soul-voluptuousness through union of all rays, the lower God starts the bellowing miracle until I am so breathless that I cannot continue reciting the poems even softly. I am therefore forced to change the systems much in the same way as externally new systems are continually started (by God's omnipotence) to slow down the attraction of rays and prevent the union of all rays necessary for sleep or complete soul-voluptuousness. Recently I found counting aloud up to a large figure of great help, but this is naturally very boring for any length of time. When severe bodily pain sets in or persistent bellowing occurs, the last remaining remedy is swearing aloud which I have to do occasionally, but which I sincerely hope will
p. 225 become less and less necessary in future.

All the above described phenomena have changed in the course of years and are still subject to change in relation to the degree of soul-voluptuousness present at a given time and the distance to which God has withdrawn. But on the whole the predictions I made years ago become truer every day; the following excerpt from Little Study XIII, in notebook *B*, already mentioned in footnote 80, may serve as proof:

16th January 1898

"In the meantime, that is to say during the years or decades which may pass until unmanning is completed, the direction of our policy is in general clear. *There is no doubt whatever that things will become easier for us with every year, every day, every week,* possible setbacks excepted, which are connected with the fact that elsewhere the necessary insight is lacking and *will probably never come about* owing to the organization of God's realms and the soul-character; therefore weak efforts will always be made to avoid the solution which is in consonance with the Order of the World".

Because of its very characteristic meaning I must devote a few more remarks to the above-mentioned question "Why do you then not shit?", however indelicate the subject may be. Like everything else in my body, the need to empty myself is also called forth by miracles; this is done by forcing the faeces in the bowel forwards (sometimes also backwards) and when owing to previous evacuation there is insufficient material present, the small remnants p. 226
in the bowel are smeared on my backside. This miracle, initiated by the upper God, is repeated every day at least several dozen times. It is connected with the idea which is quite incomprehensible for human beings and can only be explained by God's complete lack of knowledge of the living human being as an organism, that "sh....." is to a certain extent the final act; that is to say when the miracles produce the urge to sh.. the goal of destroying my reason is reached, and so the possibility afforded for a final withdrawal of the rays. Trying to trace the origin of this idea one must assume some misunderstanding of the symbolic meaning of the act of defecation, namely that he who entered into a special relationship to divine rays as I have is to a certain extent entitled to sh.. on all the world.

At the same time, however, the whole perfidy[97] of the policy

[97] In using the expression "perfidy" it will hardly be necessary to remind the reader of my previously developed ideas (the end of Chapter V; footnote 74, Chapter XI, p. 188, Chapter XIII) according to which God acts towards me in self-defence—although of His own making—and therefore considers Himself above every human and moral consideration.

conducted towards me is clear. Whenever the need to defecate is produced by miracle, some other person in my environment is sent to the lavatory—by exciting the nerves of the person concerned—in order to prevent me from emptying myself; this I have observed so frequently (thousands of times) and so regularly that one can exclude any thought of it being coincidence. The question "Why do you then not sh..?" is followed by the capital
p. 227 answer "Because I am somehow stupid". The pen almost resists writing down the fantastic nonsense that God in His blindness and lack of knowledge of human nature in fact goes so far that He assumes a human being could exist who—something every animal is capable of doing—cannot sh.. for sheer stupidity. When I do empty myself—usually in a bucket because I almost always find the lavatory occupied—this act is always combined with a very strong development of soul-voluptuousness. Liberation from the pressure of faeces present in the guts creates an intense feeling of well-being, particularly for the nerves of voluptuousness; the same happens when I pass water. For that reason all rays have always and without exception been united during evacuation and passing water; and for this very reason, namely to avoid a union of all rays, one attempts (usually unsuccessfully) to miracle away the urge.

---

p. 228

XVII

From the account in the previous chapter, the reader will have gained the impression that the trials to which I am subjected by compulsive thinking have in many respects far exceeded the measure of demands which are usually made on human capacity and human patience. To be quite truthful I must add that there were also moments which at least occasionally offered a kind of recompense for the wrong done me. Apart from knowledge of supernatural matters gained in the course of years which I would not erase from my memory for all the gold on earth, I must also mention the mentally stimulating effect compulsive thinking has had on me. Throwing into my nerves unconnected conjunctions expressing causal or other relations ("Why only",

" Why because ", " Why because I ", " Let it be then ", " At least ", etc.) forced me to ponder many things usually passed over by human beings, which made me think more deeply. All human activity near me, every view of nature in the garden or from my p. 229
window stirs certain thoughts in me; when I then hear " Why only " or " Why because " spoken into my nerves, I am forced or at least stimulated in immeasurably greater degree than other human beings to contemplate the reason or purpose behind them.

As one of many examples: while writing these lines a new house is being built in the Asylum garden and a new stove installed in the room adjoining mine. Watching this work the idea automatically arises: that man or various workmen are now occupied in doing this or that; if simultaneously with this thought a " And why " or " Why because " is spoken into my nerves, I am unavoidably forced to give myself an account of the reason and purpose of every single job. Similar things happened innumerable times in the course of years; reading books and newspapers particularly stimulates new thoughts. Being continually forced to trace the causal relation of every happening, every feeling, and every idea has given me gradually deeper insight into the essence of almost all natural phenomena and aspects of human activity in art, science, etc., than is achieved by people who do not think it worth while to think about ordinary everyday occurrences. It is often not at all easy, particularly in the case of sensations and feelings, to account for reasons (" But why ") satisfactorily; indeed most often the question why is inept, as for instance in such sentences as " This p. 230
rose has a nice smell " or " This poem has a beautiful poetical expression " or " This is a magnificent painting " or " This piece of music is particularly melodious ". Nevertheless this question is stimulated in me by the voices and moves me to think; but as I said before continual thinking is too wearying and I have though slowly learnt to extricate myself from it to some extent. Of course he who believes in the divine creation of the world can naturally always adduce as the last cause of all things and happenings the reason " Because God has created the world ". But between this fact and the individual processes of life there are innumerable intermediate links which are eminently interesting to work out. Stimulated by compulsive thinking I occupied myself a great deal with etymological questions which I must say had interested me in earlier days of health.

Finally a very ordinary event to illustrate the above: I meet a person I know by the name of Schneider. Seeing him the thought

automatically arises "This man's name is Schneider" or "This is Mr. Schneider". With it "But why" or "Why because" also resounds in my nerves. In ordinary human contact the answer would probably be: "Why! What a silly question, the man's name is simply Schneider". But my nerves were unable or
p. 231 almost unable to behave like this. Their peace is disturbed once the question is put why this man should be Mr. Schneider or why he is called Mr. Schneider. This very peculiar question 'why' occupies my nerves automatically—particularly if the question is repeated several times—until their thinking is diverted in another direction. My nerves perhaps answer first: Well, the man's name is Schneider because his father was also called Schneider. But this trivial answer does not really pacify my nerves. Another chain of thought starts about why giving of names was introduced at all among people, its various forms among different peoples at different times, and the various circumstances (profession, origin, particular physical qualities, etc.), which gave rise to them. Thus an extremely simple observation under the pressure of compulsive thinking becomes the starting point of a very considerable mental task, usually not without bearing fruit.

Another interesting phenomenon connected with the ray-communication—the real cause of compulsive thinking—is the so-called "*picturing*", which I have touched on earlier in Chapter V. Perhaps nobody but myself, not even science, knows that man retains all recollections in his memory, by virtue of lasting impressions on his nerves, *as pictures* in his head. Because my inner nervous system is illuminated by rays, these pictures can be voluntarily reproduced; this in fact is the nature of "picturing". I expressed this thought earlier (in my Little Studies XLIX of 29th October 1898) in a different form:

p. 232 "To picture (in the sense of the soul-language) is the conscious use of the human imagination for the purpose of producing pictures (predominantly pictures of recollections) in one's head, which can then be looked at by rays".[98] By vivid imagination I can produce

[98] As the continuation of the above-mentioned "Little Study" which deals with picturing in the *human* sense may be of interest it is appended here:

Picturing in the *human* sense is the representation of objects on a surface (in contradistinction to corporeal, plastic representation) *without colour* (in contradistinction to painting; or one could also say that painting is the producing of pictures in colour),

and especially *either* mere *copying* (drawing from nature), that is reproducing objects actually seen in the outer world, in which human *imagination* plays no part,

or the creation of pictures representing objects not yet existing in the outer world, for either purely artistic purposes (representation of beauty, to give oneself and others

pictures of all recollections from my life, of persons, animals and
plants, of all sorts of objects in nature and objects of daily use, so
that these images become visible either inside my head or if I wish,
outside, where I want them to be seen by my own nerves and by
the rays. I can do the same with weather phenomena and other p. 233
events; I can for example let it rain or let lightning strike—this
is a particularly effective form of "picturing", because the weather
and particularly lightning are considered by the rays manifestations
of the divine gift of miracles; I can also let a house go up in smoke
under the window of my flat, etc. All this naturally only in my
imagination, but in a manner that the rays get the impression that
these objects and phenomena really exist. I can also "picture" myself
in a different place, for instance while playing the piano I see myself
at the same time standing in front of a mirror in the adjoining room
in female attire; when I am lying in bed at night I can give myself
and the rays the impression that my body has female breasts and
a female sexual organ; I mentioned its great importance and the
reason for it in Chapter XIII. The picturing of female buttocks on
my body—*honi soit qui mal y pense*—has become such a habit that I
do it almost automatically whenever I bend down. "Picturing" in
this sense may therefore be called a reversed miracle. In the same
way as rays throw on to my nerves pictures they would like to see
especially in dreams, I too can in turn produce pictures for the rays
which I want them to see.

He who has not experienced what I have cannot form any idea
in how many ways the ability to "picture" has become of value
to me. It has truly often been a consolation and comfort in the
unending monotony of my dreary life, in the mental tortures p. 234
I suffered from the nonsensical twaddle of voices. What great
joy to be able to picture again in my mind's eye recollections of
journeys and landscapes, sometimes—when the rays behave favourably—with such surprising faithfulness and true colour that both
myself and the rays have almost the exact impression of the landscapes I want to see again as if they were actually there.

---

pleasure) or for practical purposes, that is in order to produce objects which correspond to these pictures (a model, the plan of a building, etc.),

the latter implying *imagination* (fantasy derived from *φαινεμαι*. The German word [Einbildungskraft] indicates clearly the notion of "something being *put into* the head or into human awareness", which is not present outside; hence also the term "to imagine something" [Sicheinbilden, Vorgaukeln] for *morbid* imagination, conjuring something up before one's eyes (hopes, etc.), which cannot be realized, but is used as motive for inappropriate and wrong action.

This little study is naturally deficient in style, because I made these notes when I had no idea that I might ever wish to communicate its contents to other people.

While writing these lines, I am attempting—by way of experiment—to make the shape of the Matterhorn appear on the horizon—at the point near Dittersbach from where the summit rises so beautifully—and can convince myself that I succeed up to a point with my eyes closed or open. Similarly I have innumerable times in the course of years seen shapes of people I knew enter my room or walk about in the garden, "pictured"[99] them whenever I wanted to see them; or I gave shape to cartoons, which I had seen somewhere, particularly humorous ones from the *Fliegenden Blätter*, etc. In sleepless nights I often took revenge as it were for the rays' play with miracles, by conjuring up myself all sorts of shapes, serious or humorous, sensuously exciting or fearful, in my bedroom or in the cell; the entertainment I obtained in this way was an essential means to conquer the otherwise often unbearable boredom. I often accompany my piano playing with the relevant "picturing"
p. 235 particularly when I play piano arrangements. I can produce a whole opera or parts of it by "picturing" in my mind's eye the whole course of the action, the characters, the scenery, etc.—sometimes with surprising vividness. As I mostly have dealings with miracled birds, I sometimes enjoy myself by jokingly "picturing" for them how they would appear when being eaten up by a cat, etc. Naturally "picturing" in this sense requires considerable mental exertion, and my head must be in fairly good order and I in good spirits; when these conditions prevail I can derive quite considerable pleasure if the intended pictures succeed fairly accurately. Apart from mere entertainment, "picturing" has another significance hardly less important. Seeing pictures purifies rays, as already mentioned in Chapter XI; they then enter into me without their usual destructive force. For this reason attempts are regularly made by counter-miracles to blot out what I have "pictured"; but I am usually victorious, and the pictures remain visible to me and the rays for as long as I exert my will, although admittedly they frequently become less distinct or paler. I have also to "picture" when I want to play the piano accurately, because miracles become less disturbing when I thus gain the goodwill of the rays.

Finally a not unimportant accompaniment of compulsive
p. 236 thinking is that all noises I hear, particularly those lasting some time (the rattling of railway trains, the rumbling of chain-steamers,

[99] For instance I make—in day-time or at night—Napoleon or Frederic the Great walk through my room, or the Emperor William I emerge from my wardrobe in full regalia, etc., etc.

the music of concerts, etc.), *seem* to speak the words which are talked into my head by the voices, and also those words in which I formulate my own thoughts.

In contrast to the language of the sun and of the miraculously created birds this is only a subjective feeling: the sound of spoken or developing words is communicated to the auditory impressions which I simultaneously receive from railways, chain-steamers, squeaking boots, etc.; it is far from me to assert that railways, chain-steamers, etc., really talk like the sun and the birds. This particularly disturbed the rays because (as mentioned in Chapter VII, p. 87) in their previous abode in distant celestial regions, they were accustomed to the most holy peace; all noises must therefore frighten them. Hence such continually used phrases as "If only the cursed railways would cease to speak", "If only the cursed chain-steamers would cease to speak", etc. Such sentences of course made no practical difference whatever. Indeed the idea that one could stop a nuisance by simply expressing *in words* the wish for it to stop, seems to have been one of the peculiarities of the soul-character. For example: when miracles make my face hot or my feet cold, I am continually urged to *say* aloud: "If only the cursed heat would cease" or "If only my feet weren't so cold"; whereas as a practical human being I naturally prefer to wash my face with cold water instead or to warm my feet by rubbing them. Whether this peculiarity of the soul-character is p. 237
a weakness must be answered guardedly: in the *Order of the World* souls existed only for enjoyment, not for *practical action* like human beings and other creatures of the earth. I am of course indifferent to the talking of railways and other noises; but these gained importance because they became a weapon in my hand against the falsification of my thoughts by the rays. By will-power I can keep out, if only temporarily, all vibrations from outside. Thus "I am master of all noises" as the expression goes, which enables me to force certain forms of the not-thinking-of-anything-thought on to the rays while trains and chain-steamers pass, and so achieve temporary peace for my nerves.

XVIII p. 238

Although in the preceding chapters I have reported a good deal about divine miracles, it was all about damaging effects on my

body and the interferences they created in everything I did. Obviously these are signs of an abnormal state of affairs, which arose because the Order of the World itself was out of joint. To fight an individual human being and to work destruction on his body is not the rays' task, their essential purpose is to *create*. This essential function of rays, of God's miraculous *creative* power is still evident in many ways; I will therefore proceed to expound my opinions on the basis of observations I made. I am aware that this is the most difficult subject ever to exercise the human mind, and I must anticipate that I can only make a few incomplete observations more in the nature of aphorisms. The essential secret of creation remains a closed book even for me; I have only
p. 239 an inkling which I will try to set out.

As mentioned earlier (Chapter I, footnote 11) I believe that the essence of divine creation consists in a partial self-sacrifice of rays which are sent down with the conscious will to create something in the outer world. God *wills* that something should be, and by despatching rays with this will, *what He wills immediately comes into existence*. The Bible expresses this significantly in the words "God said, Let there be light: and there *was* light"; but to understand this fully is beyond human capacity. Yet divine creative power seems to be not altogether boundless; it is somehow dependent on certain conditions connected mainly with the spatial relations to the celestial body on which creation was to take place, and therefore seems connected with drawing nearer to that body.

In order to create a complete human being—an act of creation which one must assume actually took place in the dim past—an extraordinary exertion of power was necessary, an exceptional approach to this celestial body; as a permanent state of affairs this was probably incompatible with the needs of the rest of the universe, perhaps even incompatible with the very existence of God Himself.

What applies to man naturally applies also to all higher animal life which was to be created next to already existing lower forms of animal life. One might therefore assume that all creation on any one celestial body did not come into existence as Darwin postulated
p. 240 by new species developing through gradual evolution from earlier forms, but in a series of single acts of creation by which new species were each time created as models for other species, although possibly with some recollection of their earlier forms. Each species was perhaps only created in one or a few specimens endowed from

the start with the capacity for reproduction; they could therefore in favourable conditions multiply to any number. Naturally, when a new species was created conditions had to exist which allowed that species to survive permanently; the physical conditions on the celestial body (temperature, air, water, etc.) must have reached a certain development and a population of plants and lower animal forms had to be in existence to serve the higher species as nourishment. The crowning glory of the whole of creation, however, was the human being; the plan of creation was to form him in the image of God, as a being who *after death is transformed again into God* (compare Chapter I, footnote 11).

It is impossible for me to give a detailed scientific account of the cosmogenic theory which I have sketched roughly above as I lack almost all means to do so. I have no access to scientific sources; most of the time I lack the necessary conditions of health, because while I work my head is the continual object of distracting and damaging miracles which make concentration impossible; lastly it would probably need a better intellect than mine to solve the gigantic task of proving the above conception scientifically.

I will therefore confine myself to recounting the *observations* **p. 241** which led me to this conception. My aim is to show the reader that he is not only dealing with the empty figments of a poor mental patient's fantasy—I am still considered as such among human beings—but with results which are the fruit of many years' hard thinking and based on experiences of a very special kind not known to other human beings. These may not contain the complete truth in all its aspects, but will be incomparably nearer the truth than all that has been thought and written about the subject in the course of thousands of years.

My most important observation is, that for years I have experienced direct genesis (creation) through divine miracles certainly on *lower animals* and I still experience it around me hourly. I have thus gained the certain conviction that *spontaneous generation* (parentless generation, *generatio aequivoca*) does in fact exist; not, however, in the materialistic sense which in natural science is connected with these terms, in that inorganic substances can combine by chance with one another in such a manner that an organized (living) being results; here it is used in the totally different sense that the coming into existence of such life is due to the purposeful manifestations of divine power of will or divine power of creation. The animals thus created belong to different species according to the time of day or season; apart from spiders,

the commonest are insects of all sorts, particularly flies, gnats, wasps, bees, bumble-bees, ants, earwigs, butterflies, night moths,
p. 242 moths, etc., etc. These animals always appear on definite occasions and in definite order around me; they appear so frequently that there is no doubt of their being each time newly created; they cannot possibly have existed before and only been driven into my company accidentally. For instance I can expect without fail, in fact I can *predict*, that as soon as I sit down on a bench in the garden and miracles close my eyes, which would in a short time lead to sleep through a union of all rays, *a fly, wasp or bumble-bee or a whole swarm of gnats appears* to prevent me from sleeping. These miracles are mostly started by the lower God (Ariman); but I have the impression that these relatively harmless miracles have lately also been practised by the upper God (Ormuzd); the reason, as mentioned earlier, is that even *his* hostile attitude towards me has greatly decreased since the steady increase of soul-voluptuousness.

I have most stringent and convincing proofs of the fact that these beings do not fly towards me by accident, but are beings newly created for my sake each time. I am aware that it is difficult to convince other people equally: but this is not my main purpose. At present I have not the slightest intention of making propaganda for my belief in miracles, nor for my ideas about divine matters; I am satisfied to relate my experiences and observations in the certain hope that the overall picture of the miraculous phenomena which can be observed on my person *and which probably will become more and more marked in the future*, will lead other human beings of necessity to recognize their truth—even if only in years
p. 243 to come. One will probably object that there is nothing very extraordinary in flies being about the room or wasps about in the open at certain times, etc., and that only my morbid imagination makes me believe they are divine miracles somehow related to my own person. I will therefore proceed to give some of the more important items which led me to the opposite opinion. As often as an insect of the mentioned species appears, a miracle simultaneously affects the *direction of my gaze*; I have not mentioned this miracle before but it has been regularly practised for years. Rays after all continually want to see what pleases them, and these are foremost either female beings, through which their sensation of voluptuousness is stimulated, or their own miracles, which give them the joy of having created something (compare what has been said about this in Chapter I). My eye-muscles are therefore influenced

to move in a certain direction so that my glance *must* fall on things just created (or else on a female being).

The objective reality of this event cannot be doubted after thousand-fold repetition; why should I have the slightest wish to pay particular attention to any fly, wasp or butterfly, etc., which happens to appear around me. One will in any case not dispute that I must *know myself* whether my eyes are *pulled* towards an indifferent object or whether I look at something interesting around me *of my own will.*[100] Added to this the voices p. 244
that talk to me always make these phenomena the topic of a special conversation. This happens in two ways: *either* one falsely imputes fears or wishes to my nerves, for instance, if only the cursed flies or wasps, etc., would stop, *or* one uses such an occasion for *examining* me. This is because God (as mentioned in Chapter XIII) cannot free Himself from the notion that the moment the not-thinking-of-anything occurs, that is if no ideas formulated in words emerge from my nerves, I am in a state of complete stupidity ("dementia"); but He always wishes to make quite p. 245
certain whether this is so, and with it whether the hoped-for moment has really arrived in which a final withdrawal of rays is possible.

The way this examination takes place is very peculiar and hardly understandable for anybody who knows human nature. People around me are made to say certain words by stimulating their nerves; for instance madmen throw in a certain learned term (possibly in a foreign language) which they perhaps remember from the past; these come to my ears and simultaneously the words "has been recorded" (*scilicet* into awareness or comprehension) are spoken into my nerves: for example a madman says without any connection "rationalism" or "social democracy" and the

[100] Miracles directing my gaze are practised—as mentioned in the text—on other occasions as well; lately since the rays' attitude towards me has generally become more friendly it is even done solely for my benefit. For instance I notice almost daily that when I look for a book amongst my books or for certain scores or if I am searching for a small object (a needle or small pair of scissors, etc.), which I do not notice momentarily because it is so small, miracles direct my gaze (turn my eyes) to the desired object. This phenomenon, the reality of which cannot be doubted, is in my opinion of *absolutely fundamental importance for the knowledge of divine qualities and forces.* Two conclusions can be drawn from it: *firstly* that the rays (and I know this from many other reasons too) *are able to read my thoughts* (how could they otherwise know what I am looking for at the moment); *secondly* that they must be aware of where the looked-for object is; in other words the place where such an object is is seen by God with the help of sunlight with much greater certainty and perfection than by human beings with their eyes. By the way full daylight is not necessary; even the dim light of night is sufficient; even when it is half or completely dark I am often enabled to put my hand on objects by my gaze being directed to them.

voices say "has been recorded", thereby attempting to find out whether the terms "rationalism" and "social democracy" still have a meaning for me, in other words whether I have enough reason left to comprehend these words.

It is so obstinately held that I have become stupid to such a degree that day after day one doubts whether I still recognize people around me, whether I still understand ordinary natural phenomena, or articles of daily use or objects of art, indeed even whether I still know *who I am or have been*. The phrase "has been recorded" with which I was examined, follows when my gaze has been directed towards certain things and I have seen them; they are then registered on my nerves with this phrase. For
p. 246 example when I saw the doctor my nerves immediately resounded with "has been recorded", or "the senior attendant—has been recorded", or, "a joint of pork—has been recorded", "railway—has been recorded" and especially the phrase "*Senatspräsident*—has been recorded", etc. And all this goes on in endless repetition day after day, hour after hour. *Incredibile scriptu* I would like to add, and yet everything is really true, however difficult it must be for other people to reconcile themselves to the idea that God is totally incapable of judging a living human being correctly; even I myself became accustomed to this idea only gradually after innumerable observations.

The system of examining me is similarly practised in the case of the miraculously created insects. For instance, at the present season (early September) there are many butterflies about when I walk in the garden. Whenever a butterfly appears my gaze is *first* directed to it as to a being newly created that very moment, and *secondly* the word "butterfly—has been recorded" is spoken into my nerves by the voices; this shows that one thought I could possibly no longer recognize a butterfly and one therefore examines me to find out whether I still know the meaning of the word "butterfly".

These observations will give the most sober reader the impression that remarkable things happen to me. One might of course doubt whether I *can or will* speak the truth, in other words whether I exaggerate or suffer from self-deception. But I may say—whatever one may think of my mental faculties—that I can claim
p. 247 two qualities for myself without reservation, namely *absolute truthfulness* and *more than usually keen powers of observation*; no one who knew me in my days of health or witnessed my behaviour now would dispute this.

With respect to the miraculously created lower animals (insects, etc.) I have already mentioned that there were certain differences according to season and time of day.

Not even God Himself can create whatever He likes at all times. The measure of His creative power is dependent—according to season and time of day—on the relation which exists between the sun and the earth; it seems to me that it is also dependent on the momentary condition of the weather. One must remember that, according to the ideas I discussed earlier (Chapter I and Chapter VII, footnote 44) the sun is not really a power in itself and separate from God—in a certain sense she is even to be identified with God: in other words she is the instrument nearest to earth of God's power of miracles. God can only create within the spatial relations which He established between Himself and any celestial body and the resulting conditions of light and warmth. That is why butterflies appear only in day-time, wasps, bees and bumble-bees mostly on warm days; night-moths, gnats and moths in the evening when the glow of lamps also attracts them.

Whether the same applies to (talking) birds which are created by miracle, and which I mentioned in Chapter XV, is extremely difficult to say[100B]. I have already mentioned in Chapter XV that the talking birds belong to whatever species of birds can be p. 248
expected at a particular season. But there is one essential difference: the talking birds contain remnants of previous human souls, but not so the insects created by miracle. The noise of the voices which speak into my head fuses with the noise of wasps or flies buzzing around me so that they *appear* to speak. This is certainly only a subjective feeling of the kind mentioned at the end of Chapter XVII in connection with the noises of trains, chain-steamers, etc. But I must mention another interesting detail about the miraculously created insects which confirms that they are actually newly-created beings: whether they are of a *more* or *less* molesting kind is directly dependent on whether God's *attitude* to me is friendly or not. God's attitude towards me in turn is dependent, as I have shown before, on the degree of soul-voluptuousness present in me at the time and on the distance to which He has withdrawn; the further He is removed and the smaller the degree of soul-voluptuousness, the more unfriendly His behaviour towards me. The periods of friendly and unfriendly attitudes alternate rapidly in a single day. When God was unfriendly towards me earwigs, spiders, etc.,

[100B] Compare footnote 93B, page 215.

appeared at night, and in day-time wasps, bumble-bees, etc.; in other words nasty or molesting animals which can even—by biting—cause pain; flies, moths, butterflies, etc., which caused me no unpleasantness whatsoever, appeared when God was friendly.

p. 249 In this connection I must finally mention the so-called *frightening-miracle;* this presumably was also a manifestation of God's miraculous creative power. The term frightening-miracle is not my own but originates from the voices; it indicates the originally intended *effect* of these miracles; they have been practised near me in many forms for years.

In early years there sometimes appeared when I was in bed—not sleeping but awake—all sorts of large, queer, almost dragon-like shapes, immediately next to my bed, and almost as big as my bed; they were so close that I could almost have touched them with my hands. The " black bears " and the " white bears " mentioned in Chapter VI, which I saw repeatedly in Flechsig's Asylum, belonged probably to the same category of " frightening-miracle ". Frightening-miracles have for years appeared quite suddenly very near me in the shape of dark shadows in day-time or at night when I am on the corridor, play the piano, etc. They still occur almost daily; at times they assume a human shape. I can even provoke the frightening-miracle or something very like it: if I put my hand in front of a white surface, perhaps the white-painted door of my room or the white glazing of the stove, I can see very peculiar distortions of shadows obviously caused by certain changes in the light rays of the sun. I am quite certain that these phenomena are not only my subjective sensations (" hallucinations " in the sense of Kraepelin's PSYCHIATRY, p. 110), as with every frightening miracle my attention is particularly drawn to it by directing my
p. 250 gaze (turning my eyes). This happens particularly when I play the piano: left to my own free will my thoughts would certainly rest on the score in front of me or on the feelings aroused by the beauty of the music. But my eyes are turned quite suddenly so that my gaze is directed to a shadow created on the door or somewhere near me. I presume—naturally one can go no further than to presume—that the " frightening-miracles " are perhaps to be regarded as the very first beginnings of divine creation, which in certain circumstances could be further condensed to " fleeting-improvised-men " and from there lead up to the creation of real human beings or other permanent beings. They of course lost their frightening *effect* on me as I grew accustomed to them with

the years; nowadays they are only a nuisance when they suddenly divert my attention from what really interests me.

In the next chapter I will discuss certain other aspects of God's nature and the essence of divine creation.

XIX p. 251

In the previous chapter I expressed my opinion that *spontaneous generation* (parentless generation) does actually occur; as proof I adduced my observations on the miraculously created insects. But I have to make some reservation to guard against misunderstanding. I can perhaps best express this reservation as follows: spontaneous generation occurs *again* on our earth since conditions contrary to the Order of the World have arisen; probably spontaneous generation has not occurred on our earth for thousands of years. "Spontaneous generation" is basically nothing other than a literal term for what I have called—in accordance with the language of the Bible and other religious sources—creation through divine miracles.

The fundamental view I gained about God's relation to His creation is this: God exercised His power of miracles on our earth —as probably on any other celestial body which had reached the same degree of development—only until the ultimate aim of His creation was attained with the creation of the human being. From
then on He left the created organic world as it were to itself, and p. 252
interfered directly by miracle only very rarely, if at all, in very exceptional cases (compare Chapter I). In general He diverted His activity to other celestial bodies and to drawing up to Blessedness the souls of departed human beings; He Himself retired to an enormous distance.[101]

[101] I believe I can remember having read somewhere sometime in one of the sources of our religion the sentence: "The Lord—*scilicet* when the work of His creation was finished—went away"; this sentence seems to be a figurative expression of what I wanted to convey. For a long time I assumed that this sentence was contained somewhere in the Bible; but having succeeded in getting a copy of the Bible, I found it was not there, in any case not in the report of the Creation in Genesis where I looked for it. Whether it is perhaps somewhere else in the Bible would have to be answered by theologians. I believe that this formulation of the idea did not originate in my own head. Should it therefore not be contained in our religious sources, I would have to assume that I received this sentence from the voices on some occasion which I have forgotten.

I cannot be expected to furnish scientific proof of this fundamental idea; I do not intend writing a scientific treatise on the history of the evolution of the universe. I only wish to relate what I have experienced and learned, and draw a few legitimate conclusions in the light of this knowledge. I expect confirmation of my fundamental idea mainly from my own personal fate and fortune as they will develop in the future; the time will come when other human beings will also have to recognize as a fact that my person has become the centre of divine miracles. I would then have to leave to other people to elaborate scientifically the conclusions I have hinted
p. 253 at and perhaps to correct some details. I will now return to my theme.

I assume that the whole work of creation on a celestial body consisted in a succession of single acts of creation, in general advancing from lower to higher forms of organic life. This idea is of course not new, indeed is common knowledge among those who have lately occupied themselves with the history of evolution. The point at issue is only whether to believe in blind accident as the cause of evolutionary development, which in some odd way leads to more perfect forms, or whether one must acknowledge an "intelligent cause" (God) working with a conscious will towards the development of higher and higher forms. That the development is goal-directed (Du Prel) must be granted even by scientists otherwise inclined to attribute the "tenacity of deistic notions" to the lack of intellect of the majority of people. All that is recorded in my book has led me to the certain knowledge of the existence of a living God. This entitles me to examine the relation between God and His created world from a totally new point of view in the light of the supernatural impressions I received.

As already mentioned in Chapter I, I know as little as other human beings whether the celestial bodies themselves (fixed stars, planets, etc.) were also created by God; I must therefore leave open whether the "Nebular Hypothesis" of Kant–Laplace is correct. With regard to the organic world it seems to me that one must make a fundamental distinction between the mode of
p. 254 creation of the plant world and of the animal world. One can of course assume that minimal parts of God's nerves (rays) were transformed through the act of creation into the shape of *animal* souls which, however low, would still have the *one* quality of *self-awareness* in common with divine rays. But it is incomprehensible, at least for human beings, that divine rays could enter into *plants* which, even if considered in a way as living, yet lack all

self-awareness. One might assume that the plant world could have been created in certain favourable conditions by the mere reflection of rays which fall on to the earth with sunlight; perhaps God came nearer the earth while creating an organized animal world, say on Venus. This might at the same time have resulted in calling a plant world to life on the earth, which was then less developed. But I must confess that I have received no divine intimation about this; if therefore I were to continue this discussion I might lose myself in fruitless speculations in which any student of natural science might prove me wrong. I am on much safer ground when I assert that the *capacity* to transform themselves into *animals* of all kinds, ultimately even into a human being, is the *latent potential* of divine rays; they can create these creatures out of themselves.

In this respect I command the most extraordinary experiences and observations. Above all I want to mention that the rays (nerves) of the upper God, when they are thrust down in consequence of my nerves' power of attraction, often appear in my head p. 255 *in the image of a human shape*. I am by coincidence in the fortunate position to be able to point to a really existing picture instead of having to describe these things in words; this picture is surprisingly like the picture I often see in my head. It is the painting "Liebesreigen" by Pradilla contained in the 5th volume of "MODERN ART" (Berlin, published by Richard Bong); in the left hand upper corner of this picture a woman is seen, descending with arms stretched before her and folded hands. One has only to translate her into a male person to get a fairly accurate picture of what appears in my head when the nerves of the upper God come down. Head, chest and arms were distinct; the arms swung to one side, almost as if these nerves were trying to overcome an obstacle to their descent—the nerves of Flechsig's soul crowding the heavenly vault—see Chapter VIII. The rays of the lower God (Ariman) also quite frequently create in my head the picture of a human face which (as soon as soul-voluptuousness is present) starts to smack its tongue, like human beings when eating something they like, or in other words, if they have the impression of sensual enjoyment.

I must return here once again to the "little men" mentioned earlier (Chapters VI and XI). I often observed that in certain conditions souls (rays) appeared as diminutive human shapes in my head or somewhere on my body; one must assume therefore p. 256 that the capacity to be transformed into human shape or to become a human being, is an innate potentiality of divine rays. An entirely new light is thus shed on the well-known word of the Bible: "He created man in His image and in the image of God created He him." It appears that this passage from the Bible has to be understood *literally*, which no human being has so far dared to do.

Presumably man was the highest God could create. All other created beings form only a long preparatory series with which God aimed at His ultimate goal: the creation of the human being. It would of course have been absurd to create human beings only, because human beings depend for their maintenance on many lower animal forms which serve as nourishment or for other purposes. The capacity to create the highest form, the human being, of necessity included the capacity to create lower animal forms. Man could only be created when the soil was prepared for him. In the long series of animal forms created before him one can discern more and more the approximation to the structure of the human being.

When God had created each single species His work of creation *with respect to that species* had ended; when He created the human being the *whole* work of creation was accomplished. Every single species was able to preserve itself by being provided with the conditions under which it could live, by the capacity to reproduce and by the continued warmth of the sun. To what extent the various species and their individual members succeeded was depen-
p. 257 dent on their power of resistance and their individual abilities, but was no longer subject to direct intervention by God.

I will add here a few remarks to those made previously (Chapter XIII, footnote 81) about the relationship of God's omnipotence and omniscience to human freedom of will.[103] Mankind has always been occupied with the question whether God knows the future, and if He does, how this can be reconciled with the undoubted freedom of the human will. For a correct perspective one has to remember that for God in a sense there is neither past nor future; *for Himself* God has nothing to expect by way of fate or fortune from the future; He is at all times the same; this is implied in the notion of eternity. But put in a different way, the question whether

[103] Intimation about God's relation to human freedom of will from the outset played an important role in one of the first visions I ever had (about the beginning of March 1894); as far as I can remember, in the *very first* vision in which God, if I may express it so revealed Himself to me. Unfortunately I can no longer remember details as it was long ago and I have since had so many other visions. But I do remember that I told Professor Flechsig on the following morning something about the content of this vision and that I had a conversation with him on this topic.

God knows the future *of the beings He has created*—both species and individuals—can best be answered with a few examples. I therefore raise the question: does divine omniscience exist with respect to the future in the sense that Gods knows in advance:

(1) To what age every single individual of the millions of living human beings will live? p. 258

(2) Whether and which flies will be caught by a spider in its web within a certain space of time?

(3) Which of the hundreds of thousands of numbers in a lottery will be the winner?

(4) What the terms will be of a possible peace to be concluded in the present war between Japan and the major European powers against China?

These examples, I believe, illustrate exactly the way in which for centuries scholastic philosophy of the Middle Ages treated predestination and related questions. Really one has only to raise these hypothetical questions to recognize that it would be absurd to answer them in the affirmative. All the examples concern matters of the highest interest for an individual or a nation, even vital questions; yet for God they are all of them equally insignificant. God has provided for all the species He created (indirectly therefore also for the individuals belonging to them) the necessary conditions for self-preservation; it is left to these beings themselves whether they make good use of them and succeed; God therefore cannot possibly know in advance.[104]
This of course does not exclude that God bestowed a special p. 259
interest on the higher forms of life He had created, particularly on the preservation of the human race as a whole, or single human individuals. He could thus, in suitable cases and very exceptionally, even subsequently intervene directly by miracle.

[104] But I have to add that with respect to example (3), theoretically God could, if he wished, *determine* the number which is to win in the lottery. As in similar miracles I experienced on myself and saw in my environment, it would not be impossible to direct the gaze of the person (an orphan) drawing the ticket from the urn or even his muscles directly to the number God wishes drawn. God can, if He wishes, acquire the knowledge where the various numbers lie in the urn. I conclude this from events mentioned in footnote 100, i.e. that God apparently knew where a little object was actually lying which I needed and could not immediately see. But of course such a lottery-miracle (if I may use this expression for short) will never be practised, because there can be no motive for God using His power of miracles simply to help an individual without particular merit to a stroke of luck. In other words God in this and other cases does not *know* the future, but *could* always *get to know it* if there were a sufficiently strong motive for Him.

Everything I have said so far in this chapter refers to *conditions in consonance with the Order of the World.* But through my case fundamental changes have come about in these conditions, the significance of which not even I can fully assess. As God was forced to draw nearer the earth again and remain permanently relatively close to it—perhaps neglecting at the same time other celestial bodies and certainly thereby suspending the founding of new states of Blessedness—the earth has once again become the permanent scene of divine miracles. It seems impossible for rays to remain in a state of absolute inactivity; to create (to produce
p. 260 by miracle) is after all their nature. As for the time being in any case, they could not possibly fulfil the tasks which were theirs within the Order of the World, the power of miracles was diverted, indeed became a purposeless demonstration of power achieving nothing.

Miracles are directed in the first place against my person and against all objects I use; miracles affect the behaviour of all human beings around me, rays influence their nerves to speak, to cough, to sneeze, even to pass wind and to relieve themselves, etc. and all other natural functions; miracles also affect all living animals around me; even the neighing of horses, the barking of dogs, etc. is produced by influencing their nerves. Finally miracles are used to create anew lower animals (insects etc., as mentioned in the last chapter); all to no purpose whatsoever, as living animals and human beings can do these things anyhow, and the newly created insects belong to a species which in any case already exists in vast numbers, so that there is no need to call them into life afresh.

The enactment of miracles therefore amounts as far as they concern me to a useless torment, as far as they concern other people and animals to a senseless game. Even for God Himself this situation is—as stated before—fraught with certain evils. His joy over newly created things can last only a short time and soon gives way to states of anxiety; this is evident from the nerves, separated from the totality of God's nerves by my power of attraction, coming down to me with cries of " help ". Whether
p. 261 and how it will be possible to bring these conditions, so unpleasant for all parties, back again into their normal channels and into consonance with the Order of the World, I can only speculate about; but I will add a few more relevant considerations at the end of the book.

XX p. 262

I wish to add another point in connection with God's inability to understand the living human being as an organism and to judge his thinking correctly, which has in many ways become important to me. I can put this point briefly: *everything that happens is in reference to me.* Writing this sentence, I am fully aware that other people may be tempted to think that I am pathologically conceited; I know very well that this very tendency to relate everything to oneself, to bring everything that happens into connection with one's own person, is a common phenomenon among mental patients. But in my case the very reverse obtains. Since God entered into nerve-contact with me exclusively, I became in a way for God the only human being, or simply the human being around whom everything turns, to whom everything that happens must be related and who therefore, from his own point of view, must also relate all things to himself.

This completely absurd conception, which was at first naturally incomprehensible to me but which I was forced to acknowledge as a fact through years of experience, becomes apparent at every p. 263
opportunity and occasion. For instance, when I read a book or a newspaper, one thinks that the ideas in them are my own; when I play a song or an opera arrangement for the piano, one thinks that the text of the song or opera expresses my own feelings. It is the same naive ignorance which is found among uneducated people who visit the theatre, namely the idea that what the actors speak actually renders their own feelings or indeed that the actors themselves are the persons acted. Of course it is only amusing when, for instance, while I am playing the aria from ' The Magic Flute ' " Oh I feel it, it has vanished, gone for ever, love's delight ", or " The vengeance of hell boils in my heart, death and despair flame around me ", I hear voices in my head which presume that from now on I have really lost all happiness for ever, or that I am actually in the grip of dsepair, etc. One must not underestimate how my patience has been tried for years through having to listen to the most terrible rubbish which consists of throwing in questions: " Why don't you say it (aloud)? " and " Has been recorded ". It is so nonsensical, that for a long time I was in doubt whether God Himself could be responsible, or whether it was attributable to some lower soul-less creatures created on distant planets in the

fashion of the "fleeting-improvised-men", thence to be employed for the writing-down and the questioning business.

I have often discussed the reasons for and against this idea in my "Little Studies", where anybody interested can read details. I am inclined to believe, without finally committing myself, that it is
p. 264 the distant God Himself who causes the nonsensical questioning business, and that He is ruled by the same error which underlies it.[105] This ignorance of human nature and of the human mind is really no greater here than in the other phenomena, in which I must assume that God Himself has a hand, e.g. in the matter of evacuation, to express myself briefly (see end of Chapter XVI); in the assumption that to think nothing is identical with dementia, and in taking the nerve-language as the real language of human beings (Chapter XIII) etc., etc.

That God cannot claim infallibility *since He entered into a relationship with me which is contrary to the Order of the World*, is proved to my satisfaction, as *He Himself* must have determined the whole policy pursued against me, and thus have started the systems of writing-down, not-finishing-a-sentence, tying-to-celestial-bodies etc. But this policy aims at the impossible. Yet for a full year I was concerned for my reason, being then still totally ignorant of the effects of the miracles and the terrors they caused beyond all human experience. In the last five years, however, I have come to realize that the Order of the World does not provide even God with the means to destroy a human being's reason. Nevertheless, even now God allows Himself to be led by the opposite policy,
p. 265 which amounts to possibly "forsaking me"; in pursuit of this policy He continually starts new systems and gives me proof of it day after day. Even now He cannot rid Himself of these faulty notions. But I must emphasize again that I do not think that this is in any way irreconcilable with belief in God's eternal wisdom in that sphere of action which is allotted to Him within the Order of the World.

It is demanded of me to relate to myself everything that happens or is spoken by human beings, particularly during my regular walks in the garden of the Asylum. Hence my stay in the Asylum's garden has always been very troublesome, and led in previous years to scenes of violence between myself and other patients.

[105] Earlier (Chapter IX, pp. 128–129) I stated the contrary opinion. This is because these matters, by their very nature, make any absolutely final opinion impossible; hence I vacillate even now as new impressions seem to favour first one conception and then the other.

Soul-voluptuousness has for long been so strong in my body
that a union of all rays can be expected at any moment, and so
the necessary conditions for sleep fulfilled; for years therefore
I could not sit quietly on a bench for as long as two minutes, where
I would have fallen asleep—particularly if tired after a more or
less sleepless night—without the so-called " interferences " starting
(compare Chapter X), which enable the rays to withdraw. Sometimes these " interferences " are practised in the harmless fashion
of insects being produced by miracle (as described in Chapter XVIII);
sometimes in other ways, by patients of the Asylum starting to talk
to me or making some other noise near me. There can be no doubt p. 266
that this is due to the nerves of the human being concerned being
stimulated by miracles, because each time it happens (Chapter VII
and Chapter XV) I simultaneously feel a more or less painful blow
on my head.

Because the patients[106] consist mostly of madmen of low
education and rough humour, vulgar words are usually uttered.
which the rays wanted me also to relate to myself. Sometimes
they even caused me to be actually attacked, without any exchange
of words, as for instance by a certain Dr. D. while I was quietly
playing chess with another patient. I always tried, whenever
possible, to ignore the insults hurled at me as coming from madmen.
But ignoring these things has its limits; when the lunatics come
too close to me or continue their insulting behaviour without
paying any regard to the contempt I show them by my silence,
nothing remains for me but to answer back in the same manner,
if I want to avoid showing myself up as a coward. But as on such
occasions one word often leads to another, it used to end in actual
scenes of violence in which, incidentally, I always had the satisfaction
of knocking my attacker to the ground—despite violent miracles
being simultaneously enacted against my knee-cap to make fighting
impossible for me.

For some years I have luckily been able to avoid open blows,
nevertheless even now every walk in the garden calls for a
tremendous exertion of tact and moderation on my part if real p. 267
scenes of scandal are to be avoided. For even now the method of
setting the lunatics on me with insulting forms of speech continues,
and at the same time the stupid twaddle of the voices " Has been
recorded ", " Why don't you say it (aloud?) ", " Because I am
stupid ", or even " Because I am afraid ", etc., tells me that it is

[106] All their names are of course also " written-down ".

still God's purpose that I relate these insulting forms of speech to myself.

For years therefore I made it my habit to take my chessboard into the garden on afternoon strolls and spend at least the greater part of the time playing chess, so as to maintain peace and order if possible and at the same time to offer God persistent proof that my reason was intact. I even carried this through for short periods during the winter in the most bitter cold, when I had to play chess standing up; while I play chess there is a certain amount of peace. I am exposed to the same nuisances even in my room, where the whole time—in the form of so-called "interferences"—other patients come in for no purpose; the connection of all this with supernatural matters is beyond dispute.

All these events together with other considerations made me decide about a year ago to work for my discharge from this Asylum within measurable time. I really belong among educated people, not among madmen; as soon as I move among educated people, as for instance at the table of the Director of this Asylum, where I have taken meals since Easter 1900, many of the evils caused by miracles fade away, particularly the bouts of so-called bellowing, because during such times I have the opportunity by taking part
p. 268 in an open conversation to prove to God that my mental powers are undiminished. Although I have a nervous illness, I do not suffer in any way from a mental illness which would make me incapable of looking after my own affairs (§6 B.G.B. for Germany) or which would allow my detention in an institution against my will on the grounds of administrative law.[107]

When I therefore learnt some years ago that I had been placed under temporary tutelage as early as 1895, I approached the authorities last autumn (1899) demanding a decision as to whether the temporary tutelage was to be made permanent or whether it could be rescinded. Contrary to my expectations, a formal order for my tutelage was made in March 1900 by the District Court Dresden, based on a medical expert's report from this Asylum and a court hearing of January of that year. Because I considered the grounds for the decision unsubstantiated I brought an action in accordance with procedure against the Prosecuting Authority, to have my placing under tutelage rescinded. The decision of the Court, the

[107] I wrote an essay at the beginning of this year entitled "Under what circumstances can mental patients be held in public institutions against their will?", and tried to get it accepted for publication in a law journal. Unfortunately the editors of the journal refused it on the grounds of lack of space. In case the present work should ever be published I intend adding this essay in the form of an appendix.

Country Court Dresden, is still outstanding, but can be expected in the course of this year. There is no need to give details of the case up to now, because the files of the District and Country Court Dresden contain complete records, should wider circles become interested in my case. They also touch on my religious views. p. 269

Almost imperceptibly the threads of this chapter have led me back from considerations about the nature of God to my own affairs. I want therefore to add a few more remarks about them. The circumstances of my outward life have lately changed markedly for the better, I would like to say have become more worthy of human dignity, particularly my treatment by the authorities of the Asylum; perhaps not least because my written works showed that after all in my case one may be dealing with manifestations which lie outside the field of usual scientific experience. My bodily state is difficult to describe; usually there is a very rapid change between high grade bodily well-being and all sorts of more or less painful and disagreeable states. The feeling of bodily well-being rests upon soul-voluptuousness which is at times highly developed and so strong that especially when I am in bed, it requires only a little exertion of my imagination to attain such sensuous pleasure as gives a pretty definite foretaste of female sexual enjoyment in intercourse.

I will come back to this point in greater detail in the next chapter. On the other hand as a result of the miracles practised against me all manner of painful states occur alternately (namely whenever God withdraws again), almost without exception quite suddenly and vanishing equally regularly after a short time. Besides the ones I have mentioned I also suffered from sciatica, cramp in the calves, states of paralysis, sudden attacks of hunger, and suchlike; earlier on lumbago and toothache were frequent. Sometimes the lumbago was so painful (while I was still sleeping in the padded room), that I could only lift myself from the bed with simultaneous cries of pain—half *voluntarily* uttered; the toothache was also at times so severe that it made every mental activity impossible. Even now I suffer from almost uninterrupted headaches of a kind certainly unknown to other human beings, and hardly comparable to ordinary headaches. They are tearing and pulling pains and are caused by the attempt of rays, tied-to-celestial-bodies, to withdraw from me when soul-voluptuousness has become very strong. The bellowing miracle usually occurs at the same time and causes, when it is often repeated, a very unpleasant concussion of the head; if it occurs while I am eating I must be very careful not to p. 270

spit out what I have in my mouth. This rapid change in my condition gives the overall impression of madness and my whole life therefore carries this stamp, the more so as my surroundings are made up mostly of madmen who themselves add to all sorts of mad things happening.

I can rarely remain long at any one occupation; headaches come on when I read for any time, write or do something similar, and
p. 271 make a change of occupation necessary. I am therefore frequently forced to fill my time with trifles; I then feel *physically* at my best (apart from playing the piano). I have had to keep myself busy in the past years with menial jobs, such as sticking things together, filling in pictures with paints, and suchlike; particularly helpful for my bodily well-being are those jobs which count as feminine occupations, for instance sewing, dusting, making beds, washing up, and so on. Even now there are days when apart from playing the piano I can occupy myself only with such trifles, that is to say when the state of my head precludes a more fitting occupation requiring *mental* effort. My sleep is on the whole very much better than before; I have already mentioned that sometimes I cannot remain in bed because of persistent states of bellowing (which alternate with high-grade sensuous pleasure). Even this year I have several times been forced to leave my bed from midnight or 1 a.m. onwards, and sit up until the morning by artificial lighting (which has now been provided), or in the height of summer without; in about a third of all nights this was necessary from 3 or 4 a.m. onwards. My sleep is often disturbed by dreams; from their tendentious content ("being retained on the side of men" in contrast to cultivating "feminine feelings") I can frequently recognize the influence of the rays. But rarely do dreams now have the character of visions, i.e. the peculiar vividness of impressions.

The talk of the voices I hear changes continually, it varied even during the short time while I was writing this book. Few of the previously used phrases are heard now, and hardly ever those referring
p. 272 to the "not-thinking-of-anything-thought". The talk of the voices has slowed down even more since my description of it in Chapter XVI, so that it is almost nothing more than a *hissing* in my head; I could hardly distinguish individual words, if—I must say unfortunately—I did not always know in advance from experience what senseless phrases to expect.

I think it likely that changes of the kind described, which are all connected with increased soul-voluptuousness, will continue;

and for the same reason the miracles enacted against me will in the future also change further. Most troublesome now are the states of bellowing—next to an occasional bad head—by which I have been visited for two or three years, and which have in the last year been an almost unbearable plague. Whether one can expect them to improve in the future I dare not prophesy; but if I could take up residence outside this Asylum I believe, for reasons given earlier, that these things would improve.

XXI

p. 273

So far I have hardly attempted to adduce factual proof of the reality of the miracles which I assert happened, nor of the truth of my religious ideas. Quite apart from the frequently mentioned states of bellowing,[108] a great deal of proof is provided by the condition of my body, which on examination shows recognizable feminine characteristics convincing to everybody. I will therefore use this chapter to discuss this subject particularly; I will preface it with the information, partly in excerpt, partly in full, which I sent earlier to the Directors of this Asylum.

Since the District Court of Dresden decreed on the 13th March 1900 that I was to be placed under tutelage, I sent p. 274 a note on the 24th of the same month to the Directors of this Asylum in which I set out some of the more important points on the basis of which I was going to contest this decision, as in fact I have since done. I stated as my reasons that in any future proceedings the Director of the Asylum would be asked for a further expert report about me, and that it was therefore important to acquaint him with my own opinion about the nature of my illness, so as to draw his attention to certain points before the report was made. From my note of 24th March 1900 the following passage is relevant:

" It is of course far from my purpose to wish to convince other people by means of a reasoned argument of the *truth* of my so-called

[108] At the time this note is being added (February 1901), these states of bellowing occur every morning, when I leave my bed, get dressed and wash, or otherwise bare my body (even in the bath), and lead to such extraordinary scenes that it is my opinion that every educated person would be convinced that supernatural things were happening to me. Unfortunately at that particular time of day I am only surrounded by uneducated attendants or lunatics. I consider it likely that in the course of time there will be a further change in these manifestations.

'delusions' and 'hallucinations'. I am fully aware that at the present moment this would be possible only to a very limited extent. Whether in days to come a transformation of my body altogether beyond the sphere of human experience, will not in itself furnish proof, the future alone can decide. There is only one point I wish to explain now:

> that I would at all times be prepared to submit my body to medical examination for ascertaining whether my assertion is correct, that my whole body is filled with nerves of voluptuousness from the top of my head to the soles of my feet, such as is the case only in the adult female body, whereas in the case of a man, as far as I know, nerves of voluptuousness are only found in and immediately around the sexual organs.

Should such an examination confirm that I am correct in what
p. 275 I assert, and should medical science thus be forced to admit that such phenomena on a male body cannot be explained in a natural human way, then the 'delusion' of my body being to a large extent subject to the influence of divine miracles must appear in a very different light even to a wider circle of people."

I followed this first note with a second on 26th March, which I render in its original form:

> As a sequel to my representation of 24th March, I beg to ask a favour of the Director of the Asylum. That note explains why the development on my body of nerves of voluptuousness is of central importance to me both in regard to my religious ideas and as the main issue on which I intend to contest the order of the District Court placing me under tutelage.
>
> It would therefore be of great interest to me to obtain information on the following points:
>
> (1) Does the science of neurology acknowledge the existence of special nerves whose function it is to *conduct the sensation of voluptuousness* (nerves of voluptuousness or sensory nerves—an expression I heard Professor Weber use the other day—or whatever the scientific term may be)?
>
> (2) Is it correct, as I maintain, that such nerves of voluptuousness exist over the whole female body whereas in the male in the sexual organs and their proximity only; do I therefore mention a fact known to neurology or would it be regarded as erroneous in the present state of that science?

I would be most grateful for an explanation either in *writing* p. 276
or perhaps by the loan of a book dealing with neurology in a scientific manner, from which I could make the necessary excerpts myself.

Your humble servant,
Signed.

I followed this up with a third note on 30th March as follows:

Following my note of 26th March to the Director of the Asylum concerning the nerves of voluptuousness, Professor Weber was kind enough last night to grant me an interview and to lend me two books from the medical library. I now return once again to the aforementioned questions, not for the sake of my personal interest alone, but also because I consider that the transformations observable on my body may possibly lead to new scientific insights in this field.

If I understood Professor Weber correctly, the science of neurology does not recognize the existence of special nerves as carriers of sensuous pleasure; he also contradicted the view that such nerves are *palpable* from outside, as little as nerves in general. On the other hand he did not dispute the fact that the feeling of
sensual pleasure—whatever its physiological basis—occurs in the p. 277
female to a higher degree than in the male, involves the whole body, and that the mammae particularly play a very large part in the perception of sensuous pleasure. This fact can in my opinion only be explained in that some organs (whether they be called tendons or nerves or anything else) cover the whole female body more extensively than the male body. For myself I am *subjectively certain* that my body—as I have repeatedly stated in consequence of divine miracles—shows such organs to an extent as only occurs in the female body. When I exert light pressure with my hand on any part of my body I can *feel* certain string or cord-like structures under the skin; these are particularly marked on my chest where the woman's bosom is, here they have the peculiarity that one can feel them ending in nodular thickenings. Through pressure on one such structure I can produce a feeling of female sensuous pleasure, particularly if I think of something feminine. I do this, by the way, not for sensual lust, but I am absolutely compelled to do so if I want to achieve sleep or protect myself against otherwise almost unbearable pain.

I felt exactly the same string or cord-like structures on my sister-in-law's arm during a visit (after my attention had been drawn to this point) and I presume therefore that they are present on every female body in the same way.

I also believe I am justified in thinking that these structures
p. 278 give the female skin its peculiar softness, which is also unusually noticeable on my body.

I have to add that the female characteristics which are developing on my body show a certain periodicity at increasingly shorter intervals. The reason is that everything feminine attracts God's nerves. Hence as often as one wishes to withdraw from me, one attempts to make the female characteristics which are evident on my body recede by miracle; the effect is that the structures which I call "nerves of voluptuousness" are pushed a little under the surface, that is to say are not so distinctly palpable on the skin, my bosom becomes a little flatter, etc. But when after a short time the rays have to approach again, the "nerves of voluptuousness" (to retain this term) become more marked, my bosom bulges again, etc. Such changes occur at present in as short a period as a few minutes.

The Director of the Asylum can hardly doubt that with these expositions I am pursuing not only my personal interests but also those of science; in uncovering these things which are in my opinion connected with supernatural matters, I trust I have not laid myself open to the reproach of having touched upon issues of which as a man I have to be ashamed.

Your obedient servant,
Signed.

I want to add a few further remarks to the above.

p. 279 Of course I do not doubt that the information Professor Weber gave me during his conversation with me, which I mentioned in my note of 30th March, is really representative of the present state of knowledge in the science of neurology. Nevertheless, I cannot forego expressing my conviction, with the humility a layman should show in such matters, that the string or cord-like structures described above, observable on my body, are in fact *nerves*, so that specific nerves of voluptuousness do exist, serving specifically to conduct the sensation of voluptuousness. The proof lies for me in the fact that these structures, as I know definitely, are by origin nothing but erstwhile nerves of God, which can hardly have lost their qualities as nerves through having entered my body; proof is also that I can provoke the *actual sensation* of voluptuousness at any moment by gentle pressure on these structures. I may be excused therefore for retaining the term nerves of voluptuousness.

For more than six years now my body has been filled with these nerves of voluptuousness through the continuous influx of rays or God's nerves. It is therefore hardly surprising that my body is filled through and through with nerves of voluptuousness to an extent which cannot be surpassed even by a female being. The outward appearances show a regular periodicity, as already mentioned in my note of 30th March, according to whether God has withdrawn to a greater distance—if thoughts are lacking which the rays must find in me—or has been forced to draw nearer to me.

When the rays approach, my breast gives the impression of a pretty well-developed female bosom; this phenomenon can be p. 280
seen by anybody who wants to observe me *with his own eyes.* I am therefore in a position to offer objective evidence by observation of my body. A brief glance however would not suffice, the observer would have to go to the trouble of spending 10 or 15 minutes near me. In that way anybody would notice the periodic swelling and diminution of my bosom. Naturally hairs remain under my arms and on my chest; these are by the way sparse in my case; my nipples also remain small as in the male sex. Notwithstanding, I venture to assert flatly that anybody who sees me standing in front of a mirror with the upper part of my body naked would get the undoubted *impression of a female trunk*—especially when the illusion is strengthened by some feminine adornments. I will not hesitate to add, that once I am outside this Asylum, I would grant an opportunity for observing my body to any serious specialist whose motive is scientific interest and not mere curiosity; I *myself* would however *not instigate* such an examination. If similar phenomena have never previously been observed on a male body, as I maintain, I believe I have thus furnished proof which must arouse serious doubt among serious men as to whether what has so far been attributed to hallucinations and delusions is not after all reality, and therefore my whole belief in their miraculous nature and my explanation of the phenomena on my person and on my body not also founded on truth.

I consider it my right and in a certain sense my duty to cultivate p. 281

feminine feelings which I am enabled to do by the presence of nerves of voluptuousness. In order not to lose through such a confession the respect of other people whose opinion I value, I shall have to enter into further detail.

Few people have been brought up according to such strict moral principles as I, and have throughout life practised such moderation especially in matters of sex, as I venture to claim for myself. Mere low sensuousness can therefore not be considered a motive in my case; were satisfaction of my manly pride still possible, I would naturally much prefer it; nor would I ever betray any sexual lust in contact with other people. But as soon as I am alone with God, if I may so express myself, I must continually or at least at certain times, strive to give divine rays the impression of a woman in the height of sexual delight; to achieve this I have to employ all possible means, and have to strain all my intellectual powers and foremost my imagination.

I have frequently referred in this book to the close relationship which exists between voluptuousness and everlasting Blessedness. Voluptuousness can be considered as part of everlasting Blessedness and is in a sense inherent in man and other living beings. In this light Schiller's 'Ode to Joy' is almost visionary and reminiscent of divine inspiration: "Voluptuousness is given even to the worm, but it's the Cherub who stands before God". Nevertheless there is an essential difference. Voluptuous enjoyment or
p. 282 Blessedness is granted *to souls* in perpetuity and as an end in itself, but to *human beings* and other living creatures *solely as a means for the preservation of the species.* Herein lie the moral limitations of voluptuousness for human beings. An excess of voluptuousness would render man unfit to fulfil his other obligations; it would prevent him from ever rising to higher mental and moral perfection; indeed experience teaches that not only single individuals but also whole nations have perished through voluptuous excesses. *For me such moral limits to voluptuousness no longer exist, indeed in a certain sense the reverse applies.* In order not to be misunderstood, I must point out that when I speak of my duty to cultivate voluptuousness, I *never mean any sexual desires towards other human beings (females) least of all sexual intercourse*, but that I have to imagine myself as man and woman in one person having intercourse with myself, or somehow have to achieve with myself a certain sexual excitement etc.—which perhaps under other circumstances might be considered immoral—but which has nothing whatever to do with any idea of masturbation or anything like it.

This behaviour has been forced on me through God having placed Himself into a relationship with me which is contrary to the Order of the World; although it may sound paradoxical, it is justifiable to apply the saying of the Crusaders in the First Crusade to myself: *Dieu le veut* (God wishes it). God is inseparably tied to my person through my nerves' power of attraction which for some time past has become inescapable; there is no possibility of God freeing Himself from my nerves for the rest of my life—although His policy is aimed at this—except perhaps in case my unmanning were to become a fact. On the other hand God demands p. 283
constant enjoyment, as the normal mode of existence for souls within the Order of the World. It is my duty to provide Him with it in the form of highly developed soul-voluptuousness, as far as this is possible in the circumstances contrary to the Order of the World. If I can get a little sensuous pleasure in this process, I feel I am entitled to it as a small compensation for the excess of suffering and privation that has been mine for many years past; it also affords some small recompense for the manifold painful trials and tribulations which I have to suffer even now, particularly when soul-voluptuousness diminishes. I know that I do not offend against any moral duty, but am merely doing what sense dictates in these irregular circumstances; for the effect on the relationship to my wife, see my remarks in Chapter XIII, footnote 76.

It is naturally impossible for me to spend the whole day or even the greater part of it with voluptuous ideas or to direct my imagination to them. It would be beyond human nature to do this; human beings are not born only for voluptuous pleasure, and therefore mere voluptuousness as the sole purpose of life would be as unnatural for me as anyone else. On the other hand, continual thinking, uninterrupted activity of the *nerves of intellect* without any respite, such as the rays impose on me through compulsive thinking, is equally incompatible with human nature. The art of conducting my life in the mad position I find myself—and I do not mean here the relationship with my environment but the absurd relation between God and myself which is contrary to p. 284
the Order of the World—consists in finding a fitting middle course in which both parties, God and man, fare best; in other words, if divine rays find soul-voluptuousness in my body which they can share —which alone makes *entering my body acceptable to them*—while I retain the necessary rest for my nerves of intellect, particularly at night, and the capacity to occupy myself in a manner commensurate with my intellectual needs.

This cannot be achieved without some unpleasantness for both sides, both being forced to behave in a manner really contrary to their nature. Soul-voluptuousness is not always present in full measure but periodically recedes, partly because God takes withdrawal action, partly because I cannot constantly cultivate voluptuousness. Yet every mental activity as well as indulging in man's natural right of thinking nothing (particularly when out walking) is always accompanied by a considerable decrease in bodily well-being. To find necessary rest from intellectual activity particularly sleep at night, also in daytime for instance after the main meal and in the early morning on awakening, I feel I am entitled to make my physical condition bearable even to the extent of obtaining a feeling of sensuous well-being by cultivating voluptuousness in the above sense.

The experience of years has confirmed me in this view; indeed
p. 285 I believe that God would never attempt to withdraw (which always impairs my bodily well-being considerably) but would follow my attraction without resistance permanently and uninterruptedly, if only I could *always* be playing the woman's part in sexual embrace with myself, *always* rest my gaze on female beings, *always* look at female pictures, etc.

I also wish to mention that the lower God (Ariman) in fact confirmed this, when some time ago he recommended a certain mode of behaviour in a number of phrases incorporated in the writing-down-system and spoken by the rays. Particularly such sentences as "voluptuousness has become God-fearing" and "excite yourself sexually" were often heard from the voices emanating from the lower God. Clearly the usual ideas of morality have been reversed in my relation to God. Voluptuousness is permissible for human beings if sanctified in the bond of marriage it serves the purpose of reproduction; but in itself it never counted for much. In my relation to God, however, voluptuousness has become "God-fearing", that is to say it is the likeliest satisfactory solution for the clash of interests arising out of circumstances contrary to the Order of the World.

As soon as I allow a pause in my thinking without devoting myself to the cultivation of voluptuousness—which is of course unavoidable as nobody can either think all the time or always cultivate voluptuousness—the following unpleasant consequences
p. 286 mentioned earlier occur: attacks of bellowing and bodily pain; vulgar noises from the madmen around me, and cries of "help" from God. Mere common sense therefore commands that as far

as humanly possible I fill every pause in my thinking—in other words the periods of rest from intellectual activity—with the cultivation of voluptuousness.

XXII

p. 287

I have arrived at the end of my work. I have by *no means exhausted* the experiences and supernatural impressions I received during almost seven years of nervous illness; but I think I have rendered sufficient of the circumstances to allow an understanding of my religious views and to explain certain peculiarities of my conduct. It only remains for me to say a word about the future.

"What will come of this cursed affair ?" and "What will become of me ? should he "[109] (*scilicet* say or think)—such are the questions which have for years been spoken into my head by the rays in endless repetition; even if they rest on falsifications and do not render *my* own thoughts, yet they give a hint that even God is aware of a thoroughly mismanaged affair. The answers which the rays themselves give to these questions, that is to say falsely p. 288 ascribe to my nerves (" A new race of human beings from the spirit of Schreber " and " I don't know, should he ", etc.) are so childish that I need not dwell on them any longer. My own conception is as follows.

It is of course impossible to predict with certainty what will become of me or in what way one can guide back into normal channels the circumstances contrary to the Order of the World in which God apparently finds himself towards the whole earth in consequence of my nerves' attraction. Such is the confusion that there is no analogy in human experience and no provision seems to exist in the Order of the World to deal with such a situation. Who would want to predict the future in such circumstances ? All I can say with absolute certainty is something *negative, namely* that God will never succeed in his purpose of destroying my reason. I have been absolutely clear on this point for years, as mentioned above (Chapter XX, p. 264); with it the main danger which seemed

[109] " He " in the above sentence, as in many others, naturally refers to me. Perhaps the sentence should be completed with " he who alone remains of interest to us (the rays) " or something similar. My name is apparently not mentioned on purpose because one seems to suffer from the illusion that a time must come when my own identity will no longer be known to me.

to threaten me during the early years of my illness is removed Can there be any prospect more terrible for a human being so highly gifted in such various ways, as I may say of myself without conceit, than the prospect of losing one's reason and perishing an imbecile? Hence anything which might befall me seemed more or less trivial, once I had gained the absolute conviction through
p. 289 years of experience that all attempts in this direction were predestined to fail, as within the Order of the World not even God has the power to destroy a person's reason.

Naturally I have also occupied myself with the question of my future in a *positive* way. For several years after I had completely changed my ideas (described in Chapter XIII) I lived in the certain expectation that one day my unmanning (transformation into a woman) would be completed; this solution seemed to me absolutely essential as preparation for the renewal of mankind, particularly while I thought the rest of mankind had perished. Indeed, I still regard this as the solution most in accordance with the essence of the Order of the World. Unmanning for the purpose of renewing the race has in all probability actually occurred several times in earlier periods in the history of the universe (compare Chapter V), perhaps on our earth, perhaps on other planets. Many miracles enacted on my person (compare beginning of Chapter XI), as well as the filling of my body with nerves of voluptuousness, also unequivocally signify unmanning. But whether in the conditions *contrary* to the Order of the World (tying-to-celestial-bodies, etc.) which God established after the appearance of tested souls, unmanning can really be completed I dare not predict; it is even more difficult to predict the future since I have had to correct my earlier view that mankind had perished. It is therefore possible, indeed probable, that to the end of my days there will be strong indications of femaleness, but that I shall die as a man.

This raises the further question, whether I am at all mortal and
p. 290 what could possibly cause my death. From what I experienced of the restorative power of divine rays on my body (compare earlier discussion of this) I believe that ordinary illnesses, even external violence cannot possibly cause my death. If for instance I were to fall into water or wished to put a bullet through my head or chest—ideas I of course no longer harbour—I would expect temporary signs corresponding to those of death by drowning or unconsciousness following a bullet wound which would be fatal in other people. But as long as contact with rays remains, it can hardly be denied that I would be revived again, the action of the heart and

circulation restarted and the destroyed inner organs and bones restored. One has only to remember how in the first years of my illness I often lived deprived of, or with seriously injured internal organs, with parts of my skeleton destroyed, which in others would hardly be compatible with survival. The forces which then restored my destroyed organs are still active, and therefore I can hardly imagine that I could die from such causes as mentioned above. The same applies to possible death from natural causes, i.e. illness. Therefore it appears that I could only die from what is commonly called senility. Even science cannot say what death from senility really is. Although the external appearances can be described, p. 291
the real cause has as far as I know not been found: there is as yet no certain answer to the question why a human being must die beyond a certain age. As far as I can see all created beings are only allotted a certain measure of vitality which when exhausted leads to failure of vital organs. I therefore imagine that although the rays can remedy any damage done to a body which retains its vital powers, they cannot replace these vital powers themselves.

The other aspect of this question is what is to become of God —if I may so express myself—should I die. I am certain that the whole relation into which God brought Himself to our earth and to other human beings rests at present upon the particular relation which exists between Him and me. Hence should my person disappear through death, this relation would have to change; whether this change would be obvious to other human beings I cannot say. Perhaps one would then of necessity be forced to measures which would ensure the return of the normal Order of the World (such as discontinuing the tying-to-celestial-bodies, complete suppression of the remaining tested souls, etc.), measures which so far one has not had the will power to carry through. Only in this way, I believe, will God be able to resume once again the functions which are His duty within the Order of the World, in particular to resume His task of founding anew states of Blessedness. That my nerves would be among the first to be raised to a state of Blessedness I consider as almost certain in view p. 292
of the relation which for years has existed between me and God. What detailed measures God would have to adopt after my death I feel I can hardly as much as speculate on, as it would mean abolishing those arrangements which are contrary to the Order of the World and of these I attained only a somewhat hazy notion.

As regards the form my life will take until my death I believe I can expect in measurable time and without any particular difficulty a certain amelioration in my external circumstances, suspension of my tutelage, discharge from the Asylum, etc. Whatever people may think of my " delusions ", they will sooner or later have to acknowledge that they are not dealing with a lunatic in the ordinary sense.

But not even this would afford me compensation for the sufferings and privations of the *last seven* years. I have the impression therefore that in my future life some *great* and *magnificent satisfaction* is in store for me—not provided by human beings but somehow as a logical development arising out of the situation itself. While still in Flechsig's Asylum, when I had my first glimpses of the miraculous harmony of the Order of the World, and also suffered wounding humiliations and was daily threatened by horrifying dangers, I coined this phrase for the rays: *there must be an equalizing justice and it can never be* that a morally unblemished human being with feet firmly planted in the Order of the World should have to perish as the innocent victim of other people's sins in a struggle carried on
p. 293 against him by hostile powers. This sentence, for which I had only little evidence at the time and which was mostly intuitive, proved in the course of years correct almost beyond my expectation. The scales of victory are coming down on my side more and more, the struggle against me continues to lose its previous hostile character, the growing soul-voluptuousness makes my physical condition and my other outward circumstances more bearable. And so I believe I am not mistaken in expecting that a very special palm of victory will eventually be mine. I cannot say with any certainty what form it will take. As possibilities I would mention that my unmanning will be accomplished with the result that by divine fertilization offspring will issue from my lap, or alternatively that great fame will be attached to my name surpassing that of thousands of other people much better mentally endowed. Such thoughts may seem fantastic and chimerical, perhaps even ridiculous considering the pitiful and restricted circumstances in which I still lead my life. Only he who knows the *full* measure of my sufferings in past years can understand that such thoughts *were bound* to arise in me. When I think of my sacrifices through loss of an honourable professional position, a happy marriage practically dissolved, deprived of all the pleasures of life, subjected to bodily pain, mental torture and terrors of a hitherto unknown kind, the picture emerges of a martyrdom which all in all I can only compare with the crucifixion of Jesus Christ. On the other hand there is the
p. 294 immense background of the picture of which my person and my

personal fate only form the foreground. If it be true that the continuation of all creation on our earth rests entirely on the very special relations into which God entered with me, the reward of victory could only be something very extraordinary for my loyal perseverance in the struggle for my reason and for the purification of God.

I come to the last point of my work. I consider it possible, even likely, that the future development of my personal fate, the spread of my religious ideas and the weight of proof of their truth will lead to a fundamental revolution in mankind's religious views unequalled in history. I do not underestimate the dangers which might arise from the overthrow of all existing religious systems. But I trust the victorious powers of truth will be sufficiently strong to cancel out any damage caused through a temporary confusion of religious feelings.

Even if many, particularly Christian dogmas hitherto accepted as true, would have to be revised, the absolutely certain knowledge that a living God exists and the soul lives on after death could only come as a blessing to mankind: And so I close in the hope that in this sense favourable stars will watch over the success of my labour.

POSTSCRIPTS

TO THE "MEMOIRS"

POSTSCRIPTS—FIRST SERIES p. 297

(October 1900—June 1901)

I

CONCERNING MIRACLES

(October 1900)

The miracles directed against me naturally continue without interruption. The longer they last the more they take on the character of a comparatively harmless prank, for reasons previously mentioned. A small example may show what I mean.

On 5th October 1900 while being shaved I received a small cut, which had quite frequently happened before. Walking through the garden afterwards I met the Government Assessor M.; he noted at once the inconspicuous little piece of sponge covering my cut (of about this size ○) and asked me about it; I told him truthfully, that the barber had cut me.

This little event is extremely interesting and instructive for me
as I know its deeper connections. There can be no doubt that the
cut was the result of a divine miracle emanating from the upper
God, as I have learnt from countless similar events. Needing an p. 298
"interference" in the sense previously mentioned, God acted on
the muscles of the barber's hand to give it a rapid movement which
caused the cut.

The Government Assessor M. at once started to talk of this small wound, because God (in the conditions contrary to the Order of the World) likes to make the effects of His miracles on me the subject of conversation; this seems to flatter the rays' peculiar vanity.[110] The miracle affected the Government Assessor M. apparently in a twofold manner; namely his eye muscles which led him to observe the cut and the piece of sponge above my lip, and also his nerves (his will) which led him to ask the cause of the injury. The question was framed in something like these words: "What is that on your mouth?"

I have made innumerable similar observations of the miracles causing my mouth, my hand, the tablecloth or the napkin to be

[110] In this they resemble human beings. Human beings also are always pleased when recognition of their achievement or industry, etc. is remarked on.

dirtied when I was eating. These seemed particularly frequent during my wife's or sister's visit, for instance when drinking cocoa in their presence. The miracles caused cocoa to be spilt on my mouth, my hand, the tablecloth or napkin, and without fail my wife or sister made some reproachful remarks.

p. 299 I have similar experiences when eating at the Director's table or in other circumstances. Plates simply break in two without any rough handling, or objects which the servants or others present or even I myself hold (for instance my chessmen, my pen, my cigar-holder, etc.) are suddenly flung to the floor, where those that are breakable naturally break into pieces. All this is due to miracles; for this reason the damage caused is made the topic of conversation by people around me, usually some time afterwards.

II

p. 300 CONCERNING THE RELATION OF DIVINE TO HUMAN INTELLIGENCE

(11th October 1900)

I think one is entitled to assert that divine intelligence equals *at least* the sum total of all the intelligences of previous generations of human beings. For God assimilates all human nerves after death and thus unites the sum total of their intelligences in Himself while gradually divesting them of those recollections which are of interest only to the individual but of no use as part of a universally valuable intelligence.

I am for instance in no doubt that God is acquainted with the idea of railways. How did he achieve this knowledge? God (conditions prevailing which are in consonance with the Order of the World) gains *only* the *external impression* of a travelling train, as of all other events on earth; there would always have been the possibility that by means of nerve-contact with a human being acquainted with the nature of railways He could get further
p. 301 information about their purpose and function. Yet it is hard to imagine why He should want to. In any case in the course of time the nerves of whole generations of human beings, who were all familiar with the significance of railways, accrued to God. In this way God achieved a knowledge of railways.

Is one therefore to assume that God attains His wisdom only through the intelligences of previous human generations?

Obviously everything speaks *against* such an assumption. If God Himself created man and all other living beings, one cannot assume that His intelligence is due to what He receives from man. One cannot avoid postulating an intrinsic divine wisdom particularly in the sphere of creation. But it is not altogether incompatible with His knowledge about creation that God gains the insight He certainly possesses into human affairs, human intellectual life, human language, etc., only through assimilating countless human nerves.

This assumption is irrefutable because God uses human language in talking to me, particularly German (as when circumstances in consonance with the Order of the World still prevailed He used the basic language when communicating with souls), even in cries of "help", or when the lower God Ariman partaking in soul-voluptuousness, gives *expression to genuine feeling* with the words "I am pleased".

III

CONCERNING PLAY-WITH-HUMAN-BEINGS p. 302

(January 1901)

Since writing my Memoirs I have made many more observations on the so-called "play-with-human-beings" (compare Chapter VII and particularly Chapter XV of the Memoirs). I have gone for almost daily walks and excursions into the town and surroundings of Pirna, have several times been to the theatre, attended Divine Service in the Asylum, and once even visited my wife in Dresden. In this way I naturally saw a great number of other people, in Dresden the whole bustle of city life. All this made it undeniable that manifestations of life in human beings (and animals) are not exclusively caused by the influence of rays, but that such manifestations of life can also come about independent of the influence of rays—a fact I had thought probable even before. (Compare Chapter XV of the Memoirs, where I pointed out that this question was still mysterious.[111]) For instance, when I p. 303
listen to a performance in the theatre or to a sermon in Church I cannot really maintain that every word spoken by the actors on

[111] When one remembers that for six years I was locked up within the walls of the Asylum, and apart from brief medical visits and a few visits from my relatives, saw only mentally deranged patients and uneducated attendants, it will be understandable why the above question and what is connected with it was obscure to me.

the stage or by the parson in the pulpit is caused by their nerves being influenced by miracles; naturally I have no doubt that even had I myself not been there the performance in the theatre or the Divine Service in Church would have taken place just the same. Yet my observations on these and many similar occasions have convinced me that my presence is not without influence on the behaviour of other human beings; in order to bring about the "interferences" (compare Chapters X and XV) necessary for the withdrawal of the rays the people around me are made the objects of miracles. This was least noticeable during my visits to the theatre and the Church. The reason is that at these occasions God Himself was in a sense present in the theatre and the Church (that is to say He shared by way of nerve-contact all my visual and auditory impressions during the performance in the theatre and Divine Service); and the rays, always inquisitive, were so absorbed in watching the spectacle that their tendency to withdraw was minimal. However, even here some "interferences" occurred, confined to a few soft words from the people in the Church or
p. 304 theatre or to attacks of coughing on the part of the actors or the individuals making up the public in the theatre or the congregation in the Church.

I was certain that these phenomena were caused by miracles, because at other times my head started to ache (compare Chapter XV of the Memoirs) and the voices to talk simultaneously. I experience the same during every excursion into the streets of Pirna or its environment, when I visit shops or restaurants; even total strangers who are in the same room with me in public houses in the surrounding villages on purpose use words in their conversation which have a bearing on the writing-down-material mentioned in Chapter IX. But I must add that the writing-down-material has increased to such an extent that it now includes almost all the words used in the human language. One is tempted therefore to think that it may be sheer coincidence. Nevertheless the continual reiteration of certain words is sufficiently obvious to leave no doubt of the deliberate stimulation of the corresponding human nerves to use these words. Equally significant is the wordless silence which occurs in my environment at certain times (compare Chapter XV of the Memoirs) particularly when I play the piano and read the text to the music, that is to say when I recite the words in the nerve-language, or when I read a book, a newspaper or part of my Memoirs, etc. with concentration, even when I occasionally sing aloud. One would expect the attendants

to continue going about their usual occupations along the corridor
and patients to leave their rooms as usual. This however is not p. 305
the case; but they do so regularly in the twinkle of an eye (at
first sight) as soon as I stop whatever I am doing and indulge in
thinking nothing, or if soul-voluptuousness becomes so strong
by the union of all rays that withdrawal action is called for and
to that purpose an " interference " produced. I can only explain
it in this way: although the persons concerned have themselves
the *ability* to act the way they do, nevertheless they would not do
so at that moment had they not received the impulse to such action
from the rays, e.g. leaving their room, opening my door (*frequently*
done purposely by patients), etc.

IV

CONCERNING HALLUCINATIONS p. 306

(February 1901)

By hallucinations one understands, as far as I know, stimulation
of nerves by virtue of which a person with a nervous illness believes
he has impressions of events in the external world, usually perceived
through the sense of seeing or hearing, which in reality do not exist.
Science seems to deny any reality background for hallucinations,
judging from what I have read for instance in Kraepelin,
PSYCHIATRY, Vol. 1, p. 102 ff. 6th Edition. In my opinion this
is definitely erroneous, at least if so generalized. I admit that in
many, perhaps most cases, the objects and events which hallucinated
persons believe to have observed exist only in their imagination.
Such for instance is the case when people suffering from delirium
tremens, as even I as a layman know, see " little men " or "little p. 307
mice " which of course do not really exist. The same may be
presumed for many of the other visual and auditory hallucinations
discussed by Kraepelin. (Compare Vol. 1, p. 145 ff. 6th Edition.)
But serious doubts in such a rationalistic and purely materialistic
(if I may say so) attitude must arise in cases where one is dealing
with voices " of supernatural origin " (compare Kraepelin, Vol. I,
p. 117, 6th Edition). I can of course only speak with certainty
of myself when I maintain that an external cause for these sensations
exists; however, it is suggestive that there have been or are similar
cases. In other words, those sensory impressions which are
supposed to be solely subjective (illusions, hallucinations, or as the

laity call them, sheer figments of imagination) may in other cases also have some objective basis, even if incomparably less than in my own case; that is to say they are brought about by supernatural factors.

In order to make myself clearer I will try to describe more closely the auditory and visual impressions I receive as " voices ", " visions ", etc. But I wish to stress again as in other places, (Chapter VI of the Memoirs), that I do not object in the least to considering a *morbidly excited nervous system* a necessary condition for the development of all such phenomena. Human beings who are fortunate enough to enjoy healthy nerves cannot (as a rule
p. 308 anyway)[112] have " illusions ", " hallucinations ", " visions ", or whatever expression one wants to use for these phenomena; it would therefore certainly be desirable if all human beings remained free from such experiences; they would then subjectively feel very much better. But this does not imply that the events resulting from a diseased nervous system are altogether unfounded in objective reality or have to be regarded as nervous excitations lacking all external cause. I can therefore not share Kraepelin's astonishment which he expresses repeatedly (for instance Vol. I, pp. 112, 116, 162, etc. 6th Edition) that the " voices ", etc., seem to have a far greater power of conviction for hallucinated patients than " anything said by those around them ". A person with sound nerves is, so to speak, *mentally* blind compared with him who receives supernatural impressions by virtue of his diseased nerves; he is therefore as little likely to persuade the visionary of the unreality of his visions as a person who can see will be pursuaded by a really blind person that there are no colours, that blue is not blue, red not red, etc. With this preamble I will now proceed to discuss the nature of the voices that talk to me and the visions I receive.

The " voices " manifest themselves in me as nervous impulses, and always have the character of *soft lisping noises* sounding like distinct human words—with the only exception of one night, at the beginning of July 1894 (see beginning of Chapter X). Both their content and the rate at which they are spoken have changed considerably in the course of the years.

p. 309 The most important points about them have already been mentioned; predominant is their absolute nonsense as the phrases are stylistically incomplete, and the many terms of abuse which

[112] As possible exceptions I would instance the cases of vision-like experience related in the Bible.

aim at provoking me; that is to say to make me break the silence necessary for sleep. If it is true that provoking voices are also heard by other auditorily hallucinated persons,[113] as noted by Kraepelin, Vol. I, p. 116, 6th Edition, I must state one fact which I believe makes my case characteristically different from all similar cases, so that no comparison can be made between the stimulation of my senses and the hallucinations occurring in other people; they must therefore have an entirely different cause. I presume, although not accurately informed on the matter, that other persons hear *voices only intermittently*, in other words that the hallucinations occur only at intervals with *pauses* free from voices. Such pauses never occur in my case; since the beginning of my contact with God—with the sole exception of the first weeks when there were still " unholy " times as well as " holy " times p. 310
(compare the end of Chapter VI of the Memoirs)—that is to say for about almost seven years—except during sleep—*I have never had a single moment in which I did not hear voices.* They accompany me to every place and at all times; they continue to sound even when I am in conversation with other people, they persist undeterred even when I concentrate on other things, for instance read a book or a newspaper, play the piano, etc.; only when I am talking aloud to other people or to myself are they of course drowned by the stronger sound of the spoken word and therefore inaudible to me. But the well-known phrases recommence at once, sometimes in the middle of a sentence, which tells me that the conversation had continued during the interval, that is to say that those nervous stimuli or vibrations responsible for the weaker sounds of the voices continue even while I talk aloud.

The tempo in which one speaks has slowed down almost beyond imagination as mentioned in Chapter XVI of the Memoirs and even since then. I have already given the reason: the more my body's soul-voluptuousness has increased—and it is increasing rapidly and constantly through the uninterrupted influx of God's nerves—the more slowly one must let the voices speak so as to bridge the vast distances between my body and their celestial abode with p. 311

[113] When Kraepelin, Vol I, p. 116, 6th Edition, reports that provoking voices are heard by hallucinated persons as coming from grunting pigs, affronting or barking dogs, crowing cocks, etc., he is in my opinion dealing with the same phenomena which I considered in Chapter XVII of the Memoirs at the end of the discussion on the *subjective feelings* caused by the *seemingly* talking chain-steamers, railway trains, etc. It is obviously only a simultaneously heard *sounding* of external noises added to the nervous impulses perceived as voices, so that these noises *seem to* echo the words spoken by the voices. These have to be clearly distinguished, in my case at any rate, from the *genuinely* talking voices of the birds, the sun, etc.

their few meagre ever-recurring phrases available.[114] The hissing of the voices is now best compared to the sound of sand trickling from an hour glass. I can distinguish individual words hardly at all or only with the greatest difficulty. Naturally I do not trouble to do this, on the contrary I try to ignore what is spoken. However, when I do hear individual words from well-known phrases, I cannot prevent my memory supplying the continuation (well-known to me by thousandfold repetition) so that the "automatic-remembering-thought", as this phenomenon is called in the soul-language, itself causes my nerves to vibrate till the sentence is finished. But while at first I felt this tremendous slowing down as increasing nervous impatience (compare Chapter XVI), it actually led to steady improvement. As long as I listened to the voices and indeed had to automatically, it was extremely painful for me to endure a delay of several seconds in the expected continuation of a sentence. But the slowing down has recently become still more marked and the voices, as stated, degenerated into an indistinct hissing. I have therefore been able to get so used to it that instead of doing something (like playing the piano,
p. 312 reading, writing, etc.), which anyhow drowns the voices, I simply *count* 1, 2, 3, 4, etc. in the nerve-language; this gives me a break in thinking (the so-called not-thinking-of-anything-thought). I achieve at least the *one* result, that a swear word must then be spoken which *distinctly* sounds in my mind's ear and which I then allow to be talked into my nerves as often as I like. The regular swear word in these circumstances is so vulgar that I will not commit it to paper; anybody interested could gather it from my many scattered notes. As soon as the "inner voices" are thus silenced, the rays must approach again and I hear words from the talking birds impinging on my ears *from outside*. What they say is naturally immaterial to me; one will readily understand that—having got used to it through the years—I am no longer hurt when the birds I feed shout at me (or more correctly lisp at me) "Are you not ashamed" (in front of your wife)? and suchlike. All this again exemplifies the truth of the saying that every nonsense carried to extremes destroys itself in the end—a truth which the lower God (Ariman) repeatedly affirmed in the phrase "All nonsense cancels itself out".

[114] "If only you had not committed soul-murder"; "He must be done by now"; "Fancy such a person was a *Senatspräsident*"; "Are you not ashamed then", *scilicet* in front of your wife; "Why do you not say it", namely aloud? "Do you still speak", *scilicet* foreign languages? "That was now really" *scilicet* namely too much according to the soul-conception, etc., etc.

Visual stimuli (visual hallucinations) are in my case almost as *persistent* as *auditory stimuli* (voices, auditory hallucinations). With my mind's eye *I see* the rays which are both the carriers of the voices and of the poison of corpses to be unloaded on my body, as long drawn out filaments approaching my head from some vast distant spot on the horizon. I can see them *only* with my mind's eye p. 313
when my eyes are closed by miracles or when I close them voluntarily, that is to say they are then reflected on my inner nervous system as long filaments stretching towards my head. I see the same phenomena with my *bodily* eye when I keep my eyes open; I see these filaments, as it were, from one or more far distant spots beyond the horizon stretching sometimes towards my head, sometimes withdrawing from it. Every withdrawal is accompanied by a keenly felt, at times intense, pain in my head.[115] The threads which are pulled into my head—they are also the carriers of the voices—perform a circular movement in it, best compared to my head being hollowed out from inside with a drill.

It is easy to imagine that very unpleasant sensations can be connected with this; yet bodily pain itself has been of secondary importance at least during the last years. Human beings get used to many kinds of bodily pain, which at first are very frightening and p. 314
almost unbearable. Hence the pain I still have to suffer every day—alternating regularly with periods of voluptuousness—has latterly not been so severe as to hinder me seriously from undertaking some intellectual activity or a quiet conversation with other people, etc. Much greater nuisance is caused by the states of bellowing which regularly accompany the withdrawal of the rays. Naturally I consider it beneath my dignity to have to bellow like a wild animal because of miracles enacted on me; furthermore the bellowing itself when repeated leads to equally painful concussion of the head. Nevertheless at certain times I have to allow the bellowing as long as it is not excessive, particularly at night when other defensive measures like talking aloud, playing the piano, etc. are hardly practicable. In such circumstances bellowing has the advantage of

[115] Apart from my head, pain is also caused on other parts of my body where the poison of corpses is unloaded. All parts of my body are affected; sometimes my belly (this always with the simultaneous question: "Why do you not sh . .") is filled with foul matter producing an acute call to stool, even occasionally sudden diarrhoea; sometimes I feel stabbing pains in the lungs, in the seminal cord, paralysis of the fingers (particularly when playing the piano and writing), sometimes more or less severe pains in the lower extremities (knee-cap, thighs, swelling of the feet so that my boots become too tight) when walking, etc., etc. Not all miracles are due to the unloading of the poison of corpses, often they are caused directly by the power of the rays themselves, as for instance closing the eyes, all states of paralysis, etc.

drowning with its noise everything the voices speak into my head, so that soon all rays are again united. This allows me to go to sleep again or at least to stay in bed in a state of physical well-being when, in the early morning, the time for getting up approaches but my sitting-room cannot yet be used because of the necessary airing, cleaning, etc.

I must always be guided by a *purposeful thought*, essential for human beings, but apparently incomprehensible to the rays; I
p. 315 must ask myself every moment: Do you now want to go to sleep or rest or follow some intellectual occupation or carry out some bodily function, for instance empty yourself, etc? To accomplish any purpose the union of all rays is usually necessary, even for emptying myself (as mentioned at the end of Chapter XXI of the Memoirs) because despite talking a great deal about "Sh....," one always tries to force back the need to empty myself by means of miracles, as its satisfaction causes soul-voluptuousness. I must therefore put up temporarily with such evils as bellowing when I want to go to sleep, empty myself, etc., to be able to do *in concreto* what is indispensible for one's bodily well-being; emptying in particular which one tries to prevent by miracles, I now achieve best when I sit on a bucket in front of the piano and play until I can first piss and then—usually after some straining—empty my bowels. However incredible this may sound it is true; for by playing the piano I force the rays trying to withdraw from me to approach, and so overcome the opposition put up against my efforts to empty my bowels.

I wish to add some interesting points concerning *visions* (visual hallucinations). The first is that the filaments aiming at my head and apparently originating from the sun or other distant stars do *not* come towards me in a straight line but in a kind of circle or parabola, similar perhaps to the way the chariots in the games of the
p. 316 old Romans drove round the *Meta*, or a special variety of skittles where the ball fastened to a string is first thrown around a post before it strikes the ninepins. I clearly saw this circle or parabola in my head (with my eyes open in the sky itself); the filaments which function as carriers for the voices do not as a rule come from the direction of where the sun actually is in the sky (although they issue at least partly from it) but from a more or less opposite direction. I believe I am justified in connecting this with the previously (Chapter IX of the Memoirs) discussed "tying-the-rays-to-celestial-bodies". The rays' direct approach must be prevented or at least slowed down by some mechanical means; otherwise

they would simply shoot down into my body, drawn to it by the enormously increased power of attraction, and still further augment the soul-voluptuousness in my body; in other words God would hardly be able to contain Himself in heaven, if I may so express it. When this happens bright spots of light appear in my head, or when my eyes are open, in the sky itself—at present at comparatively short intervals. It is the same vision I previously called the Ormuzd sun (Chapter VII, footnote 44 of the Memoirs) because I thought the spots of light were the reflections of some tremendously distant celestial body which, owing to its tremendous distance, appeared to the human eye only as a tiny disc or spot of light like the stars. After innumerable similar observations in the course of years, I feel inclined to modify this view. I now feel justified in assuming that the spots of light are particles of rays broken off from the totality of the upper God's (Ormuzd) nerves; they are thrust down to me as pure God's rays whenever the *impure* ray p. 317
filaments laden with poison of corpses are exhausted. I base this conception on the fact that I usually become aware of the spots of light together with an *auditory impression* of cries of help. I am forced to assume that the cries of help come from these rays or nerves of God being thrust down in a state of anxiety; because of their purity this impresses the human eye as light. I have no doubt that these are the nerves of the upper God, for reasons which would lead too far afield here. I even believe I have now found a satisfactory explanation of why cries of help are only audible to me and not to other people (compare Chapter XV of the Memoirs). It is presumably a phenomenon like telephoning; the filaments of rays spun out towards my head act like telephone wires; the weak sound of the cries of help coming from an apparently vast distance is received *only by me* in the same way as telephonic communication can only be heard by a person who is on the telephone, but not by a third person who is somewhere between the giving and the receiving end.

V

CONCERNING THE NATURE OF GOD p. 318

(March and April 1901)

My experiences in the last seven years and the innumerable manifestations of the divine gift of miracles on myself and my environment, have often made me think about the question how one is to imagine the spatial conditions of God's existence, if I

may so put it. The most important points have already been given in Chapter I of the Memoirs. From the remarks in the previous paragraph it will be seen that I recently gave up the assumption of a special Ormuzd sun, from which I previously started (Chapter VII, p. 88). On the other hand, I retain the conception, at least as a hypothesis, that the light and warmth-giving power of the sun and all other fixed stars is not their own innate property *but is derived in some way from God.* The analogy with the planets would then, as mentioned, have to be made with great caution, for I am
p. 319 absolutely certain that God speaks to me through the mediation of the sun and in the same way creates or works miracles through her mediation. One would have to assume the totality of divine rays or nerves being either spread over single points of celestial space or —of course still further distant than the remotest celestial bodies we can perceive with our most powerful telescopes—filling the whole of space. The latter seems to me the more probable; it appears almost a postulate both of eternity and of that tremendous display of power, which still manifests itself at so enormous a distance in creative activity in general and—while conditions contrary to the Order of the World prevail—in individual living beings by their being influenced by miracles. This influence by miracles has become absolutely certain fact for me after experiences repeated a thousandfold; its truth leaves not the slightest room for doubt. My further remarks on the subject are naturally hypothetical, and I only put them on paper so as to provide future generations with further food for thought.

In general I must maintain my previously developed ideas of God's incapacity to understand adequately the living human being as an organism (Chapters V, XIII and XX of the Memoirs) in the circumstances contrary to the Order of the World which arose from nerve-contact being established with one single human being, namely myself. My subsequent experiences confirmed what was said there. God, Who under normal circumstances maintained contact only with souls and with corpses—in order to draw up their nerves—completely misunderstands the needs of an actually living body and treats me like a soul, sometimes like a corpse,
p. 320 and thinks He can force upon me the souls' mode of thinking and feeling, their language, etc., and demand from me continual enjoyment or continual thinking, etc., etc.

This is the basis of the innumerable misunderstandings which must be presumed on God's part, and of the almost unbearable mental tortures I have had to endure through the years. While

God can *perceive* something through my mediation (sharing my visual impressions), *while soul-voluptuousness is present* in my body and *affords enjoyment*, or while my mental activity produces *thoughts formulated in words*, God is to a certain extent satisfied. His tendency to withdraw from me is then either absent or almost so. The need to withdraw from me periodically has only become necessary I must presume because of the arrangements contrary to the Order of the World which were introduced some years ago (tying-to-celestial-bodies, etc.). But continual enjoyment or continual thinking is impossible for a human being. As soon therefore as I indulge in thinking nothing without simultaneously fostering the cultivation of voluptuousness in the previously mentioned sense, withdrawal of the rays accompanied by more or less unpleasant manifestations at once sets in (painful sensations, attacks of bellowing, and noise around me). My eyes are then regularly closed by miracle in order to rob me of visual impressions, because these would otherwise attract the rays.

In consequence of the constant increase in soul-voluptuousness which makes all "inner voices" cease, the reapproaching of rays now occurs at shorter and shorter intervals (frequently only a matter of minutes) depending on which externally organized "system" is involved. States of voluptuousness then occur, p. 321
which must lead to sleep when I am in bed; but *length of sleep* according to human needs is by no means always afforded. Even now there are nights in which I wake up after a short sleep and am exposed to attacks of bellowing. If these last some time without my falling asleep again, I naturally ask myself whether it would not be better to leave the bed and occupy myself in some way, perhaps even smoke a cigar. What course of action to adopt depends naturally on the time. I very much dislike deciding to leave my bed in the middle of the night or in the very cold. If daybreak seems near and I think I have had enough sleep, then of course getting up is no great sacrifice; under such circumstances I usually feel very well out of bed; but naturally, once I am up, I have renounced sleep until my return to bed. Getting up can only be achieved with acute, at times severe pains; before Christmas these were for some time so intense (like lumbago) that I could sit up and get out of bed only with the help of an attendant, who at my request was sleeping in the adjacent room for a few nights.[116]

[116] (Added June 1901). While adding these lines, the manifestations have again changed. Immediately after leaving bed, signs of paralysis occur in my trunk (shoulder-blades, etc.) and in my thighs, which although not particularly painful

p. 322 Since God entered into exclusive nerve-contact with me, and I thus became the sole human being on whom His interest centres, the highly important question arises, whether His capacity to see and hear is confined to my person and to what happens around me. I dare not answer this question yet; but the experiences of the future will most probably afford me reliable indications for a positive or negative answer to this question. It is unquestionable that the light and heat emanating from the sun is spread now, as before, over the whole earth; but it is by no means impossible that seeing, which is a faculty of rays (that is of the totality of God's nerves) is confined to my person and immediate surroundings—like one
p. 323 used to say for many years after the 1870 war about the foreign policy of the French, that they stared at the gap in the Vosges as if hypnotized. The sun herself is not a living or seeing being; but the light emanating from her is or was the means by which God can

---

are so severe that for a time I am completely bent and can hardly walk upright. These manifestations, like all which are dependent on miracles, are quite transient; usually after a few steps I can walk normally again and accomplish quite considerable feats of walking during the day; I have of late repeatedly made excursions including going up the Porsberg, the Bärenstein, etc. I regret very much that these events are not made the object of detailed scientific observation; anybody watching me get up in the morning would undoubtedly think it impossible for the same person to be capable of any physical exertion during the day. Yet I can understand that the doctors, to whom I have repeatedly extended written invitations to make observations of the events at my bedside, do not feel the urge to investigate more closely. For what would they do if they could not avoid the impression of something miraculous occurring with me, incompatible with the usual run of human experience? Should they as much as consider the possibility of miracles, they would have to fear laying themselves open to ridicule by their colleagues, by an irreligious press and in general by our age of disbelief in miracles. Besides, one would expect them to feel a certain natural reserve when faced with matters which appear inexplicable to them; any *obligation* to closer examination exists still less as they can always maintain that if it is really a question of miracles, medical science is neither called for nor capable of explaining the nature of such phenomena.

Remarkable things also happened when, since the beginning of this month, I started to bathe in the Elbe, first in the basin for non-swimmers, and then yesterday (21 June) for the first time in the Elbe itself, which is only for experienced swimmers. While bathing in the basin pretty severe signs of paralysis occurred several times—but always vanished rapidly; they did not frighten me; they affect only a single extremity and as I am an experienced swimmer I can in case of need always swim on my back or make do without an arm or a leg, even without both for a short while. In any case I am never fully incapacitated, moving is only more difficult. Yesterday while bathing in the open Elbe miracles increased tremendously my rate of breathing, and caused my whole body to shiver as soon as I sat on a floating log; the signs of paralysis were less marked, but again very noticeable during later bathes in the open. All these things are subject to constant change and will probably become increasingly weaker in future. I know exactly how far I can trust myself and I am therefore not afraid to bathe in deep water despite all these happenings; but one may imagine that, all the same, peculiar feelings must arise in a human being who expects a miracle to be enacted against him at any moment while swimming in deep water, making it difficult for him to move.

perceive all things which happen on earth. In any case miracles occur only on my person or in my immediate vicinity. I have again received striking proof of this in the last few days which I think is worth mentioning here. The 16th of March—I believe I am not mistaken in the date—was the first day this year with a spring-like temperature and bright sunshine. I went into the garden p. 324 in the morning where I now remain only half to three-quarters of an hour, as my stay there usually turns into almost uninterrupted bellowing—except when I have an opportunity for loud conversation; but this hardly ever arises as my environment consists almost entirely of lunatics. I was very tired as I had had a poor night; I sat on a bench, and started to *count* (in the nerve-language) 1, 2, 3, 4—as I always do when I am not occupied—in order to drown the incoming voices. My eyes were closed by miracles and shortly after sleep descended on me. Thereupon a wasp appeared immediately in front of my face in order to startle me just as I was going to sleep—this event was repeated *three times running* in my short stay (perhaps half an hour) in the garden, during which I changed benches. I believe I am justified in stating that these were the only wasps present in the garden on that particular day, as I saw no others while walking about in between sitting down. The wasps were a miracle of the upper God (Ormuzd), as I know from evidence which would take us too far afield here; in the previous year they had still been miraculously produced by the lower God (Ariman), while the miracles of the upper God were at the time distinctly hostile in character (inciting of lunatics, etc.). The following afternoon several gambolling mosquitoes were similarly produced by miracle in front of my face while I sat in the garden of the inn of the neighbouring village of Ebenheit during an excursion; and again they appeared *only* in my immediate vicinity.

This morning (19th March), the same weather conditions p. 325 prevailing as on the 16th of March, I decided to provoke the wasp miracle during my walk in the garden. I sat down on a bench and the usual happened: first the closing of my eyes and then the bellowing miracle. I for my part *counted* in silence and waited for what was going to happen next. But now the " interference " was practised in a different form: while I quietly sat on a bench and only occasionally let out the bellowing sound produced by miracle, a patient approached me whom I could not possibly have noticed before as my eyes were once again closed by miracles. He hit me a pretty smart blow on my arm without any provocation; I naturally got up and countered his rude action with a few loud words. The patient concerned had previously been unknown to me; I subsequently discovered his name was G. by asking an attendant. This small event, though insignificant in itself, may illustrate also the tremendous demands which throughout the years of my stay in the Asylum's garden have been made on my tact and my moderation; for as mentioned earlier (Chapter XX) such verbal and physical attacks used to be very frequent and their deeper cause was always the same: the influence of rays.

I have mentioned in several places that the rays are "*essentially without thought*", or that they lack thoughts. This idea did not arise in me spontaneously, but rests on statements I received and still receive from the voices themselves; even now the hackneyed reeled-off phrases are followed every two minutes by the phrase: "The leading idea is missing". Something real must be at the
p. 326 bottom of this phrase and I think it worth while discussing briefly what is meant by it. The rays' essential lack of thoughts is by no means to be taken in the sense that God Himself has lost His original wisdom or even that it has diminished. If this were the case clearly He would no longer be able to initiate decisions in the nerves of human beings in my environment, nor make them speak by miracle about matters within their educational standard, etc.; He would no longer be able to direct my gaze by miracle, nor to examine me, etc., etc. (compare Chapter XVIII of the Memoirs), all of which still occur all the time.

Therefore I think one can assume that the wisdom which from the beginning was God's own is inherent equally and to the same extent (but limited in the same way as far as the *living* human being is concerned) in the totality of rays when they are a *quiescent* mass; the idea behind the phrase "essentially without thoughts" refers only to rays *moving* towards a single human being—a *state* contrary to the Order of the World arising from my nerves' power of attraction. I must state again that I was never in *direct exclusive contact* with divine rays or nerves, but between myself and God there were always so-called intermediary instances whose influence had always to be eliminated first before God's pure rays could reach me. These were, and in part still are, the "tested souls", which had been very numerous (compare Chapter VIII and Chapter XIV of the Memoirs) and those remnants of the erstwhile "fore-courts of heaven" which had been spared in order to slow down the attraction; I must assume that these are identical with certain
p. 327 nerves of those birds which, as "talking birds", have spoken to me since then without interruption.

All these intermediary instances, that is to say the remainder of Professor Flechsig's tested soul and those remnants of the "fore-courts of heaven" put into birds' bodies, have completely lost their former intelligence which was equal to, or higher than, the human. They have become completely devoid of thoughts in a manner comparable to what is called "forgetting" in human beings. For human beings are incapable of remembering for ever all impressions received in life; many impressions, particularly the less important, are rapidly lost. Something similar (of course immensely magnified) seems to happen or have happened with those souls which—instead of entering into God, gradually losing their personal memories and thus fulfilling their destiny as departed souls according to the Order of the World—remained individual souls and flutter around independently without merging with God and without becoming reunited with the divine intelligence. Such an event was not envisaged in the Order of the World and could only come about through the circumstances contrary to the Order of the World which had arisen between God and myself. All these independent souls melted away to perhaps only one or a few nerves, completely lost the capacity to think and apparently only retained that degree of sensibility which allows them to appreciate or enjoy sharing the voluptuousness which they meet in my body. They have even lost the capacity for independent speech, with the exception of those birds which in moments (twinkle of an eye) of sharing the voluptuousness in my body are still capable of the words "cursed fellow" or "Oh cursed p. 328
something"—which proves conclusively that they are remnants of souls which used to speak the basic language.

I can clearly recognize the genuine feeling expressed in these words in contrast to the phrases "drummed-into" their nerves (compare Chapter XV of the Memoirs, footnote 92) both by their effect—real voices do not cause me pain or any other damage but help to increase soul-voluptuousness—and by their *sound*, and particularly by the *tempo* in which they are spoken. The genuine words follow with a rapidity peculiar to all nerves and become more distinct from the drummed-in phrases as the tempo of the latter slows down. But the nerves without thoughts must also speak in order to slow down their approach. As they however lack thoughts of their own, and as there are no beings with thoughts of their own at the places (on stars, celestial bodies) where they are loaded with poison of corpses (one may picture these beings which are also responsible for the writing-down system either as

human shapes like the "fleeting-improvised" men, or in some other way) the quiescent totality of divine rays can (when they approach) only give them or drum into them to speak what they have read as my own undeveloped thoughts (usually by falsifying them to their opposite); or remarks about the miracles to be enacted on me; or one has to fall back on the writing-down-material (representing essentially my own thoughts); or finally when all else has been reeled off and one only meets the not-thinking-thought
p. 329 in me, one resorts to the ultimate phrase: "The leading idea is missing", to which is added "Why do you not say it", namely "aloud", etc., etc. This is the rough picture I formed of the thousandfold repetition of the rays "being-essentially-without-thoughts"; naturally one is only dealing with suppositions, because full insight into the true state of affairs is beyond human capacity here as in all supernatural matters; but I think what I have said gives a fairly accurate picture.

I have other reasons for believing that God Himself, or in other words the totality of quiescent rays, retained a superior intelligence, probably a wisdom vastly exceeding all human intelligence. This is evidenced by a number of the phrases, not genuine but "learnt by rote" or "crammed-in", used by the lower God (Ariman) (mentioned in Chapter XIII and Chapter XXI of the Memoirs: "It is hoped that voluptuousness has reached a certain degree"; "The lasting results are on the side of the human being"; "All nonsense cancels itself out"; "Excite yourself sexually"; "Voluptuousness has become God-fearing", etc., etc.).[117] I must admit that only years later did I recognize the truth of these sentences; at
p. 330 first I was sceptical of some of them, for instance a phrase of the lower God years ago (in 1894 or 1895) meant to direct my behaviour and repeated frequently: "The motto must be 'as far as I am concerned'". It meant that I was to stop worrying about the future and—trusting in eternity—quietly leave my personal fate to the natural development of things. But at the time I could not accept the advice to brush all my experiences aside with a carefree "as far as I am concerned"; from a human point of view I must add, this was understandable.

The miracles menacing my mind and my body at that time were too terrifying, the damage wrought on my body too terrible

[117] These forms of speech by the way are now no longer used by the voices; by continual repetition they became a kind of "not-thinking-of-anything-thought" and thus they were no longer able to slow down the attraction. But because I remember them I sometimes call them purposely to mind.

(compare Chapter XI of the Memoirs) for me to feel unconcerned about my future. Every human being when in danger of his life, is concerned for the future. But in the course of time I got used to them; this, coupled with the salient point, namely that I had no need to fear for my reason, allowed me to make "as far as I am concerned" my motto, and regard the future in this spirit. Even now things are unpleasant at times: some days and nights I can hardly endure because of attacks of bellowing, mental torture caused by the chatter of voices, and bodily pain. These reverses are always of short duration; they are instituted to p. 331
counteract increased soul-voluptuousness and are due to the "systems" used against me being made more severe. When soul-voluptuousness is found greatly increased in my body, one attempts to slow down the attraction, to withdraw to greater distances and so prevent the union of all rays which lead to voluptuousness or sleep. To achieve this the "systems" used against me are more rigorously applied regarding the distribution of the talking voices and ray filaments, the content of the voices' talk, etc. This effect, however, never lasts; increased soul-voluptuousness soon triumphs and a more agreeable bodily and mental state follows for a time. What I said about the slogan "as far as I am concerned" applies equally to the other sentence "all nonsense cancels itself". When I heard this sentence from the voices many years ago—I have not heard it lately—I could not believe it. I remembered that in history nonsense did in fact rule individuals and whole nations for long periods of time, and led to catastrophes which could afterwards not always be made good. Nevertheless experience of several years has convinced me of its truth. A human being who in a certain sense can say *that eternity is in his service*, can afford to ignore all nonsense in the certain knowledge that ultimately a time must come when nonsense exhausts itself and a sensible state of affairs returns.

I have discussed these phrases at length because they are of great value as proof that superior divine wisdom years ago recognized certain truths in this (as in many other matters) which only p. 332
became clear to me much later. I find it extremely difficult to reconcile this superior wisdom with the ignorance shown in other directions, such as the completely absurd (as the outcome shows) policy pursued against me, etc.[118] This question has exercised my

[118] Its absurdity was recognized by the lower God (Ariman) himself (as mentioned in Chapter XIII of the Memoirs) with the phrase: "These are the results of the famous soul-policy".

mind for years almost without a break, yet I must admit that I will never find a complete solution and that it will always remain a mystery. For I must reaffirm that God does not know the living human being in the circumstances contrary to the Order of the World which have arisen between Him and myself. He must, earlier at least, have thought it possible to destroy my reason or make me demented. He may have started with the mistaken idea that in any case He was dealing with an already almost demented, perhaps also morally unworthy person; this idea may at the same time have served to silence His scruples about pursuing such a policy against me. Such misjudgment of my mental and moral state was possible in former years, probably because withdrawal and drawing nearer occurred only at longish intervals.

These periods have become very much shorter owing to rapid increase of soul-voluptuousness; ignorance apparently soon gives way to better insight. Yet it appears that souls have an irresistible tendency to withdraw if they do not find in my body that enjoyment (Blessedness)—if only momentarily—which is the soul's form of existence within the Order of the World; or perhaps they
p. 333 are forced to withdraw, because a state of affairs contrary to the Order of the World was instituted. One might have realized that withdrawal would not be successful in the long run, but that an approach had to follow with the rays being thrust down to me with cries of "help", that is to say in a state of anxiety.

This phenomenon can only be explained by the character of souls being completely different from that of human beings. Manly contempt of death, as expected of men in certain circumstances such as soldiers and especially officers in war-time, is not in the souls' nature. In this respect they are like little children who cannot forego their sweets—soul-voluptuousness—for even a moment. At least this seems to be true of those rays on whom, as the most closely concerned, the decision to withdraw rests. Hence, since the miracles have largely lost their earlier terrifying effect, God appears in almost everything that happens to me ridiculous or even childish. I am consequently often forced in self-defence to *mock God* with a loud voice; I simply have to do this at times to convince that distant place which tortures me so often unbearably with attacks of bellowing, with nonsensical twaddle of voices, etc., that one is not dealing with a dement, but with a human being in full command of the situation. But I must
p. 334 stress again that all this is only an episode which I trust will come to an end at the latest with my death; in other words that only I,

and no other human being, have the right to mock God. For other human beings God remains the Almighty Creator of heaven and earth, the ultimate cause of all things and their future salvation, Who should be worshipped and highly revered—even if a few traditional religious beliefs do need modification.

VI

CONSIDERATIONS ABOUT THE FUTURE: MISCELLANEOUS p 335

(April and May 1901)

What I said in Chapter XXII of the Memoirs about a satisfaction which awaits me, or a reward I may expect for the pains and privations I have suffered, assumes a more and more concrete form according to new observations. Even now, a few months later, I believe I can say more about the nature of the reward. At present, however, my life is an extraordinary mixture of states of voluptuousness, painful sensations and other annoyances, among which I count, besides bellowing, the stupendous noise frequently made around me. Every word spoken to me in conversation is still combined with a blow against my head; the pain it causes is sometimes pretty severe when the rays have withdrawn to too great a distance. This can be very exhausting, particularly after bad p. 336
sleepless nights; it is worse still when other pains are simultaneously caused by miracles, for instance toothache.

On the other hand there are periods every day, when I float in voluptuousness so to speak, i.e. when an indescribable feeling of well-being corresponding to feminine feelings of voluptuousness pervades my whole body. It is by no means always necessary to let my imagination play on sexual matters; on other occasions too, like reading a particularly moving part of a poem, playing a piece of music on the piano which particularly pleases me aesthetically, or enjoying nature during an excursion into the country, the state of well-being which is based on soul-voluptuousness creates moments when, as I may truly say, I experience a kind of foretaste of Blessedness. At present these feelings are only short-lived: at the very moment of the height of voluptuousness, headache or toothache is produced by miracle to prevent fully developed voluptuousness, which irresistibly attracts the rays. How the *whole* person feels in such a state is difficult to describe; at times I enjoy the highest voluptuousness up to my neck, while my head is in a bad way.

I think, however, I can prophesy that in the future the painful sensations will diminish and states of voluptuousness or Blessedness prevail. Soul-voluptuousness increases steadily, hence rays entering my body have more and more the impression of voluptuousness;
p. 337 even now one is increasingly unsuccessful in inflicting pain on my body as a means of reducing voluptuousness. The *intention* however remains, as I gather from what the voices simultaneously say, that one intends to "affect my eyes by miracles", i.e. inject the poison of corpses into them, or produce toothache, that is to say unload the poison of corpses into my teeth, etc.; but lately the rays have less and less often reached those parts of my body, while the induced feeling of voluptuousness in other parts of my body prevails; the poison of corpses meant for my eyes or my teeth is then unloaded without any harm on some other part of my body, perhaps on my bosom or on my arms. From all this I believe I can predict for the not too distant future that in my lifetime I will enjoy in advance that Blessedness granted to other human beings only after death. This state of Blessedness is mainly a state of voluptuous enjoyment, which for its full development needs the fantasy of either being or wishing to be a female being, which naturally is not to my taste. I must however submit to the necessity of the Order of the World which forces me to accept these ideas, if my bodily state is not to be made unbearable by pains, by bellowing produced by miracle, and by insane noise.[118A] A substitute of the highest significance for the loss of opportunities of using my mental powers in other ways in the service of mankind and thereby achieving honour or fame in the eyes of men, is the knowledge of God and divine matters I have gained through the continuous contact with divine rays. With it I harbour the hope that I will be
p. 338 the middleman, through whose personal fate the knowledge I have gained will spread fruitfully far and wide, and that in this way it will be granted me to help mankind to correct views about the relationship between God and the world, and the revelation of religious truths and salvation, even long after my death.

How all this will work out when I die—and this must be expected to happen sometime—I naturally cannot say. According to the views expressed in Chapter XXII of the Memoirs I think I could only die from senility. I harbour the wish that when my last hour finally strikes I will no longer find myself in an Asylum, but in

[118A] I would have to modify this to a certain extent now.

orderly domestic life surrounded by near relatives, as I may need more loving care than I could get in an Asylum. I also consider it likely one will be able to observe some extraordinary phenomena at my sick- or death-bed, and I therefore express the wish that men of science from various branches of human knowledge will be given the opportunity to attend; perhaps they will be able to draw important conclusions concerning the truth of my religious ideas. At the moment I am still far from my aim of being released; the decision of the Lower Court placing me under tutelage as mentioned in Chapter XX of the Memoirs has been confirmed (by the judgment of the District Court at Dresden of 15th April 1901). I still do not know the grounds on which this judgment is based and therefore cannot say whether I will proceed by appealing to a Higher Court; in any case I am absolutely certain that I will achieve the suspension of my tutelage and with it my discharge from this Asylum, if not in the immediate future then in the course of a few years.

I will add a few remarks not directly related to the foregoing and p. 339
only put in here because they are too short for a separate chapter.

Stimulated by the supernatural impressions which I received, I have thought a good deal about *folklore* and *superstition* in the course of the years. These and the mythology of earlier peoples now appear to me in a quite different light. I think that there is a grain of truth in most folklore, some presentiment of supernatural matters which in the course of time dawned on a large number of people, naturally much augmented by deliberate elaboration of men's fantasy, so that the grain of truth can now hardly be shelled out. Had I sufficient literary resources at my disposal, I might attempt to investigate a number of items of folklore from this point of view.

Lacking such help I will confine myself to two examples. Well known is the superstition of ghosts stalking the midnight hour, which is the spirits' only opportunity for communion with human beings and which forces them to return to their graves at the stroke of one. In my opinion this superstition is based on the correct belief that dreams are not always only vibrations of a sleeping person's nerves uninfluenced from outside, but under certain circumstances are caused by communion with departed souls

p. 340 (*nerve-contact*, preferably made by a dead relative, see Chapter I of the Memoirs). The hour after midnight as the time of deepest sleep is therefore with some justification taken as the most favourable time for such intercourse. As a second example I will mention the idea which is bound up with the phrase that the *devil can crawl through a keyhole*. In my opinion this belief is correctly based on the fact that no mechanical obstacle made by man can prevent the entry of the rays. I experience at every moment on my own body that this is so; no wall however thick, no closed window can prevent the ray filaments penetrating in a way incomprehensible to man and so reaching any part of my body, particularly my head.

In case this book should reach publication, I am well aware that there is one person who could feel hurt by it. It is Professor Flechsig in Leipzig. I have already discussed this in detail in a memorandum of 4th February 1901 of this year to the Director of this Asylum, the wording of which I reproduce here:

"It is known to the Director of the Asylum that I am thinking of publishing my Memoirs and hope to do this after the order placing me under tutelage is rescinded.

For a long time I was in doubt whether publication was permissible. I am fully aware that with respect to certain
p. 341 sections of my Memoirs Professor Flechsig in Leipzig could feel urged to prosecute me for libel or even demand the withdrawal from circulation of the whole book as constituting a punishable offence (§40, Str.G.B.). Nevertheless I have at last decided to proceed with publication.

I know I am free from any personal animosity against Professor Flechsig. I have therefore only mentioned such matters concerning him in my Memoirs, which in my opinion are essential for understanding my thesis. I might erase the perhaps somewhat offensive and unessential footnote (erased) of my Memoirs in case of publication. I hope that Professor Flechsig's scientific interest in the content of my Memoirs will outweigh possible personal susceptibilities. If this should not be the case, the importance I place on the publication of my work, in the hope of thereby enriching science and clarifying religious views, is so great that I would run the risk of prosecution for libel and the threatened financial loss in case of a possible withdrawal of my book from circulation.

I do not make this communication to the Director of the Asylum to obtain an opinion whether a penalty is considered p. 342 possible, but only to *furnish new proof* once again of how carefully I consider the consequences of any of my actions in advance, and so to demonstrate how little one is justified in maintaining that I am incapable of managing my affairs.

Sonnenstein, 4th February, 1901.

Your most obedient servant,
(signed)

I wish to add a few more remarks.

I have to presume Professor Flechsig must retain at least some recollection of the external events connected with my stay at the University Nerve Clinic in Leipzig of which he is the Director. I dare not say that he himself has ever become aware of the supernatural things with which his name is connected; the voices mentioned *and still daily mention* his name in this connection—despite my personal relations with Professor Flechsig having long receded into the background, so that any continued interest on my part could only be aroused from outside. I have admitted the possibility that in his capacity as a human being he was and still is aloof from these events; but it remains mysterious how, while a human being is still living, his soul can have a separate existence outside his body. That such a soul or at least part of such a soul existed and *still exists*, is nevertheless certain from my many direct observations. I must therefore *recognize the possibility* that what I reported in the first part of my Memoirs in connection with the p. 343 name Flechsig, refers only to Flechsig's soul as distinct from the living human being Flechsig; its separate existence is certain but cannot be explained in a natural way. It will be appreciated that I do not wish in any way to attack the honour of the living Professor Flechsig in my intended publication.[118B]

[118B] Besides repeatedly revising my work after the termination of the proceedings regarding my tutelage, I cut out, altered and tried to tone down my expressions so much that I believe the question of insulting content no longer arises. I trust I have thus removed everything which in the medical expert's reports, in the judgments of the First and Second Instances and in my own written presentations to the Court was thought could possibly lead to prosecution.

VII

p. 344 ## CONCERNING CREMATION

(May 1901)

The organized movement for cremation which has become pretty lively lately, started certain thoughts in me which might be of interest to others. The objections raised by devout religious people against this way of dealing with bodies deserve most serious consideration in my opinion, for one may ask whether the person submitting his body to cremation thereby renounces a reawakening in the life beyond or deprives himself of the attainment of Blessedness.[119] *Not even the soul is purely spiritual, but rests on a material*
p. 345 *substrate, the nerves.* Therefore if the nerves are totally destroyed by cremation the ascension of the soul to a state of Blessedness would be precluded. As a layman in the physiology of nerves I cannot state definitely whether this premiss is true. But I am certain that this question is quite different from cases where a human being died by burning through accidental fires, or in the Middle Ages by the burning of heretics and witches. Death by fire under such circumstances is probably largely death by asphyxia, and one can hardly speak of a total destruction of the body; even the soft parts are probably mostly only charred; certainly a total destruction of bones and nerve endings within them (particularly in the skull) does not take place. These cases are therefore hardly comparable to modern cremation, where in special crematoria by means of excessive heat, cutting off atmospheric air, etc., total destruction is methodically aimed at and probably achieved, so that nothing remains of the human being after death but a small heap of ashes. It is at least probable that in this process a physiological or chemical change takes place in the nerves which precludes their reawakening in the life beyond.

In view of this the advantages of cremation from the aesthetic, sanitary, or economic points of view which are often stressed must in my opinion recede far into the background. Even the last-named advantage is a most precarious one; particularly the intended

[119] That a continued existence after death or a state of Blessedness exists in the Order of the World seems to me absolutely beyond doubt (compare particularly Chapter I of the Memoirs). This is naturally not contradicted by the fact that as long as the circumstances contrary to World Order persist in the relation between God and my person, the founding of new states of Blessedness is suspended (compare end of Chapter II and end of Chapter V of the Memoirs).

gain by saving cemeteries, etc., would probably be cancelled out by the tremendous costs of cremation—if one thinks in terms of the p. 346
custom becoming general. It is not likely that the majority of people would give up the old custom of burial for centuries to come. It is also very unlikely that the time will come when every small village or every small district has its own crematorium. However, the morally decisive question will always remain: whether modern cremation is compatible with the hope of a future state of Blessedness.

I know well that many people are tempted to gloss over this question with indifference. It is not always only a matter of unbelief, of deliberate adherence to atheism. Repugnance to the idea of a person's body decomposing after death in some people overrides every other consideration; hazy notions about the nature of the new existence to be expected in the life beyond not infrequently cause, particularly in pessimistic people, a mood in which they talk themselves and others into being unconcerned about a life after death; as if they were quite happy for death to bring everything to an end, and for all traces of them to vanish utterly so as not to remain behind as objects of diminished interest for other people. But I believe I am not far wrong in supposing that such moods never last longer than till such time as the terrors of actual death come tangibly near. Some consolation and hope are essential for a human being who, perhaps subject to a long and painful illness, is faced with the certainty of impending death; terrible may be the sufferings of a dying person who thinks he has deprived himself of every hope because of his attitude to religious matters, and thereby excluded himself from the consolations of religion. In the case of a p. 347
person who has arranged for cremation, the torturing doubt may be added whether he himself has not contributed to the loss of all hope. Happy the man I would exclaim, who in such circumstances is still able to cancel his cremation, which he may have arranged in a carefree mood while in good health!

Whether the clergy should be allowed to give the Church's blessing at a cremation or speak a few words of comfort out of consideration for the sorrowing mourners, will be answered differently according to individual feeling. But there can be no doubt that the position of the faithful clergyman in such circumstances is extremely difficult. He cannot help feeling that the person who ordered the cremation showed by his decision a gross indifference in a matter important for the question of continued existence after death; furthermore probably all clergymen will appreciate the doubts I have raised whether a state of Blessedness is possible at all after total destruction of the nerves.

One must not be deceived by the objection that it is incompatible with the idea of God's omnipotence to believe that cremation could influence the possibility of resurrection after death. God's omnipotence is not absolute and without limitation; for instance God cannot achieve the same degree of Blessedness for a child's soul or the soul of a human being sunk in sin, as He can for the soul of a mature man of an intellectual significance equivalent to that of our great men of art and science, or for the soul of a morally worthy man. Therefore the possibility remains that a human
p. 348 being, by his own doing, can exclude himself from the possibility of resurrection after death, such as would be his due within the Order of the World. Human freedom of will is here as elsewhere not limited by God's omnipotence (compare Chapter XIX of the Memoirs); human beings can use this freedom of will to achieve results which not even God can reverse.

p. 349

POSTSCRIPT, SECOND SERIES

(October 1902)

There is little to add to the foregoing.

My outward circumstances, the rescinding of the order of my tutelage and my impending discharge from this Asylum, have been discussed in the Preface. I note with satisfaction that my prediction at the beginning of Chapter XXII of the Memoirs was confirmed shortly afterwards.

Miracles and the talking of voices continue as before. The slowing down of the voices has progressed further so that the words are hardly understandable (Chapter XVI of the Memoirs and Postscript No. IV); but the voices are still *continuous*, as noted in No. IV of the Postscripts. The miracles continue to take on a more and more harmless character. Only occasionally, particularly when I am in bed, severe cramp and paralysis occur especially in the lower extremities and back; they are intended to hinder me from
p. 350 getting up or changing my position in bed; or for the same purpose acute pain in the bones particularly of the lower legs. But I still suffer frequently (several times a day) from *tearing headaches* which come and go with every withdrawal of the rays; they have already been described in Postscript No. IV, and are still sometimes so intense as to make consecutive reading or similar activities impossible.

The sensation of temporary thinning and furrowing of the bony substance of my skull persists, and can hardly be only subjective. Sleep is almost normal considering my age; on the whole I sleep quite satisfactorily, mostly without artificial sleeping drugs.

The attacks of *bellowing*, although not completely gone, are less severe, particularly because I learnt to counteract them successfully when they might be a serious nuisance to other people. Apart from reciting poems it is apparently sufficient simply *to count* in the nerve-language in order to convince God of His erroneous idea that He is dealing with a person deprived of his ability to think, i.e. who is demented. Therefore bellowing does not occur as long as I count continuously. This is particularly important at night because with bellowing precluded by counting I usually achieve sleep, and when I do waken I soon fall asleep again. This success cannot always be achieved. It is not easy for a human being to count for hours. Therefore even if by counting continually for some time I cannot fall asleep and I stop counting, at that very moment the bellowing miracle commences and when frequently p. 351
repeated in bed becomes unbearable. Although much more rarely, I must still sometimes leave my bed and carry on some occupation to demonstrate that I am a thinking person. By continual counting I can also prevent bellowing almost completely in public places, in the theatre, in an educated environment, etc. or during pauses when not carrying on a conversation aloud. I may have to make some little noise like coughing, clearing the throat or yawning somewhat ill-manneredly, none of which is likely to give particular offence. But while going for walks along country roads, through open fields, etc., I make things easy for myself when no one else is about. I simply let the bellowing happen; sometimes it continues for five or ten minutes almost without interruption, during which time I feel physically perfectly well. If it gets too bad I speak a few words out aloud, even when alone, preferably about God, eternity, etc., in order to convince God of the error of His oft-mentioned idea. A witness of such bouts of almost continuous bellowing would however hardly be able to understand the connection and might really think he is seeing a madman. Although I carefully watch whether people are about in such circumstances, I am really unconcerned, because I know that at any time one single word spoken aloud would be sufficient to prove my complete mental clarity.

It has already been mentioned that the miracles concerned with damaging my body are increasingly harmless; frequently only a

p. 352 kind of practical joke is played with the things I most commonly use. But my bodily condition is not even now always an enviable one; the tearing headache caused by the withdrawal of the rays, the unceasing talk of voices causing mental unrest, accelerated breathing, miraculously produced tremors, palpitation, etc. make a quiet occupation at times extraordinarily difficult. However, nothing I suffer now is worth mentioning in comparison with the destruction carried out on my body in the first years of my illness (compare the account given in Chapter XI of the Memoirs).

All the same this development of things causes contradictory feelings in me. Whereas of course I can only welcome feeling incomparably better personally, yet I realize that the prospect of convincing other people of the reality of the miracles becomes fainter, the less the miracles leave externally perceptible traces. The latter point of view is almost as important for me as the former, because I can only see a real purpose in my life if I succeed in putting forward the truth of my so-called delusions, so that other people will be convinced and mankind gain a truer insight into the nature of God.

During the first years of my illness it would in my opinion have been an easy matter by a thorough examination of my body with the help of medical instruments and above all with Roentgen-Rays (not then discovered) to demonstrate the most obvious changes in my body, particularly the injuries to my internal organs which in
p. 353 other human beings would have been fatal. This would be much more difficult now. If it were possible to make a photographic record of the events in my head, of the lambent movements of the *rays coming from the horizon*, sometimes very slowly, sometimes—when from a tremendous distance—incredibly swiftly, then the observer would definitely lose all doubt about my intercourse with God. But unfortunately human technique has not yet the necessary apparatus for investigating such sensations objectively. I am certain that this is *not only* a question of pathological phenomena—of tremendous inner excitement of the apperceiving brain apparatus, as Dr. Weber expresses it in his report of 5th April 1902; particularly the divine cries of " help " (Chapter II and Chapter XV of the Memoirs and the end of Postscript No. IV) which I hear absolutely clearly hundreds of times every day at short intervals, cannot possibly be hallucinations. Furthermore, not only the visual and auditory hallucinations, but also events occurring in my environment on lifeless objects, on other human beings and animals, make me certain of the special relationship in which I stand to God. I

can clearly distinguish how far other people's actions do or do not rest on miracles. The latter have been of course more numerous recently since I have been more in contact with other people; but the former—those resting on miracles—still number hundreds every day. I can recognize them quite definitely:

(1) by the pulling, jerky sensation, sometimes combined with severe pain which I feel in my head;

(2) by my gaze being directed (Chapter XVIII of the Memoirs, footnote 100), consisting of my eyes regularly being turned to the p. 354
spot at which such action takes place;

(3) by the examining question "has been recorded" which regularly goes with it (compare Chapter XVIII of the Memoirs), by which one tries to ascertain whether I still comprehend the expressions used (particularly such as indicate a higher educational level or belong to foreign languages, etc.).

To me therefore it is *unshakable truth*, that God *reveals Himself anew* daily and hourly through the talking of voices and the miracles.[120]

Even if I have therefore to admit that the chance of objectively demonstrating the miracles and my contact with God has not improved with the years, I hope nevertheless that enough remains to afford definite clues in a future scientific examination. In general I p. 355
want to refer to my exposition in the proceedings before the Country Court in my appeal against the judgment of the District Court, an excerpt of which I will therefore insert as Appendix C. Apart from what the future may bring, I again stress the following as characteristic signs hardly capable of a natural explanation:

(1) the attacks of bellowing very different from the noisy outbursts of *catatonic* patients. Among paranoiacs—to which category I am supposed to belong—they seem to be very unusual:

[120] I need hardly say that "to reveal" is here used in a sense somewhat different from its ordinary meaning. Usually when one speaks of divine revelations in religious tradition, one thinks of God manifesting Himself *deliberately* to certain human beings chosen by Him especially to teach divine matters and to spread the insight thus gained among mankind. This is not so in my case. God does not reveal Himself to me deliberately; the knowledge of His existence and His powers declares itself to me *independent of His will and for no particular purpose* through miracles which He enacts on me and through the voices in which He speaks to me. It is true that in the first years of my contact with God some information was imparted to me (partly in words, partly in the form of visions) apparently serving as instruction, but mainly to give me directives for my own behaviour (compare Chapter XIII of the Memoirs). For some years such didactic communications have almost completely ceased; only very occasionally are there vision-like events in dreams which give the impression of a purposeful instruction. But I cannot decide whether this is actually the case or whether it is only due to my nerves playing on me.

Dr. Weber, in his report of 5th April 1902, could only mention one single case where apparently something similar was observed in a paranoiac;

(2) the closing of my eyes by miracles and their subsequent opening for a single moment (at sight); of which it would be easy to determine that neither my own will nor weakness of my muscles is in any way concerned;

(3) the quite abnormal and apparently completely motiveless acceleration of breathing which occurs even when I am perfectly quiet, lying in bed or on the couch, etc.;

(4) the presence of nerves of voluptuousness over my whole body which I must maintain are present despite contradictory statements in Dr. Weber's report of 5th April 1902, as the subjective feelings caused by them—particularly when softly pressed—belong
p. 356 to the most definite experiences which I have daily and hourly, and as the periodic swelling of my bosom could hardly be missed by a thorough examination. At regular intervals, that is to say at every reapproach of the rays which leads to their union, voluptuousness streams so mightily into me, that my mouth is filled with a sweet taste; while lying in bed it would require a very special effort on my part to ward off this feeling of voluptuousness, as it would in a female person expecting an embrace.

Of happenings to inanimate objects I only wish to refer again to two: the snapping of my piano strings and what happens to my musical instrument (symphonion).

Snapping of piano strings is not as frequent as before, but happened nevertheless at least half a dozen times every year. That the reason cannot lie in " my careless treatment of the instrument ", as Dr. Weber in his report of 5th April 1902 suggests, seems perfectly obvious. One may compare my previous discussions in Chapter XII of the Memoirs and number I of my grounds of appeal (Addendum C.) What I said there about the impossibility of *piano strings snapping* through heavy hitting on the *keys* will, I believe, be credited by every expert.

I bought the above-mentioned symphonion and simple musical clocks, mouth organs and suchlike in order to drown the talk of the voices which was sometimes hard to bear, and so procure at least temporary rest. As often as I use the symphonion it becomes
p. 357 the object of miracles and so-called " interferences " (compare Chapter X of the Memoirs) are practised on it and extra sounds, buzzing noises and repeated heavy knocking are produced in the instrument.

I frequently took the opportunity to let the doctors and clergymen of the Asylum witness these events. They cannot be due to a peculiarity of *my own* musical instrument because exactly the *same* happens to musical machines in restaurants, etc., when these are wound up in my presence by third persons or I set them in motion myself by inserting a coin. Unfortunately I am almost always alone when I go for walks, and not accompanied by a scientifically trained observer; I could frequently have convinced such a person of the correctness of my statement. Yet I would not like to say definitely whether these miracles on musical machines will be observable in the future, because the objects of the miracles continually change. Nevertheless I hope that in future there will be occasion to prove the striking events on my symphonion and other musical instruments. The (simple) musical clock which I previously used was by the way long ago made unusable by miracles; its defective condition can still be seen.

I can do no more than *offer my person as object of scientific observation for the judgment of experts.* My *main motive in publishing this book* is to invite this. Short of this I can only hope that at some future time such peculiarities of my nervous system will be p. 358
discovered by *dissection of my body,* which will provide stringent proof. I am informed that it is extremely difficult to make such observations on the living body.

Finally a few more remarks about *God's egoism,* which I mentioned in different places in the Memoirs (compare end of Chapter V, Chapter X, footnote 66). I have no doubt that God, in His relation to me, is ruled by egoism. This might be calculated to confuse religious feelings as God Himself would then not be the ideal Being of absolute love and morality, as most religions imagine. But, considered in the right light, this does not detract from God's grandeur and sublimity, which are intrinsically His and which must be faithfully acknowledged by all human beings.

Egoism, particularly in the form of the instinct of self-preservation, which at times demands the sacrifice of other beings for one's own existence, *is a necessary quality of all living beings*; individuals cannot do without it, if they are not themselves to perish; in itself it therefore does not appear reprehensible. *God is a living Being* and would Himself have to be ruled by egoistic motives, if other living beings existed who could endanger Him or in some way be

detrimental to His interests. *In circumstances in accordance with the Order of the World there could not be, nor indeed were there, such beings next to God;* this *is the only reason* why the question of God's egoism could not arise as long as these circumstances remained in unadulterated purity. But in my case different circumstances
p. 359 have set in as an exception; since God by tolerating tested souls—probably in connection with occurrences of a soul-murder-like character—had tied Himself to a single human being by whom He had to let Himself be attracted, albeit unwillingly, the conditions for egoistic actions were given. These egoistic actions have been practised against me for years with the utmost cruelty and disregard as only a beast deals with its prey. But success could not be permanent, because God brought Himself into conflict with the Order of the World, that is to say into conflict with His own Being and His own powers (compare Chapter V of the Memoirs, footnote 35). Consequently, as I firmly believe, this irregular state of affairs will be finally liquidated at my death at the latest. In the meantime I find immense consolation and encouragement in the knowledge that God's hostile opposition to me continues to lose in virulence and the struggle against me becomes increasingly conciliatory, perhaps finally to end in complete solidarity. This (as already mentioned in Chapter XIII of the Memoirs) is the natural sequel of the steadily increasing soul-voluptuousness of my body. Soul-voluptuousness lessens the antipathy to being attracted; this is because one regains in my body after a short interval, that which had to be relinquished owing to the attraction: namely the state of Blessedness or soul-voluptuousness, in other words complete well-being of the nerves condemned to find their end in my body. This also shortens the periodicity of drawing nearer and appears to me to allow God to recognize at ever shorter intervals that " forsaking me ", " destruction of my reason ", etc. must come to nothing; therefore eventually it is only a question of making life as bearable as possible for both
p. 360 parties in the emergency which has arisen because of attraction. I myself have never been an *adversary of God,* even if from time to time I had to mock God aloud for reasons given; it would be absurd for a human who once acknowledged God to say such a thing of himself.

The whole development therefore appears as a *glorious triumph for the Order of the World,* in which I think I can ascribe to myself a modest part. If anywhere, then the beautiful sentence applies to the Order of the World, that all legitimate interests are in harmony.

APPENDIX

p. 361

IN WHAT CIRCUMSTANCES CAN A PERSON CONSIDERED INSANE BE DETAINED IN AN ASYLUM AGAINST HIS DECLARED WILL?[121] p. 363

The answer to the above question offers not inconsiderable difficulties as only a few or no explicit regulations exist in law, and what can be described as existing law must mainly be derived from general principles.

In illustration I will start with a practical example. My neighbour, Mr. N., complains incessantly about unlawful deprivation of his liberty, calls for the Public Prosecutor and the Mayor, and believes he can expect them to intervene against the administration of the Asylum for depriving him of his liberty.

Objectively, of course, the case is one of confinement in the sense of § 239 Str. G.B. However, it is a criminal offence only if the confinement is unlawful; hence, as Oppenhof states in his commentary—the only work on criminal law within my reach at the moment—deprivations of liberty in the course of exercising educational, correctional or domestic rights, or a duty as for instance professional, official or supervisory are excluded. A Public Prosecutor or an examining magistrate who keeps in provisional custody or commits for trial a person charged or accused in accordance with the regulations of the law, and equally the authorities of a prison executing a penalty of imprisonment p. 364
inflicted by a Court, naturally do not act unlawfully. The same applies to the administration of a Public Asylum for the Insane, if within its competence it orders the confinement of a person handed over to the Asylum or arranges for further limitations of such a person's liberty. Before discussing the extent and limits of this competence it will first be discussed how this applies to Private Establishments for the Insane.

The admission of a person to a Private Establishment for the Insane and his stay therein is dependent on such a person's expressly or implicitly declared will, unless he is held in tutelage; the request of relatives may in certain circumstances be of practical value to protect the administration of the Asylum against the reproach of acting arbitrarily; in itself it is of no legal significance.

[121] This essay was written early 1900, at the time of my complete isolation from the outside world, and therefore almost totally without the opportunity of using literary sources.

On the other hand one can maintain that if somebody allows himself to be admitted to a Private Asylum, he thereby submits from the beginning to limitations of his liberty such as result from the regulations of the establishment or from necessary measures taken by the chief physician in the exercise of his duties for the physical and mental well-being of the patient. Limitation of possible excursions, the allotment of certain rooms in the Asylum, etc., must be accepted by the person admitted without his being able to complain of unlawful deprivation of liberty even if his opposition is met by force. Likewise, immediate discharge cannot be demanded at the instance of any sudden impulse (*ad nutum*); the Director of the Asylum would be in his right to ignore such demands, if in his professional opinion he believes them to be only *inconsistencies of will* due to the patient's morbid frame of mind, which can be presumed not to be lasting. It is different, however, if
p. 365 a patient *not kept under tutelage* declares his will to be discharged from the Asylum *persistently and in a manner testifying his careful consideration*, for instance for the purpose of being transferred to another Asylum or being nursed by his family. The mere subjective opinion of the chief physician that the patient would be better left in his hands than anywhere else, would not entitle the former to restrict the patient in any way in the choice of his future residence. An exception would only arise if the patient's mental state had assumed a character which would make his being at liberty dangerous either to himself or others, in particular when suicide is suspected. In this case the chief physician would be entitled, possibly with the consent of the patient's relatives, to make preparations for his transfer to a Public Asylum, and to have the patient supervised till then against his will in the Asylum and during the transfer without laying himself open to the charge of unlawful deprivation of liberty. He exercises police functions, as an executive organ of the Public Authorities and is thus exempt from all criminal responsibility, as in § 127 Str. Pr. O. in the case of somebody who arrests a person caught in a criminal act.[122]

[122] This is also the reason—albeit not the only one—why the undertaking of "Private Lunatic Asylums" has been made dependent on a concession of the superior Administrative Authority in §30 of the Trade Regulations. In view of the actual power which must be invested in the Directors of such Asylums over the person of the patient, the State deems it necessary that only persons be entrusted with keeping such establishments, whose reliability is beyond doubt. The granting of such a concession, however, has not the significance of giving to the Directors of Private Asylums for the Insane the capacity of *permanent* organs of the security police, in other words they are not endowed *permanently* with the power of official authority.

The *final* custody of insane persons who might be a danger to themselves or others, is incumbent on the *Public Asylums.* Regulations about their establishment were issued for the Kingdom of Saxony in a *Directive* for the Care in a Country Asylum of Insane Persons[123] published in the form of an extract by the decree of 31st July 1893 (G.-u.V.-Bl. p. 157 ff.) But this Directive does not contain the essential *sedes materiae* in respect of the question in what conditions a person can be brought to, or kept in, a Public Asylum against his declared will. The Judge in a criminal Court could not immediately find from the Directive—although some of its stipulations may be supportive—the norm according to which to decide the question whether illegal deprivation of liberty exists. The Directive contains stipulations about the establishment and the province of respective Asylums, regulates the conditions of admission and transfer to them, obviously considers admission mainly from the point of view of a *benefit* to the person admitted (compare § 1 under 4)[124], safeguards in particular the fiscal interest in securing the maintenance costs and can therefore only be considered as a compilation of *service instructions* for Asylum officials, which has no direct legal power. To answer the question raised at the beginning, one has therefore to revert to general principles.

p. 366

p. 367

From this point of view the accommodation and maintenance of insane persons in institutions established for that purpose is part of the State's task of general care for the well-being and safety of its subjects. The State—or by delegation the municipality—provides opportunity for intellectual education through schools and other higher educational institutes, cares in special schools for the deaf and dumb, the blind, etc., for handicapped persons to obtain adequate education; keeps hospitals and infirmaries for the sick and alms-houses for needy persons, etc.; likewise the State has founded recently[125] Public Asylums with the object of medical treatment, supervision and maintenance of the insane. *The use of all such welfare institutions is however as a rule not forced upon a person;* on the contrary the persons concerned or their legal representatives are free in their choice as to whether or not they want to make use of them—

[123] In the meantime superseded by the new Directive of 1st March 1902 (G-u. V.-Bl. p. 39 ff).

[124] In the Directive of 1st March 1902, § 2.

[125] In earlier centuries, as far as I know, the insane were simply put into prisons or similar places as "demoniacs" without any question of treatment. As I have no access to literary sources in my present abode I might be mistaken. It should be easy, however, for the specialist to ascertain a possible error. It would seem according to Kraepelin, Psychiatrie, 4th Edition, 1893, p. 230 ff. that what has been said in the text is correct in its essentials (added in February 1901.)

unless special laws order something different, as for instance compulsory education. The same would apply also to Public Asylums, if apart from the furtherance of public welfare their work were not in many cases simultaneously a matter for the security police.

p. 368 One must make a distinction therefore between insane persons whose detention *is in the public interest* and those to whom this does not apply. To the first class belong all those insane persons *who through their illness could become dangerous either to themselves or others,* particularly cases of raving madness or melancholia, the latter particularly through the possibility of suicide. In general one has to count amongst the same category persons who are admitted to the Country *Home* at Colditz according to the regulation of 30th July 1893 under 2[126], namely incurable cases where patients are "deeply demented and abhorrent to look at". To the second class belong all the other cases of mental illness—of a severe or lighter character, showing perhaps only a few delusions—of whom it *cannot* be said that being at liberty would be dangerous either to themselves or others. Mental illnesses of the latter kind I would like to designate as cases of *harmless insanity* for the purpose of their position in *administrative law*—irrespective of how these diseases are classified *by scientific psychiatry*[127].

p. 369 To detain mental patients of the first category—they will for short be called *dangerous mental patients* in the following—even against their will in special Asylums, is not only the right but also the obligation of the State from the point of view of exercising security police power.

The legal right for the deprivation of liberty in a special case is therefore not different from a case in which, for example, the police detain in custody a person found drunk in the street until he is sober. It is irrelevant for the legal right depriving a person of his liberty whether it is a temporary state as in the case of drunkenness, or whether as in cases of mental derangement these states persist

[126] In the Directive of 1st March, 1902, § 2, part 2, in conjunction with Appendix 1 under B (G.V.BI.p. 38 and 64).

[127] The writer of this essay counts himself amongst the harmless mental patients in the sense described above; it is said of him that he is possessed by religious hallucinations, whereas in his own opinion these contain objective truth unrecognizable for other people. He trusts in particular to have proved with this essay that cases do in fact exist, in which clarity of logical and particularly juristical thinking is unimpaired by the presumed hallucinations, so that one cannot maintain the existence of a morbid mental derangement excluding free determination of will *in the direction of reasonable action* in the sense of § 104[2] of the German B.G.B., nor an inability to look after his own affairs in the sense of § 6 of that law.

for some time. Similar further legal considerations therefore
apply to both cases from a legal point of view. Thus, of course, the
admissibility of deprivation of liberty has to be decided by the
competent authority exercising its duties, and not according to the
ideas of the person concerned. After all it is a daily occurrence that
a drunkard assures the arresting policeman that he is totally sober.
The policeman nevertheless has the right to detain him if he is
dutifully convinced of the contrary. Similarly most mental patients
will maintain that their mental health is in no way disturbed, that
they are "unlawfully deprived of their liberty", and that there is no
danger either for them or others in the case of their discharge. But
the Director of a Public Asylum is perfectly justified all the same in p. 370
detaining them in the Asylum, even to limit their freedom still
further, whenever he believes from his scientific experience and the
nature of the particular illness that such a danger exists despite
protests to the contrary. Further, the duration for which deprivation of liberty is admissible is dependent on the persistence of its
lawful reason. The drunken person must be discharged by the
police authorities as soon as his drunkenness has passed, unless an
additional reason exists for detaining him. In the same way
discharge cannot be denied a person admitted to a Public Asylum or
his legal representative once the illness is cured or has lost the
particular character which made the patient's liberty a danger to
himself and others.

As to the second category, the *harmless* mental patients in the
above sense, no public interest in their detention arises. If they are
patients in a Public Asylum, the Asylum's administration is on the
whole in the same legal position to them as the Director of a Private
Asylum discussed above. If tutelage exists a declaration of an insane
person's intent is legally void, particularly his request to be discharged from the Asylum. For the personal care of the ward is
vested in the guardian, also in the case of persons of age, within the
limits of the purpose of this guardianship (§ 1901 in conjunction with
§§ 1897 and 1858, German B.G.B.). The formally superseded regu- p. 371
lation under II, § 5 of the law of 20th February 1882 ("the guardians
of persons placed under tutelage because of insanity and of the persons named under §§ 2 to 4 are entrusted to prevent their wards from
damaging themselves or others, and if necessary to place them into
an Asylum") has still materially and essentially to be regarded
as valid law irrespective of the change in law as given above.

If therefore the guardian or the judicial authority deems
admission of a mental patient to a Public Asylum necessary, the

insane patient himself is not heard when expressing the reverse request. But if the patient is not under tutelage or if this is later rescinded, the administration of the Asylum must respect *in the case of a harmless mental illness* the persistently pronounced will of a mental patient to be discharged from the Asylum as coming from a person capable of managing his own affairs, just like the Director of a Private Asylum as described above. In particular it cannot ignore the right of a mental patient to change his residence, particularly to be transferred to another Asylum, even to forego medical treatment altogether, on the assumption that from a medical point of view it has better insight into what is in the patient's real interests. Were one to offend against this, the taking away of liberty would indeed assume the character of an unlawful deprivation of liberty Towards harmless mental patients the Director of a Public Asylum is after all not an organ of the security police with authoritative power, but essentially only a medical adviser; *on the question of deprivation of liberty* his relation to his patients is in no way different from that of any private practitioner towards his patients.

p. 372 If one compares the conclusions reached above with the regulations of the Directive of 1893, one must not expect to find in the various regulations an express confirmation of these conclusions which have been drawn from general principles. The Directive itself as stated above is not intended to regulate the question of the conditions in which a deprivation of liberty by detention in an Asylum against the will of the patient is permitted. In any case considering the authoritative source of the Directive, it is of interest to show that nothing is contained in the Directive which would make the above principles appear doubtful. Particularly important are the regulations concerning the discharge or granting of leave in § 10 of the Directive[128]. These distinguish between cases in which discharge of a patient can be decided upon by the administration of the Asylum and those where a decision of the Ministry of the Interior must be obtained. When in § 10 under 1[129] it is stated, that the discharge *can* take place on the decision of the administration of the Asylum in the cases under *a*, *b* and *c*, this, of course, does not amount to the exclusion of an *obligation* on the Asylum's administration in certain circumstances. Such an obligation exists particularly in the case under *c*. The " competent party " who

[128] In the Directive of 1902, § 42.

[129] In the Directive of 1902, § 42, under 1, *a* to *c*, the " can take place ' has been altered to " has to be ordered ".

can request discharge is, according to circumstances, either the patient himself (if capable of managing his own affairs) or his legal representative (the parental authority, the guardian or the judicial authority) : "Doubts which the Asylum's administration may p. 373
entertain about a discharge requested from a competent party", must be founded on considerations arising from security police interests, that is to say they can only be asserted if the patient in the opinion of the Asylum's administration is considered a "dangerous mental patient" in the above-discussed sense (compare also §1 under 2 of the Directive[130]).

But if the Asylum's administration has to admit that it is not a case of that kind, but one of a *harmless mental illness*, the request must be allowed, even if in their personal opinion retention in the Asylum appears advisable "for the purpose of cure or improvement of the patient's state" (§ 1, Section 2 of the Directive[131]). Should the administration force this opinion on the patient (capable of managing his affairs) himself or on his legal representatives, whether persons or bodies, they would transgress the limits of their competence, in other words be guilty of unlawful deprivation of liberty.

The purpose of § 10, 2 of the Directive [132] seems to be to provide the Ministry of the Interior with the opportunity to forestall possible miscarriages to which the Asylum's administration might be inclined. It is of course in the public interest that the confidence in the regular administration of Public Asylums should nowhere be shaken, and to avoid a case arising in practice of criminal proceedings being brought against the Director of a Public Asylum for unlawful deprivation of liberty, or even a lawsuit for damages on these grounds.

Postscript p. 374

Only subsequently was the author's attention drawn to the Ministerial decree of 13th May 1894 regarding the accommodation of patients in Private Asylums (G.u.V.BI.p. 139 ff.) which were until then unknown to him as he himself has lived in Asylums since the end of 1893. In his opinion nothing is contained in the Ministerial decree which contradicts the opinions developed in the present essay. In any case actual force of law does not appertain

[130] In the Directive of 1902, § 1, paragraph 3.

[131] In the Directive of 1902, § 1 seems to be slightly altered for editorial reasons only.

[132] In the Directive of 1902 § 42, under 2c.

to it, and hence in a given case it is not binding *for the judge* (apart from the regulation about punishment under 9). It is obviously not intended to give greater powers with respect to deprivation of liberty to the Directors of Private Asylums than they have according to general principles; on the contrary it adds in this respect to the *obligations* arising from the general principles further (instructional) obligations, which may lead offending Directors of Asylums to a *police penalty* (applying number 9 of the regulation) and if necessary to the withdrawal of their concession. The decisive point by which the *Judge* must be guided *in the case of a possible indictment for deprivation of liberty* will always be, whether and in how far the Director of an Asylum for the Insane has to be considered *simultaneously as an official organ exercising the powers of the security police* with respect to detaining dangerous insane patients. This is the case with Directors of Public Asylums—they have *authoritative powers* much as on the railways certain officials exercise the powers of railway police, but not with the
p. 375 Directors of Private Asylums (apart from the exception of temporary care until the transfer of a patient to a Public Asylum).

Second Postscript

In the meantime the Ministerial decree of 30th May 1894 has again been superseded by another decree, concerning the admission of patients in Private Asylums of 9th August 1900 (G.u.V.BI.p. 887 ff.) and the Directive of 31st July 1893 by the Directive for the admission to a Country Asylum for the Insane of 1st March 1902 (G.u.V.BI.p. 39 ff.).

This might imply some modification *for Saxony* of what has been said in the previous essay; but these modifications are certainly not of fundamental importance. Above all it must be stressed repeatedly, that the mentioned regulations and decrees are not acts of the legislature. Therefore if ever a Court of Justice has to deal with a question of unlawful deprivation of liberty, whether in civil or criminal law, the regulations in the recent decrees and directive could in any case not be considered decisive *as such* and *by themselves*. Where for instance the decree of 9th August 1900 § 6 states with respect to so-called "*voluntary boarders*" in a Private Asylum (that is, patients who have entered the Asylum of their own free will) that the discharge of a voluntary boarder has to be allowed whether requested by himself or his legal representative "*in every case without delay*", it can certainly not be assumed that
p. 376 every delay of his release would constitute an unlawful deprivation

of liberty, on which a responsibility according to civil or criminal law of the Asylum's Director can be founded. One must keep in mind that the distinction between a patient merely "mentally ill" and an "insane patient" is an extremely difficult one and that these forms of illness shade into one another in almost imperceptible transitions.

It can therefore easily happen that the state of a "mentally ill person", who of his own free will entered a Private Asylum as "voluntary boarder" undergoes such changes during his stay in the Asylum, that his immediate discharge (because of suicidal intent) would be dangerous for the patient himself. The regulation § 5 Part 2 of the decree of 9th August 1900 cannot be adduced in such a case, because it deals only with "*publicly* dangerous" mental patients or imbeciles. Can then a certain delay of the discharge (for the purpose of informing the police or the relatives in order to transfer the patient to a Public Asylum) be charged to the Director of a Private Asylum as an unlawful deprivation of liberty in all circumstances? It appears to me that one must be extremely cautious before answering this question in the affirmative.

ADDENDA

(OFFICIAL DOCUMENTS FROM THE PROCEEDINGS REGARDING RESCISSION OF TUTELAGE)

OI 128/01 at C.J.J. 64/99[2]. p. 379

Sonnenstein, 9th December 1899.

A. *MEDICAL EXPERT'S REPORT TO THE COURT*[133]

The retired *Senatspräsident* Daniel Paul Schreber, Doctor of Law, of Dresden, was admitted to this Country Asylum on 29th June 1894 for treatment and has been here ever since.

According to the formal certificate of Professor Flechsig of Leipzig issued for the transfer of the patient to this Asylum, President Schreber had already had a serious attack of hypochondria in 1884–1885; he recovered from it and was admitted for the second time to the University Psychiatric Clinic in Leipzig on p. 380 21st November 1893. At the beginning of his stay there he mentioned mostly hypochondriacal ideas, complained that he was suffering from softening of the brain, would soon die, etc.; but ideas of persecution soon appeared in the disease picture, based on hallucinations, which at first occurred sporadically, while simultaneously marked hyperaesthesia, great sensitivity to light and noise made their appearance. Later the visual and auditory hallucinations multiplied and, in conjunction with disturbances of common sensation, ruled his whole feeling and thinking; he thought he was dead and rotten, suffering from the plague, mentioned that all sorts of horrible manipulations were being performed on his body, and that he was going through more terrible states than anybody had ever known. All that for a holy purpose, as indeed he still maintains. These morbid ideas gained so great an influence over the patient that he was inaccessible to any other impression, sat for hours completely stiff and immobile

[133] The Reports *A*, *B* and *D* follow without any comment (apart from footnotes 134 and 135). The comparison with the corresponding accounts in the Memoirs and in my grounds for appeal will show immediately that the reports contain some *factual* mistakes, inexactitudes and misconceptions. But I have no doubt that the reason lies to some extent in unreliable reports furnished by third persons (attendants, etc.).

(hallucinatory stupor); at other times they tortured him so much that he wished for death, repeatedly made attempts at drowning himself in the bath and demanded the "cyanide destined for him". Gradually the delusions took on a mystical and religious character, he communicated directly with God, devils were playing their games with him, he saw "miracles", heard "holy music", and finally even believed that he was living in another world.

In this Asylum, to which President Schreber was transferred after a short stay in the private establishment of Dr. Pierson, he showed at first mainly the same picture as in Leipzig. This physically strong man, in whom frequent jerkings of the face musculature and marked tremor of the hands were noticeable, was at first completely inaccessible and shut off in himself, lay or stood immobile and stared with frightened eyes straight ahead of himself into space;
p. 381 he did not answer questions at all or only very briefly and protestingly; but clearly this rigid demeanour was far removed from indifference, rather the patient's whole state seemed tense, irritable, caused by inner uneasiness and there could be no doubt that he was continually influenced by vivid and painful hallucinations, which he elaborated in a delusional manner. In the same way the patient abruptly rejected every communication and continually demanded to be left alone, indeed even that the whole house be cleared because God's omnipotence was being obstructed by the presence of attendants and others, while he himself wanted "divine peace". For the same reason he refused nourishment so that he had to be forcibly fed, or only took a few light dishes, refusing meat completely, and it was only with great difficulty that he was gradually made to eat regularly again. At the same time he retained his stool apparently deliberately, as far as he possibly could; he was therefore even incontinent at times[134]. Similarly for a long time it was impossible to persuade him to any activity such as reading, which he rejected because every word he read was being shouted out through the whole world. He frequently complained that there was a "loss of rays", that the doctor had "negligently emitted rays", without explaining more closely what he meant.

In November 1894 the patient's stiff posture loosened a little, he came out of himself more, became more mobile, started to speak coherently although in an abrupt and somewhat staccato manner; there now emerged undisguised, the fantastic delusional elabora-

[134] These reported soilings find their true explanation in my statements at the end of Chapter XVI of the Memoirs.

tion of his continual hallucinations; he felt himself adversely influenced by certain persons previously known to him (Flechsig, p. 382
v. W. . .), whom he believed to be present here, thought that the world had been changed by them, God's omnipotence destroyed, he himself struck by their curses; maintained that they pulled thoughts out of his body and suchlike. While he continued to refuse to read, he sometimes wrote stenographic signs on paper, occupied himself occasionally with a game of patience, and appeared to give a little more attention to events in his environment.

Very gradually the patient's excitement mounted further, disturbed his, up till then, moderate sleep and manifested itself externally, particularly by loud persistent laughter occurring to a certain extent in attacks (by day as well as by night), and by heavy hammering on the piano in a most disturbing manner. That this very striking behaviour had to be looked upon as a reaction to hallucinations, particularly to delusional ideas springing from them, became evident from some of the patient's statements, such as that the world had come to an end, that everything he saw round himself was only a sham, he himself and the persons around him only lifeless shadows. At the same time he still had hypochondriacal ideas, mentioned among others that his body was completely changed, one lung had disappeared altogether, and he could hardly breathe sufficiently to remain alive.

Subsequently, the nights in particular became increasingly restless, while simultaneously a change occurred in him in so far as the earlier continuously stiff rejecting and negativistic attitude gave place, so to speak, to a certain dualism. On the one hand the reaction against the hallucinations became increasingly noisy and intense, in the garden the patient used to stand for a long time motionless in one place, staring into the sun, at the same time grimacing in an extraordinary way or bellowing very loudly at the sun with threats and imprecations, usually repeating endlessly one and the same phrase, shouting at her, that she was afraid of him, and that she had to hide from him the *Senatspräsident* Schreber, and also called himself Ormuzd. Or he raved in his room to such p. 383
an extent, harangued for some time the "soul-murderer" Flechsig, repeated endlessly "little Flechsig", putting heavy accent on the first word, or shouted abuse and suchlike out of his window with such tremendous force even at night, that the townspeople gathered and complained of the disturbance. On the other hand he was in many respects more polite and accessible towards the doctors and other persons, even if they surprised him during such

noisy scenes, even answered simple questions about his condition, etc., though in a somewhat reserved and partronising manner, said nothing of his troubles and was able to control himself for a little while quite well; he also started to read, play chess and piano as he had done before.

In the meantime the nightly scenes became increasingly noisy unchecked by the sleeping drugs given in ever increasing doses, so that, as the medicines could not be increased without fear of causing harm, and as the whole department suffered considerably through the continual nightly disturbances, one was forced in June 1896 to segregate the patient at night in a more isolated room and carry this *out for a number of months.*[135] The patient, of course, was somewhat irritated by this, but permitted it without marked resistance, apparently realizing that his actions were pathological and causing extraordinary almost unbearable annoyance to his environment.

For some time the physical behaviour of the patient showed only little change, the peculiar very loud forced laughter and the p. 384 monotonous uttering in endless repetition of incomprehensible abusive language (for instance "the sun is a whore", and suchlike), which served apparently to a certain extent as counter-action against the hallucinations and disturbances of feeling (pain in the back, etc.), continued as before, sleep remained very deficient but nourishment was taken more adequately and he was gaining weight; even then there were early signs of a peculiar delusion which developed later: the patient was frequently found in his room half undressed, declared that he already had feminine breasts, liked to occupy himself by looking at pictures of naked women, even drew them and had his moustache removed.

However, perhaps since the spring of 1897 a change was noticed in the patient; he entered into a lively correspondence with his wife and other relatives; and it must be admitted that the letters were correctly and deftly written, and hardly showed anything pathological, but rather a certain insight, when for instance he revealed that he had been very frightened, had not been able to get himself to do anything, but that things were now much better and he was grateful to be able to find so much stimulating conversation, etc., while nevertheless the former insulting, laughing and shouting continued, and nightly isolation could not be discontinued.

Even while the patient continued to show himself little inclined to more serious conversation, and soon became restless and impatient

[135] As regards the duration, compare pages 197, 198, 201 (two and a half years).

when this was attempted, started to grimace, utter peculiar short interjections and one could see that he wished the conversation quickly finished, nevertheless the patient's occupations became more varied and more continuous; frequently it was difficult to understand how he could achieve sufficient peace and concentration p. 385
for such intellectual work during the continuous obviously intensive hallucinatory burden, to talk about the most varied matters in a relevant manner and moreover to control himself in a way which at times hid his illness. Gradually even the nightly noisy outbursts diminished, so that the patient could again use his usual bedroom and remain in it with only little support from drugs.

Without going further into all the details of the course of his illness, attention is drawn to the way in which from the early more acute psychosis which influenced all psychic processes and which could be called hallucinatory insanity, the paranoid form of illness became more and more marked, crystallized out so to speak, into its present picture.

This kind of illness is, as is well known, characterized by the fact that next to a more or less fixed elaborate delusional system there is complete possession of mental faculties and orientation, formal logic is retained, marked affective reactions are missing, neither intelligence nor memory are particularly affected and the conception and judgment of indifferent matters, that is to say matters far removed from the delusional ideas, appear not to be particularly affected, although naturally because of the unity of all psychic events they are not untouched by them.

Thus President Schreber now appears neither confused, nor psychically inhibited, nor markedly affected in his intelligence, apart from the psychomotor symptoms which stand out clearly as pathological even to the casual observer: he is circumspect, his memory excellent, he commands a great deal of knowledge, not only in matters of law but in many other fields, and is able to p. 386
reproduce it in an orderly manner, he is interested in political, scientific and artistic events, etc., and occupies himself with them continuously (although recently he seems to have been distracted from them a little more again), and little would be noticeable in these directions to an observer not informed of his total state. Nevertheless, the patient is filled with pathological ideas, which are woven into a complete system, more or less fixed, and not amenable to correction by objective evidence and judgment of circumstances as they really are; the latter still less so as hallucinatory and delusory processes continue to be of importance to him and

hinder normal evaluation of sensory impressions. As a rule the patient does not mention these pathological ideas or only hints at them, but it is evident how much he is occupied by them, partly from some of his writings (extracts of some are added), partly it is easily seen from his whole bearing.

The patient's delusional system amounts to this: he is called to redeem the world and to bring back to mankind the lost state ot Blessedness. He maintains he has been given this task by direct divine inspiration, similar to that taught by the prophets; he maintains that nerves in a state of excitation, as his have been for a long time, have the property of attracting God, but it is a question of things which are either not at all expressible in human language or only with great difficulty, because he maintains they lie outside all human experience and have only been revealed to him. The most essential part of his mission of redemption is that it is necessary for him first of all to be *transformed into a woman.* Not, however, that he *wishes* to be transformed into a woman, it is much more
p. 387 a " must " according to the Order of the World, which he simply cannot escape, even though he would personally very much prefer to remain in his honourable manly position in life. But the beyond was not to be gained again for himself and the whole of mankind other than by this future transformation into a woman by way of divine miracle in the course of years or decades. He maintains that he is the exclusive object of divine miracles, and with it the most remarkable human being that ever lived on earth. For years at every hour and every minute he experiences these miracles in his body, has them confirmed also by voices that speak to him. He maintains that in the earlier years of his illness he suffered destruction of individual organs of his body, of a kind which would have brought death to every other human being, that he lived for a long time without stomach, without intestines, bladder, almost without lungs, with smashed ribs, torn gullet, that he had at times eaten part of his own larynx with his food, etc.; but divine miracles (" rays ") had always restored the destroyed organs, and therefore, as long as he remained a man, he was absolutely immortal. These threatening phenomena have long ago disappeared, and in their place his " femaleness " had come to the fore; it is a question of an evolutionary process which in all probability will take decades if not centuries for its completion and the end of which is unlikely to be witnessed by any human being now alive. He has the feeling that already masses of " female nerves " have been transferred into his body, from which through immediate fertilization by God new

human beings would come forth. Only then would he be able to die a natural death and have gained for himself as for all other human beings the state of Blessedness. In the meantime not only the sun but also the trees and the birds, which he thinks are something like "remains of previous human souls transformed by miracles", speak to him in human tones and everywhere around p. 388
him miracles are enacted.

It is not really necessary to go further into all the details of these delusional ideas, which by the way are developed and motivated with remarkable clarity and logical precision—the description given should suffice to give an idea of the content of the patient's delusional system and of his pathologically altered conception of the world, and it only remains to mention that also in the patient's behaviour, in the clean shaving of his face, in his pleasure in feminine toilet articles, in small feminine occupations, in the tendency to undress more or less and to look at himself in the mirror, to decorate himself with gay ribbons and bows, etc., in a feminine way, the pathological direction of his fantasy is manifested continually. At the same time the hallucinatory processes, as already mentioned above, continue in unaltered intensity and they as well as certain pathological motor impulses are shown by very noticeable involuntary automatic actions. As the patient himself declares, he is very frequently forced by day and night to utter "unnatural bellowing sounds"; he affirms that he cannot control them, that it is a matter of divine miracles, of supernatural happenings, which cannot be understood by other human beings, and these vociferations, based on physical compulsion, and very annoying also for his environment, occur so unremittingly that they disturb the patient's nightly rest in the most painful way and necessitate the use of sleeping drugs.

Only in one connection has the patient in recent times shown a change in attitude; whereas previously, perhaps because of a more marked feeling of being ill, he was to a certain extent resigned to his fate, although protesting here and there against some measures, did not give any external sign of wishing to change his situation p. 389
and appeared to have little interest in his legal and social affairs, he now demands energetically the lifting of his tutelage, wishes for freer movement and more active contact with the outer world and expects definitely to return to his home in the not too distant future. These plans exercise him a good deal and have apparently even pushed the mentioned pathological ideas to a certain extent into the background.

Whether President Schreber is to be considered deprived of the use of reason in terms of the law by virtue of the above exposition of his pathological mental state, which must be labelled paranoia, is a question for the Court to decide. If, however, what has been said gives the impression, far removed from medical opinion, that the patient is prevented by mental illness from understanding *all* events objectively and correctly, from judging them by circumstances as they really are, and from taking his decisions after unimpaired sensible consideration and with free will, then clearly in this case the existing hallucinations, the delusions connected with them and built up into a system, and the irresistible impulses which rule the patient, amount to a considerable degree of impairment and continue to do so.

There is no medical objection to President Schreber being examined by the Court.

The aforementioned is attested by the undersigned acting under his oath of office.

L.S. (Signed) Dr. Weber,
Superintendent of the Asylum,
Area Psychiatrist, Psychiatric
Adviser to the Court.

Sonnenstein, 28th November 1900. p. 390

B. *ASYLUM AND DISTRICT MEDICAL OFFICER'S REPORT*

The undersigned has delayed for so long furnishing a further report about the retired President Schreber's mental state because his psychic condition has not undergone any marked change since rendering the first report, and therefore one would have to repeat in the main the previous statements, unless new viewpoints for deciding the issue one way or the other could be found.

The undersigned believes to have found such in the writings which the patient commenced some months ago and which deal in the most detailed manner with the history of his illness of many years' duration, both in its external relations and in its inner development. These writings are to be given all the more weight because in general the patient is little inclined to reveal his pathological ideas to other persons, and further because these ideas are elaborated in so complicated and subtle a manner that he himself admits that rendering them by word of mouth is difficult. In fact the "Memoirs of my Nervous Illness" as the author calls his treatise, are not only valuable from the scientific medical point of view for assessing the total character of his illness, but they also afford ample support p. 391
of practical value for the understanding of the patient's behaviour. Because the "Memoirs" have become more bulky than was visualised, their completion has taken considerable time, and only a short time ago was a complete copy received by the undersigned.

Further, as in the present state of affairs emphasis should be placed not on clinical exposition of, and an opinion on the mental illness which is doubtless present, but on trying to answer the question whether the patient is incapable, owing to his illness, of looking after his affairs—in the broadest sense of this word—the undersigned wished to attempt to establish a number of definite facts on which the Judge would be able to base his judgment on this question. The undersigned wishes to emphasise again, as he did in his first report, that it should not be considered the province of the medical expert to give the final decision whether a person is capable in consequence of mental derangement of taking care of his own interests, is capable of acting in the sense of the law; but that his task should be confined to furnishing the competent authorities with a statement of the mental condition of a person in such a way that the authorities are enabled to draw their own conclusions.

If evidence is demanded of *actual* events which would prove that the person on whom an opinion is to be given is incapable owing to mental illness of managing his affairs, or as it is put in the resolution on the evidence, would by unreasonable actions endanger his life, his health, his property or any other of his
p. 392 interests in life were he given freedom to manage his affairs, it is obviously very difficult, in fact almost impossible, to furnish such factual evidence in respect of a person who for years has been interned in an asylum owing to his mental state and therefore can interfere only very little in the shaping of his outer circumstances by his own actions. If one is dealing with a mental patient who moves in the outer world and is in direct contact with his previous circumstances of life, then actual events will be established without difficulty in the way he carries out his job, in the way he manages his business affairs, in his family life, in social intercourse, his contact with authorities, etc., which provide a definite answer to the question whether the patient owing to his abnormal mental state acts inappropriately, unreasonably and wrongly. Matters are different in the case of a patient confined in an asylum. In the nature of things his life is ordered down to the smallest detail by the authorities of the Asylum, he does not come into contact with the unending manifold demands of life; how he would conduct himself if faced with them can only be surmised from his total state. The matter could be put to the test by exposing him temporarily to those demands and placing him outside the shelter of the Asylum. Indeed such tests are carried out in some cases—mostly only when it would not matter much if the patient did compromise himself—and indeed the undersigned believed that even in the present case this method should be employed to a limited extent. But this would have required a longer interval. Neither did President Schreber show inclination to move outside the Asylum until recently, nor could this be attempted without considerable concern owing to his conduct up till now. Only since contesting his
p. 393 tutelage was the patient prepared to move about more freely; the desire to move out of the confines of his inner life and to approach the outside world again had to be gradually encouraged in him. In consideration of many circumstances, particularly the

reasonable concern of his family, it has not been possible to extend the trials in this direction as much as was planned, and although taking meals regularly at the family table of the undersigned, taking part in social occasions, joining in excursions extending as far as Dresden to the home of his wife, the carrying out of small commissions in the town, afforded the desired occasions for observing the patient's behaviour in intercourse with the outside world; nevertheless until now definite convincing results one way or the other have not been obtained. The undersigned does not however think he should delay any longer furnishing the required report, but content himself with the observations so far made.

When one considers the course President Schreber's mental illness has taken, it is not necessary as things are at present to return to the earlier phases of his illness. Without doubt they have considerable importance for understanding the total picture of the pathological process, much as every natural phenomenon can only be fully understood if considered in the light of its development; further the manner in which the patient himself regards them is important. But for the solution of the present practical question these earlier stages of the illness are not as relevant as the actual state to which they have led in the course of time and which is now open to observation in its more or less ultimate form. In line p. 394
with the patient's originally rich gifts, his mental productivity and his wide education, the manifestations of his pathologically altered mind are not, as so frequently in otherwise similar cases, poor and monotonous and their connections easily surveyed: on the contrary they present a structure of ideas so fantastically elaborated and developed and so far removed from the usual trends of thought, that it is hardly possible to sketch them briefly without rendering their inner structure incomprehensible and impairing understanding of their specific meaning. For this reason and for another to be mentioned later, I consider it useful to give the Country Court the patient's "Memoirs" complete for their consideration, with the humble request to return them later, in the belief that from them the Judge will readily obtain a clear picture of the author's mental state without any further comment.

Clearly according to observations in previous phases of his illness the patient was completely unfit to act and not in a position to look after his affairs or even to give them any interest, and this is quite evident from the patient's own account. For a long time the patient was so absorbed in the pathological events of his mental

life, his conception of things was so exclusively determined by hallucinatory imaginings, he was so completely disorientated in time, place and person, reality had been replaced by such a vast completely fantastic and false world of imagination, his emotional life had been so far withdrawn from all natural events, his will-power was either so inhibited, constrained or employed so much in warding off the afflictions of his illness, his actions finally were
p. 395 so unreasonable and doubtful, both with regard to his own personal interests and to his relations with the outer world, that there could be no question of unimpaired self-determination or sensible reasoning, rather the patient was completely under the power of overwhelming pathological influences.

In the previous report it was detailed how President Schreber's acute insanity gradually passed into a chronic state, how out of the stormy tides of the hallucinatory insanity a sediment was, so to speak, deposited and fixed, and gave the illness the picture of paranoia. As the accompanying mighty affects gradually decreased and the hallucinatory experiences lost their confusing and directly overpowering influence, the patient was able to a certain extent to put up with them and gradually to find his way back to a more orderly mental life. He did not, however, realize and recognize the actual products of his altered perceptions and the combinations built up on them as pathological, nor could he rise above the subjectiveness of his views and reach a more objective judgment of events. He could not achieve this, because the hallucinations persisted and delusions continued to be built on them; but as the accompanying effects became less strong, and common sense and orientation returned, there occurred a certain split in the totality of his ideas; the persisting pathologically altered field of his mental life became more sharply demarcated from the rest, and although in the organic unity of all psychic events the latter fields cannot remain altogether intact and a transition of seemingly partial disturbances to the whole psychic function always occurs, nevertheless it happened in this case as it usually does in paranoia,
p. 396 that when the acute illness has run its course, certain areas of feeling and thinking appear little touched by the pathological changes. Intellectual capacity in particular is little impaired, formal association of ideas appears to proceed in a regular way, and judgment about matters and affairs far removed from the delusional ideas which are retained and knit into a closed system, are mainly unclouded and correct.

That with these *changes* in the character of the illness, the total state has undergone a real *improvement*, cannot be said without qualification, however much external appearances may seem to indicate it. One could even assume the contrary: as long as the acute signs of illness lasted one could hope for a favourable outcome of the illness, whereas now when one sees the fixed result of such a process, this hope must be abandoned. Also there is a total lack, as already stated, of the most important criterion of improvement or even recovery, namely the more or less clear insight into the pathological nature of previous events. President Schreber it is true leaves open whether this or that perception could be illusory; in the main however he adheres firmly to the reality of his delusional ideas and declares the most monstrous of the events described by him as facts.

The patient's complicated delusional system has its point of origin in a most singular conception of the nature of God.

> (An exposition of the "delusional system" follows in the form of a short extract from the Memoirs; this can be omitted here because the reader has the Memoirs at his disposal.)

It is evident from this short extract and more particularly from the p. 397
patient's own account, how much even now his whole thinking and feeling are still under the influence of delusions and hallucinations and to what extent they determine his actions, causing him to defend himself against some, and to surrender completely to others of the pathological events, and to what extent his whole way of regarding the world, his judgment about human beings and everyday affairs is determined by them. It only remains to ascertain in detail as far as possible how far and to what extent the patient's pathological state influences and rules him in his relations to the outer world and the demands of everyday life.

It must be repeated that the patient's, like so many paranoiacs' intelligence and formal logical associative thinking have not apparently suffered to any *considerable* extent; the patient is in command of a great many ideas and can discourse about them in orderly fashion; his circumspection is equally unimpaired. The undersigned has for nine months had the most thorough opportunity of discussing all sorts of subjects with President Schreber during daily meals at the family table. Whatever matters were discussed —naturally apart from his delusions—whether they touched on state administration and law, politics, art or literature, social life or anything else, in all Doctor Schreber showed keen interest, detailed knowledge, good memory and correct judgment, and in ethical matters as well an attitude which one can only agree with.

Equally he was well-behaved and amiable during light conservation with the ladies present and his humour was always tactful and decent; during the harmless table talk he never brought up
p. 398 anything which should not have been introduced there but during medical visits. One could not ignore, however, that even during meal times the patient often appeared preoccupied, his attention was distracted, and he did not fully take in what was going on around him, so that frequently he brought up some matter which had only just been discussed. This preoccupation was also evident from the patient's demeanour—he either stares rigidly in front of himself or moves restlessly in his chair, *grimaces* in a peculiar manner, clears his throat more or less loudly, touches his face and apparently tries to push his eyelids upwards, which in his opinion were " closed by miracles ", that is to say closed against his will. Obviously it often requires his greatest energy not to utter the " bellowing noises ", and as soon as the table is cleared while he is still on his way to his room one can hear his inarticulate sounds.

This distraction of attention by hallucinatory experiences and his noticeable reaction to them is disturbing also on other occasions. During excursions into the neighbourhood, while joining in some festive occasion, during a visit to the theatre, the patient was able to restrain *loud* outbursts, but that at times he felt very embarrassed could be seen from his distorted face, his humming, clearing his throat, short bursts of laughter and from his whole bearing; indeed even during a visit to his wife in Dresden he could not entirely repress the noises at table, so that a sign had to be given to the servant-girl not to take any notice; and although the visit lasted only a few hours he was strikingly keen to return to the Asylum.

But not only in social relations could the influence of his
p. 399 pathological experiences act disturbingly. In its reasons for placing the patient under tutelage the District Court in Dresden mentioned among others that the patient Schreber would be quite capable of presiding over difficult legal proceedings, etc. This however must be doubted—the patient himself says that he is prevented by the " interferences " (as he presumes purposely brought about) from applying himself for any length of time to any serious and difficult intellectual work; he mentioned himself during the Court hearing that he did not consider it feasible to continue practising his profession, because the miracles happening in him attempted to distract him. Thus an observer will gain the impression from

his behaviour that efforts requiring complete mental freedom and concentration such as the above are out of the question.

Outwardly most disturbing have been for a long time what the patient himself calls attacks of bellowing, that is to say the uttering of partly inarticulate sounds, partly threats and imprecations against imaginary disturbers of his well-being (Flechsig, etc.). These noisy outbursts occur completely automatically and in a compulsive manner against the patient's will. Though he is able to repress them, if not always at any rate for a time through lively speech, making music fortissimo, and some other tricks, they sound not only throughout the greater part of the day from his living room and in the garden, causing considerable annoyance to his environment, but even at night they can often be heard for hours, causing intolerable disturbance of peace and quiet in the whole department; he sometimes even shouts down into the town without regard. Recently especially these vociferations have become very noisy, and how the patient himself suffers thereby, how helpless and powerless he feels against these "miracles" and is forced to the most nonsensical counter-actions, can be seen from the enclosed letter. To such counter-measures belong, amongst p. 400
others, that the patient (probably in order to evoke the frequently mentioned soul-voluptuousness) moves about his room half naked, stands in front of the mirror in a very low-cut vest decorated with gay ribbons, gazing at what he believes his female bosom. He exposes himself to colds by this behaviour (earlier on he also stuck his bare legs out of the window), the consequences of which he then attributes to miracles. He has, by the way, no intention of damaging himself as he also no longer thinks of suicide, because he believes that even the most serious injuries to his body cannot affect him.

It is the patient's opinion that these attacks of bellowing might improve after eventual discharge from the Asylum; but in any case he thinks he can avoid the resulting disturbances of peace and quiet which would not be tolerated in a house with other inhabitants, by finding an isolated dwelling in a garden. But as his first statement is naturally illusory, so it is equally striking that the patient in his morbid egoism does not even consider how his wife would have to suffer from all this; in fact married life with him would be almost impossible for her; not to mention the fact that he considers the nuisance caused to his present environment completely irrelevant and complains only of *his own* sufferings.

The ill-effect of the illness on marital relations is according to

his wife's information also noticeable in other ways. Earlier on the patient had offered his wife a possible divorce in view of his expected unmanning; even now when she demurs and contradicts his ideas and behaviour, he is quick to hint that she could leave him
p. 401 if she wished. Therefore in this respect also one must not overlook the impact of the pathological process.

Whether the patient, having regained his independence as he desires, could pay enough attention to his financial affairs and would always live within his means, can hardly be anticipated with certainty, because naturally for a long time he has had no opportunity to act independently in any important financial matter. As far as observations have been made in this direction, the patient has neither shown particular parsimony nor a tendency to squander, in fact while his requirements were satisfied he never enquired further about the monetary aspect, whereas he dealt with safeguarding his family's copyright in his father's book in an altogether professional manner as far as one can see. But in the face of his grand mission, pecuniary interests naturally recede into the background, and it must be regarded as doubtful how far his striving for fulfilment of his pathological wishes and hopes for the future, as expressed at the end of his Memoirs, and the dependence of his well-being on certain conditions, would lead him into material expenses far beyond his means.

The most important moment in judging the capacity of the patient to look after his affairs is and remains the fact that he lacks insight into the pathological nature of the hallucinations and ideas which influence him; what objectively are delusions and hallucinations are to him unassailable truth and adequate motive for action. It follows from this that the patient's decisions at a given moment are quite unpredictable; he may follow and turn into action what his relatively intact mental powers dictate or
p. 402 he may act under the compulsion of his pathological mental processes. In this connection I wish to draw particular attention to a very pregnant example and for this reason also I enclose the patient's "Memoirs". It is understandable that the patient felt the urge to describe the history of his latter years, to lay down his observations and sufferings in writing and to put them before those who have in this or that matter a lawful interest in the shape of his fate. But the patient harbours the urgent desire to have his "Memoirs" (as presented here) printed and made available to the widest circles and he is therefore negotiating with a publisher —until now of course without success. When one looks at the

content of his writings, and takes into consideration the abundance of indiscretions relating to himself and others contained in them, the unembarrassed detailing of the most doubtful and aesthetically impossible situations and events, the use of the most offensive vulgar words, etc., one finds it quite incomprehensible that a man otherwise tactful and of fine feeling could propose an action which would compromise him so severely in the eyes of the public, were not his whole attitude to life pathological, and he unable to see things in their proper perspective, and if the tremendous over-valuation of his own person caused by lack of insight into his illness had not clouded his appreciation of the limitations imposed on man by society.

In conjunction with the enclosures I can confine myself to what has been said above. The factual material contained therein, although for reasons given not complete, is nevertheless on the whole sufficient and reflects the state of affairs so clearly that it affords the Judge, in my opinion, the necessary basis for a judgment p. 403
as to whether and to what degree the remaining delusions and hallucinations which have been worked into a system, influence the free self-determination of President Schreber, lead to a compulsion of thoughts, wishes and actions, influence him decisively in his mood and demeanour, and whether the present mental illness is sufficient in extent and severity to prevent the patient from looking after his affairs in the widest sense.

Dr. Weber,
Superintendent of the Asylum,
Area Psychiatrist, Psychiatric
Adviser to the Court.

C. *GROUNDS OF APPEAL* p. 440

I give the following as grounds for the appeal which I have lodged:

I. CONCERNING THE EXPOSITION OF THE FACTS IN THE JUDGMENT AGAINST WHICH I APPEAL.

The facts laid down in the judgment against which I appeal do not represent in the main anything more than a reproduction of the text of the written communication handed over to the Court by my lawyer at the hearing on 16th May 1900. On the whole I agreed with the contents of this document, and did so in my letter of 24th May 1900, although several legal arguments of my lawyers, for instance those under (1) of the facts in the judgment and under (2) in the communication, I could not consider relevant. What is correct in my opinion in the document was to no little extent written by my own pen, that is to say taken from the representation which I sent to the Director of this Asylum on 24th March 1900 and of which as far as I know there is a copy in the files of the Court.

I am forced to contradict severely two statements in the judgment. Yet, I would expect no success from a rectification of the facts in the judgment in the sense of § 320 C.P.O., as I cannot p. 405
refute that my lawyer actually made the statements concerned during the hearing. My lawyer's statements are in this respect, however, based on a misunderstanding of my own opinion; the case arises therefore of a revocation of admissions in the sense of § 290 C.P.O.

The two points in question are as follows:

(1) At the very beginning of establishing the facts the judgment referring to a passage in the communication from my lawyer states:

"The appellant does not contradict that he is mentally ill".

This is incorrect; I refute most decidedly that I am mentally ill if, as is usual among laymen, this word is combined with *an idea of clouded intellect.* I made this point quite clear also in my representation to the Director of the Asylum on 24th March 1900.

I explained there that I do not argue the presence of a mental illness *in the sense of a nervous illness;* but I drew special attention to the different meanings of "mentally ill" for the medical man and legally.

I want to explain this a little more fully: I do not deny that my nervous system has for a number of years been in a pathological condition. On the other hand, I deny absolutely that I am mentally ill or ever have been. My mind, that is to say the functioning of my intellectual powers, is as clear and healthy as any other person's; it has been unaltered since the beginning of my nervous illness—apart from some unimportant hypochondriacal ideas. Therefore the medical expert's report to the Court contains, in having accepted the presence in my case of paranoia (insanity), a blow in the face
p. 406 of truth, which could hardly be worse. As I write this sentence *I do not want to offend the medical specialist in the least; I do not doubt at all that his report was given in good faith.* But this cannot prevent me, where the recognition of my legal capacity is at stake, from giving expression to my conviction of the *objective error* of the report frankly and without restraint. I will try to explain below how the report received its present content.

(2) The second error is in the sentence under (3)b of the exposition of the facts in the judgment, that I myself am convinced that my stay in Sonnenstein Asylum could only be to the advantage of my mental health. This sentence, it is true, appeared in my lawyer's communication, but led me already last summer to protest against its incorrectness; I reproduce verbatim the passage concerned from the letter which I wrote on 14th June 1900 to my lawyer:

> "As I am writing to you I do not want to omit adding that the consent which I expressed in my letter to you of 24th May of this year to the content of the communication which you have handed to the Court, requires certain modification which at that time I did not consider necessary because in my opinion it was without importance for the legal assessment of the case. I refer to the passage that I myself consider my stay in the Asylum as one which could only be to the advantage of my mental well-being. This is not quite true. I am not pursuing my release from the
> p. 407 Asylum at the moment for the only reason that having

spent six years in it, it matters little whether I spend another six or twelve months here, and in any case my return to my previous domestic life with regard to living conditions, etc., requires certain preparations. *On the other hand I do not expect any advantage to my health by extending my stay in this Asylum.* In any case there can be no question of the return of mental clarity because this has always been present undiminished; the hyperexcitability of my nerves can however not be removed by human means; it will continue to the end of my life because it is connected with supernatural matters, unless some change should occur in my body which would also open the eyes of other human beings.

Naturally, however, I do not wish to spend the whole of the rest of my life in an institution where my mental powers lie almost fallow and where I am almost totally without contact with educated people, as well as all the other pleasures of life. Should certain nuisances (like the bellowing) continue to give concern as regards my appearing in public, I would know how to restrain myself in such circumstances.

I leave it to you to decide whether a copy of this letter is added to the files for the orientation of the Court."

Since the Court in the final judgment of 13th April last was—to my greatest surprise—guided by considerations of which there were p. 408
not the slightest indications in the resolution on the evidence of 15th June 1900 which in my opinion was essentially correct (the resolution on the evidence followed almost verbatim the wording I had myself suggested in a letter of 4th April 1900—Appendix A in the file of 16th May 1900) I must express lively regret that my letter of 14th June 1900 reproduced above was not also brought to the notice of the Court. Had it been, the disputed passage could not possibly have been incorporated unchanged in the facts of the judgment.

II. CONCERNING THE GROUNDS OF THE JUDGMENT.

The grounds of the contested judgment rest mainly on the medical specialists second report of 28th November 1900; most of it was taken word for word from this report, so that in my refutation I can also limit myself in the main to a discussion of how far its conclusions are to be regarded as correct.

Only a few points are independent additions of the Court; I will try to deal with these first, before I concern myself more closely with the content of the report itself.

I accept entirely the remarks in the judgment referring to the fact that there is no reason for concern about my endangering my life if freedom over my person were granted to me, and that otherwise also my mental faculties are unclouded, and that the so-called attacks of bellowing can remain out of consideration because pure police matters could not furnish grounds for upholding my tutelage.

p. 409 Another consideration raised by the Court is to be found in the sentence at the end of the judgment, namely that I suffer from hallucinations as a result of which I believe I can see human beings before me which do not exist (" fleeting-improvised-men "). If one takes the trouble to read carefully those parts of my Memoirs dealing with this matter, this consideration at once proves invalid, as it is expressed in the *present tense* " the appellant *believes* he sees human beings before him ", etc. The whole idea of the " fleeting-improvised-men " belongs to a time which lies years behind me; it only existed during the first year or two at the most of my stay in this Asylum. This can be clearly read at the beginning of Chapter XVI of my Memoirs. I can therefore leave the question open whether my ideas concerning this matter rested only on hallucinations or on factual events. It is a question only of earlier phases of my illness as the medical specialist rightly states—perhaps on page 8 of his later report; I can only cite from the copy before me but it should not be too difficult to find the corresponding place in the original which is now in the Court file—which need not be taken into consideration in assessing the present state. I have known for a long time now that people I see before me are not " fleeting-improvised-men " but real human beings, and that I have to conduct myself towards them as a reasonable human being usually does in his dealings with other human beings. The sentence at the end of the judgment that because of these earlier ideas there is danger of my acting unreasonably, can therefore be eliminated as a notable support of the Court's decision.

p. 410 I now turn to a discussion of the medical reports. These start *a priori* from the tacit assumption that everything I reported in my Memoirs or otherwise mentioned about the connection which has arisen between God and myself, as well as about divine miracles

which happen to my person, rests only on pathological imaginings. If I wanted to give expression to my true feelings on this point of view I could only do it with Huss' cry to the wretched peasants who were carrying wood to his funeral pyre: *Oh sancta simplicitas!* I do not mean to be impertinent to the medical specialist; I would be genuinely sorry if Dr. Weber felt insulted by any of my words, for I have the highest regard both for his character and professional and scientific capacity. I know he could do no other than apply to my case the yardstick of common scientific experience. On the other hand I also hope that he will not take it amiss if I give sharp expression to my contrary view. I must state therefore: *the certainty of my knowledge of God and the absolute conviction that I am dealing with God and divine miracles towers high above all human science.* This may sound distinctly presumptuous; but I know that the basis of this conviction is not personal vanity nor morbid megalomania. Irrespective of my undoubted rich gifts in many directions I have never been blind to my shortcomings, I have never imagined myself among the foremost minds of the nation; after all it was not my merit that in consequence of a miraculous concatenation of circumstances, insight p. 411
into the true state of divine matters was granted me in an incomparably higher degree than any other human being before; I have had to pay dearly enough for this insight with the loss of my whole happiness in life for a great many years. But all the more certain for me are the results won by this insight; in fact they have become, and indeed must be, the very centre of my whole life as God even now daily and hourly, I can even say at every moment, reveals Himself anew to me in His miracles and in His language. This accounts for my continual serenity, despite all calamities to which I am even now exposed, and which anyone can observe in my contacts with other people, even with uneducated people and children—only not with lunatics; from it springs also the quiet feeling of good will which I extend even to those who in earlier years unwittingly hurt me; it also explains the immense value I place on the publication of my Memoirs. For should I thereby succeed only in arousing in other people a serious doubt whether it had not been granted me to throw a glance behind the dark veil which otherwise hides the beyond from the eyes of man, my work would certainly still belong to the most interesting ones ever written since the existence of the world.

I could not deny myself emphasizing with some vigour my basic point of view before going into all the details, because the

judgment as well as the report think they can treat me somewhat condescendingly—not entirely without justification as I have admitted myself, as both represent State Authorities. Of course I have to realize that for the time being there is little prospect of
p. 412 other people appreciating my basic point of view, least of all in the decision of the present Court case. I therefore used to consider it possible and indeed advisable to exclude every discussion of my supposed hallucinations and delusions from the points at issue in the case, the purpose of which is the contesting of my tutelage; I could not ignore the fear—as already mentioned in my letter to the Director of the Asylum of 24th March 1900—that the attention of the Court would be diverted from the decisive and only question in their competence, namely *whether I possess the capacity for reasonable action in practical life*. More recently however I have not been able to ignore the fact that it would be impossible for me to do so without a certain appreciation of my so-called delusions or my religious beliefs, and not only on the formal side of their logical sequence and orderly arrangement, but to a certain degree also regarding the question whether it is within the bounds of possibility that my delusional system, as one is pleased to call it, is founded on some truth. I have to make the attempt as regards other people, my judges in particular, not really to convert them to my miraculous belief—naturally I could only do this at present to a very moderate degree—but at least to furnish the general impression that the experiences and considerations laid down in my "Memoirs" cannot simply be regarded as a *quantité negligeable*, as empty fantasy of a muddled head, which from the outset would not justify the effort of further thought and *possible observations on my person*. Only in this way will it perhaps be possible to explain to the Court that petty considerations, ordinarily decisive for
p. 413 human beings, such as the sensibilities of others, fear of revealing so-called family secrets, indeed even fear of a penalty, can only carry very little weight in my case, where the achievement of a holy purpose is at stake, which I must regard as my life's task.

In what follows I will therefore mention (and perhaps later put to proof) a number of points which, although they cannot exactly prove the reality of the stated miracles, will I hope at least make them so far credible that one will hestitate to condemn the whole presentation as pure nonsense from the start, but rather admit that the scientific world could make them the starting point of further researches. It is true, only a few points can be made and these deal mostly with apparently insignificant external events; for it lies in the nature of the matter that by far the largest part of the supernatural impressions which I receive in overwhelming number are only perceived by myself, and cannot be observed in any external signs by other people. Nevertheless the little I wish to put forward could suffice to cause astonishment in any unbiased person.

(1) In the course of the years a quite extraordinarily large number of *strings have broken on my piano*—and I maintain through miracles. They amounted perhaps all in all to thirty or forty; the exact number does not matter much. In the year 1897 alone the bill for broken strings came to 86 Marks. Perhaps the opposing party in the case, the Royal Prosecuting Authority, will not dispute this fact; if they did I would be in a position to prove it by calling as witnesses my wife, the attendant Möbius and the music shop p. 414
C. A. Klemm in Dresden, as well as perhaps a supporting statement in a further report from the Director of the Asylum. Concerning my assertion that they could not possibly have been broken by any foolish actions on my part (hammering on the piano), I wish to point out what was said in the middle of Chapter XII of my Memoirs; in order to avoid repetition I refer the reader there. I am sure every expert would confirm that even using great force one could not break the *strings* of a piano by merely hitting the *keys*; if need be I could ask for an expert's report. If this is so, and it is altogether extremely rare for piano strings to break—it had never happened to me previously in the whole of my life and I have never heard of it happening to other people; it might happen in concert rooms where there are gross changes in temperature, perhaps in the case of excessively taut strings of *string instruments*, but even there hardly in the case of the strings of a concert grand piano—*how then can one explain the remarkably large number of such breakages which happened to my piano? Could a natural cause be responsible?*

(2) Very noticeable to my whole environment are the so-called *attacks of bellowing* which have for years—*not* in the first years of my illness—occurred very frequently. I have already described their nature in my letter to the Director of the Asylum of 24th March 1900, in that the muscles which serve respiration (the lung and thorax muscles) are by divine miracle set in motion p. 415
with such violence that *I am compelled* to let out the bellow or cry, unless I make quite extraordinary efforts to suppress it, which by

the suddenness of the impulse is not always possible, or possible only by constant attention to it. I refer the reader to (2) of Chapter XV of my Memoirs concerning the purpose which ni my opinion is intended with this miracle. That I neither simulate nor provoke the bellowing purposely—it is after all a hard burden for me too—is apparently not doubted by the medical specialist (compare the later report, pp. 28 and 31 of my copy); he recognizes that it frequently requires the greatest effort on my part to prevent the bellowing noise, and that such noisy outbursts occur completely against my will, *automatically and compulsively*. I must therefore raise the question: *has science in any way a satisfactory explanation for this phenomenon? Is any case known in the annals of psychiatry of a human being* suffering from a mental illness (paranoia), assumed to be my illness, who is at the same time recognized to be of high intelligence, with unclouded mental faculties, of tactful and decent behaviour in social conversation, with ethically correct conceptions, etc., and whose whole nature shows no tendency to coarseness in any way, in whom *such automatically caused loud outbursts or attacks of bellowing have been observed*—which the medical specialist calls humming, clearing the throat and short attacks of laughter when they occur in milder form? Naturally I have not sufficient experience of other mental
p. 416 patients, but I presume these questions must be answered in the negative. If this assumption is correct I would value confirmation by its inclusion in the report. Naturally I do not expect the medical specialist to adopt *positively* my explanation of the phenomenon, that it is the result of miracles, but even the *negative*, i.e. that one is dealing with a quite remarkable case, unique in the field of psychiatric experience, would in my opinion not be without influence on the judgment of my case, as one would thus give some credit at least to the possibility of the influence of supernatural forces. This point of view would appear all the more noteworthy if the medical specialist could further confirm that the attacks of bellowing almost never occur when I am engaged in loud conversation, am in educated company or move outside the Asylum, on steamships, railways, public places, or in the streets of the town, etc., but in the main are only observed when I am alone in my room or in the Asylum's garden among lunatics with whom conversation is impossible. If science had to admit that here also it lacks adequate explanation, then one could not avoid attributing a certain importance to *my* exposition of the matter. According to this it is a question of miracles; all these

phenomena are easily explained by the rays (in other words God) being as a rule only tempted to withdraw from me when I am not thinking or when visual impressions which particularly attract the rays are not available in me. Such visual impressions are never lacking during excursions in the streets of the town for instance where I can look at shop windows, and where there are always many people about, particularly female persons, etc. (compare p. 417
for details the first third of Chapter XV of my Memoirs, also Postscripts III and V of the Memoirs near the beginning of the last paragraph).

(3) In the new medical report (page 28 ff. of the copy before me) it is stated—a point with which I completely agree with certain reservations—that I appear even at meal times "preoccupied", stare rigidly in front of myself (more correctly sit with eyes shut), "grimace" in a peculiar manner, and in particular that I try to push my eyelids upwards; the medical expert thus admits that these had previously been closed and he can hardly mean that I push my eyelids up with my hands, but by using the muscles contained in the eyelids.

The medical expert deals with these "hallucinatory processes" and the "striking reaction" caused by them only from the point of view to what extent these "pathological processes" constitute a disturbance in social relations. For me they have an incomparably greater significance: *as signs which other people can also observe*, of my whole musculature being exposed to certain influences which can only be ascribed to forces working from outside, in other words to divine miracles. I could add other phenomena to those mentioned by the medical expert, for instance that at times I suffer from *being hard of hearing for a few minutes*, that at times even when I remain quite still a severe acceleration of respiration occurs, so that literally I have to gasp for air and my mouth is kept open in a most unnatural manner, etc., etc. All these events can be noticed by p. 418
anybody observing me attentively; it therefore sometimes requires an enormous mental effort to join in social conversation freely and good-humouredly; no human being has any idea of what goes on at the same time in my head and in my whole body.

But it is not unknown to me that hallucinations, that is to say auditory stimuli causing voices to be heard, and convulsive twitchings, that is to say cramp-like contractions of the musculature particularly of the face, are not exactly rare accompaniments of a morbid nervous state. But I believe I can maintain, and count on confirmation from the expert's report, that the manifestations in my case deviate so markedly from what is usually observed, that one could hardly avoid regarding their cause also as something essentially different.

I have dealt in detail with my hallucinations in Appendix IV of my Memoirs, and I refer to it at this juncture. From the medical specialist's report I notice with some satisfaction that he himself attributes a certain *reality* to my hallucinations, in so far as he apparently does not doubt that the "voices" described in my Memoirs are in fact perceived by me. The only difference of opinion then is whether the subjective sensation of hearing voices is caused *only* by pathological functioning of my own nerves, or whether some external cause acts on them, in other words whether the sound of voices is, so to speak, a trick on the part of my own nerves, or whether some being outside my body
p. 419 speaks into me in the form of voices. Equally the question may be raised concerning "grimacing", the pulling of faces, closing of my eyes, etc., whether it is only a pathological state of my nerves causing muscular contractions or whether there is some external stimulus acting on my body. *In essence it is one assertion versus another.* Mere rationalism will naturally deny from the start that divine miracles are the cause. But happily rationalism, in Goethe's words, "What cannot be accounted for, does not count", is almost nowhere in science the guiding principle. I who cannot prove the miracles but only wish to put other people in a frame of mind to believe in the *possibility* of supernatural influences in connection with my person, I would be satisfied if the medical specialist were to affirm that in my case these phenomena have a characteristic and distinct stamp hitherto unknown in scientific experience. I presume that hallucinations of the kind described have never previously been observed except in my case, particularly the incessant talking of voices which cannot be silenced by any mental distraction, is something totally unheard of, as are the muscular contractions *against the patient's will* (as even the medical expert admits) which force him to shut his eyes, to utter bellowing noises, markedly accelerate his breathing even while at rest, etc. I would also like to see this assumption confirmed in a definite medical statement, unless it can be shown to be incorrect. It would be of particular value to me if the medical expert could
p. 420 also confirm that closing of my eyes—against my will—occurs regularly and *immediately* as soon as I am silent after taking part in a loud conversation, in other words when I indulge in thinking nothing.

(4) I am convinced that certain manifestations can be observed on my body which are totally inexplicable by the common run of scientific experience; I might consider demanding a physical examination by the doctors of this Asylum or other doctors, perhaps including if feasible the application of Röntgen-rays in order to ascertain this state of affairs. The matter concerns mainly, but not exclusively the so-called nerves of voluptuousness with which I have dealt in detail in Chapter XXI of my Memoirs. There is a passage in the later report of the medical expert (p. 22 of my copy) where it is stated that "I thought I could feel nerves of voluptuousness on my body like those of a female body, although science does not acknowledge the presence of nerves of voluptuousness". I cannot really tell whether the medical expert was only *relating my own* statement in this matter or whether he was expressing *his* opinion that science does not acknowledge the existence of special nerves of voluptuousness which are differently distributed in the male and female body. In any case it appears to me that this is merely *a play with words* without any bearing on the issue itself. Surely the medical expert would hardly wish to doubt —at least I have understood him to that effect in a verbal conversation, and besides consider it a scientifically established fact—that the nervous system of the female sex shows certain characteristics over the whole body particularly the bosom, connected with the sensation of voluptuousness, quite different from those of the male sex.* It is immaterial what one calls these charac- p. 421
teristic structures; if as a layman in neurology I chose the wrong expression, it would not matter much. I assert therefore that on my body, particularly on my bosom, there are present the properties of a nervous system corresponding to a female body and I am certain that a physical examination would confirm this. The conclusions to be drawn from this are considered in detail in Chapter XXI of my Memoirs.

At this point I wish to mention, in order to avoid any misunderstanding (which I will deal with more closely later), that I would demand such an examination *for purposes of the present Court case only*, that is in order to obtain rescinding of my tutelage. As soon as I shall have achieved my freedom, though I would permit

* To elucidate this matter further, the following questions might be raised: what are the physiological peculiarities of the female bosom, particularly what is its swelling due to in the years of beginning puberty? Is it only a strengthening of the musculature, collection of fat and suchlike, or is the explanation not rather to be found in a development of *the nervous system in the female bosom* which is specifically different from that of the male sex?

such an examination *at the request* of selected experts, I would never initiate it myself and much less spend as much as one penny of my fortune upon it.

(5) The medical expert acknowledges (p. 9 in my copy of the later report), that the " emanations of my pathologically altered psychic state " are not, as commonly in similar cases, meagre and monotonous, but show a fantastically formed intricate structure
p. 422 of ideas very different from the usual way of thinking. Pursuing this remark, I plan to submit my Memoirs for examination to specialists from other fields of experience, particularly theologians and philosophers. This would serve a double purpose, firstly to prove to the judges that my " Memoirs ", however strange much of their content may be, could yet form an appreciable stimulus to wider scientific circles for research in a most obscure subject and make it understandable how lively my wish must be to have them published. Secondly, I would then welcome the expert opinion of men of science in the mentioned fields so as to ascertain whether it is probable, even psychologically possible, that a human being of cool and sober mind as I used to be in the eyes of all who knew me in my earlier life, and besides a human being who, as mentioned at the beginning of Chapter VI of my Memoirs, did *not have a firm belief in God and the immortality of the soul* before his illness, should have *sucked from his fingers* so to speak the whole complicated structure of ideas with its enormous mass of factual detail (for instance, about the soul-language, soul-conception, Chapter I and Chapter XII of the Memoirs, etc., etc.). Does not rather the thought impose itself that a human being who is able to write on such matters and attain such singular ideas about the nature of God and the continued existence of the soul after death, must in fact have had some particular experiences and particular impressions from which other human beings are excluded?

The above is not intended as a formal application at present for
p. 423 such an expert report. For I cannot hide from myself the big expenditure in time and money which it would involve. Should the Court of Appeal decide to suspend my tutelage without it, I would naturally much prefer it. Should they, however, not be inclined to do this—and I will be able to orientate myself about this during the verbal hearings at some of which I hope to be present —I would reserve my right to make such an application.

The matters discussed in the foregoing section have really only the importance of an arabesque around the real core of the question under decision, namely whether in consequence of my presumed mental illness I lack the capacity of looking after my affairs.

Turning to this question I must first make some more remarks about the characterization of my personality in the report. I acknowledge gratefully the medical expert's good will in doing justice to my whole personality; I am further indebted to him for not sparing the trouble of thoroughly studying my " Memoirs "; it enabled him to give in his report a substantially correct summary of at least some of my main ideas. It was probably unavoidable that a few small errors and misunderstandings crept in, considering the inflexibility of the material; I do not have to enter into these more closely as they would hardly influence the Court's decision in any way.

On the whole I believe I am justified in asserting that the medical p. 424 expert has only come *to know me really well in the last year*, that is to say since I have taken my meals regularly at his family table; his opinion about me after another six months of such contact would probably again be much more favourable than at the time of writing the last report. Before that time (that is to say perhaps before Easter 1900) the medical expert only became acquainted with the pathological shell, as I would like to call it, which concealed my true spiritual life. Nothing in these words is meant as a reproach for the treatment I received earlier on in the Asylum. I admit that during the first years of my stay in this Asylum I might have given the impression (although it was deceiving) of an imbecile unfit for social contact. I can also understand that the doctors retained this opinion which they had formed, for many years after my behaviour had in many ways long shown a change in my mental state. It is impossible in a large asylum to devote uninterrupted and detailed observation to every single patient; in view of the intransigence I showed in the first years in this Asylum it was in fact difficult to get any correct impression of my mental life. Nevertheless the statement in the report is not quite correct (p. 7 of my copy) that I showed no inclination " until such time ", that is to say until the demand for a new report was made (June 1900), to move outside the Asylum and that the " desire " to approach the outside world again had to be gradually " encouraged " in me. There seems to be a small inaccuracy in memory here. I can prove from documents that in an exposition p. 425 I personally gave to District Court President Schmidt, my official guardian, during a visit by him on 8th October 1899, I complained that for five years I had not been allowed outside the walls of the Asylum even for the small walks allowed to many other patients. In order to be loyal I sent a written copy of this exposition to Dr. Weber in a letter of 27th November 1899. Yet, after that I had to wait four to six months before being invited to take meals at the family table and being given the opportunity of an excursion outside the Asylum (by carriage). I repeat I have no wish to recriminate about the past; I can however not allow the statement to go uncorrected that it was only my fault that one did not get to know me sooner as a human being in full possession of his mental powers and able to conduct himself correctly in decent society. In my opinion this would have *been quite feasible since at least the beginning of the year* 1897.

In any case even the medical specialist himself, according to his report (p. 27 of my copy), is now convinced that one need not worry about letting me take part in social intercourse, as well as in occasions where a great number of persons are gathered together, as at theatre, Church, etc. The pathological events (grimacing, clearing my throat and suchlike), which at times are noticeable even on such occasions, are as experience shows, not of such severity as to be very disturbing to other people.

The medical expert added to his account concerning my social
p. 426 behaviour a further passage in which he somewhat contradicted the District Court at Dresden, which concluded in its decision of 13th March 1900 that I was capable of directing the most difficult Court cases, of drawing up a judgment to which no objection could be taken, etc. I quite agree with the medical expert that what the District Court at Dresden says in this connection requires certain modification, but I wish to bring out more clearly than the report does in what it has to be modified. In my opinion I am capable *in written expression of my thoughts* of meeting every demand which my previous position as Judge of a Higher Court could make on me; even now I would credit myself with the capacity of drawing up any judgment or any other document which comes up in the course of a Judge's work, to the satisfaction of the highest standards. For all miracles are powerless to prevent the expression of ideas in writing; the occasional attempt to paralyse my fingers, though making writing somewhat more difficult, does not prevent it, and attempts at disturbing my thoughts are easily overcome by putting them down in writing during which one has a great deal of time to collect one's thoughts. Things which

I *have written* have therefore, since writing materials were again placed at my disposal and I was inclined to write, revealed *at all times* even in the first years of my illness a human being completely clear mentally. Things are somewhat different in expressing thoughts verbally. Here the miracles practised against my organs of respiration and speech, in conjunction with attempts to disturb my thoughts, produce a marked interference. As I am still simultaneously preoccupied with hallucinations—the hearing of voices p. 427
—I agree with the medical expert that such intense intellectual concentration as is demanded in directing verbal Court proceedings, taking part in consultations of the Court, etc., would only be possible for me with great difficulty. It is therefore not a question of a lack of intellect, but that certain influences make prompt verbal expression of thoughts difficult; these in my opinion are due to miracles, but according to the medical expert to purely pathological processes.

So much to round off the total picture of my mental state which the medical expert furnished in his report. It now remains to answer the question of whether my assumed mental illness makes me incapable of looking after my affairs, that is to say, to act reasonably in practical life.

In this connection I wish to mention again first that in my opinion the *onus of proof* lies with my opponent, the Public Prosecutor. As the law does not recognize mental illness in itself as grounds for placing a person under tutelage but presumes a mental illness of such kind that the person concerned is in consequence thereof prevented from managing his affairs reasonably, it is strictly speaking the duty of him *who requests* that a person be placed under tutelage to furnish the Judge with the required factual proofs. To advance vague apprehensions and generalities, such as that it is " completely unpredictable ", if freedom to dispose of my person and my fortune were returned to me, whether I might be led to *some* unreasonable actions through my delusions and hallucinations, is insufficient for treating a human being of my high mental and moral status, which one is forced to recognize, legally like a child under the age of seven. It would rather have to be proved *on the* p. 428
evidence of factual experience gathered in the last few years that and in what way a tendency to unreasonable action in consequence of my delusions and hallucinations has been manifested. It is true that the possibilities for gathering such experiences are not present to the same extent in a person detained in an asylum as in a person who is free. Nevertheless it is *not my fault that for years I have*

been detained in the Asylum and denied leave, after the real reason, that is to safeguard myself and other people from danger, had passed; on the other hand the increasingly greater freedom of movement which I have had for more than a year has in my opinion given sufficient evidence that one need have no fear of unreasonable actions if freedom of decision over my person and my fortune were fully restored to me. I have since then shared hundreds of meals at the Director of the Asylum's family table, have gone on smaller and greater excursions on foot, by steamship or railway, to public places of entertainment, to shops, to Church, theatre and concerts, not infrequently without being accompanied by an attendant from the Asylum, and have been in possession of a certain, if limited, amount of money. *Nobody will have noticed on these occasions the slightest sign of unreasonable action on my part.* It never occurred to me to molest other people by telling them
p. 429 of my delusions and hallucinations; as an example, I think I can maintain that the ladies who sit at the family table of the Director of the Asylum have not the merest inkling of the existence of these delusions and hallucinations, unless by chance they learnt of them some other way. It is true I gave some hints to my wife and my relatives, both verbally and in writing. But this would be sufficiently justified by the close relationship which should exist among married couples and near relatives and which does not allow one to hide from the other party anything that fills one's emotional and spiritual life. Even this information was never pressed upon them, but mostly in answer to their special enquiries. The *only thing* which could be counted as somewhat unreasonable in the eyes of other persons is, as mentioned by the medical expert, that at times I was seen standing in front of the mirror or elsewhere with some female adornments (ribbons, trumpery necklaces, and suchlike), with the upper half of my body exposed. This by the way happens only when *I am alone*, never as far as I can avoid it within sight of other people. The small acquisitions needed (also some sewing material and suchlike), which for the most part were obtained for me by Asylum officials, cost hardly more than a few marks, and therefore from the purely financial point of view do not come under further consideration. I have *very good and important reasons* for this behaviour, however stupid or even despicable it may appear to other people. When I need mental peace I achieve by it—one cannot play the piano, read, write or occupy oneself in some other way intellectually the whole day—a marked decrease in the *states of bellowing* which are so excessively

annoying to myself and my surroundings. The connection between the two will not be evident to other people without further explanation; anybody interested is referred to Chapter XXI of my " Memoirs ". As far as I am concerned this p. 430
circumstance has been proved to my satisfaction beyond any doubt through several years' experience, so that I cannot heed other people's judgment as to whether or not these measures are appropriate. Even if people think the advantage exists in my imagination only, as doubtless many naturally will, they can at worst only see in this behaviour an incomprehensible *whim*, the *absolute harmlessness* of which cannot be denied—except perhaps in relation to my wife, a matter to which I will return in greater detail—as neither for myself nor for other people is it connected with any disadvantage. The danger of catching cold which the medical expert considers possible, certainly does not arise at usual room temperatures, as the example of ladies in *decolleté* sufficiently shows.

My wearing female adornments, etc., has obviously greatly influenced the opinions expressed about me in the medical report and the judgment; I have therefore had to deal with it somewhat at length. But it is the *sole* point with regard to which it can be said now, and could perhaps be said in the future with a certain degree of truth, that my behaviour towards the outer world and particularly other human beings is influenced by my delusions and hallucinations. And so I come to that sentence in the report which in my opinion is its mainstay and therefore for me also the main issue which I contest. The medical expert says, four pages before the end of the report in my copy:

> " The most important moment in judging the capacity of the patient to look after his affairs is and remains the fact that p. 431
> everything which objectively seen appears as delusions and hallucinations is for him (a) unshakable certainty and (b) adequate motive for action ".

I have to confirm the first part (a) of this statement, namely that my so-called delusional system is unshakable certainty, with the same decisive " *yes* " as I have to counter the second part (b), namely that my delusions are adequate motive for action, with the strongest possible " *no* ". I could even say with Jesus Christ: " My Kingdom is not of this world "; my so-called delusions are concerned solely with God and the beyond; they *can* therefore *never in any way influence my behaviour* in any worldly matter, if I may use this expression—apart from the whim already mentioned,

which is also meant to impress God. I do not know how the medical expert arrived at the contrary conclusion, namely that my delusions are sufficient motive for action; at least I do not think I have given any grounds for this belief either in my behaviour or in the written expositions of my " Memoirs ". In them I have repeatedly emphasized that I would practise what might appear to other people extraordinary behaviour only " *as far as consideration for my environment permits* " (Chapter XIII of my Memoirs near the beginning) or " *while alone with God* " (Chapter XXI of the Memoirs, in the middle). What the law subsumes under the term " affairs ", that is looking after all interests of life particularly pecuniary ones, *cannot* be affected by my delusions and hallucinations. I have no intention whatever as the medical expert
p. 432 imputed and before him the lawyer Mr. Thürmer, to make pecuniary sacrifices to propagate my belief in miracles, to have the nerves of voluptuousness in my body verified or to increase the " material well-being " which rests on them. Whoever thinks this is possible has not really entered into my inner spiritual life; but naturally I do not intend any reproach with this statement, because a full understanding is really impossible for other people. The certainty of my knowledge of God and divine matters is so great and unshakable that it is completely immaterial to me what other people think of the truth or probability of my ideas. I shall therefore—other than for the purpose of this legal action—never undertake anything by way of spreading my experiences and beliefs among people except publishing my Memoirs; apart from this I will not move a finger in order to prove them or make them seem likely. In this my point of view is like Luther's: " If it is man's work it will perish; if it is the work of God it will last ". I will quietly await whether unequivocal events will not compel other people to accept the truth of my delusions. The same applies to the " material well-being " mentioned by the medical expert or as I call it the increase of bodily well-being dependent on soul-voluptuousness. This must of necessity fall into my lap by itself without my having to do anything to bring it about; indeed it could hardly be expedited by advertisement. Particularly it would never occur to me to replace the few rags or cheap trinkets which make up my so-called female ornaments by anything which could appear even to a poor servant girl as
p. 433 real ornaments or jewellery. I have not bought or made these objects for my pleasure, but in order to create a certain impression on God, and for this cheap almost valueless articles suffice.

I trust one will believe all my assurances about my future behaviour, as I have never given occasion for doubt in the sincerity of my love of truth. With it, in my opinion, all those fears are removed which could have exercised the minds of the medical expert or the judges when it was stated that my behaviour was " completely unaccountable " and that my delusional ideas might yet cause me to act unreasonably *in some directions not more closely specified*. Therefore, only two possible points remain for upholding my tutelage which are specially dealt with in the Court's judgment, namely that if my liberty to dispose of my person and my fortune were restored to me " my relationship with my wife would be destroyed ", and that I would compromise myself in front of other people or expose myself to the danger of a penalty through publishing my Memoirs. I want to go into these two points in greater detail in the following:

(A) Concerning the first cause for apprehension, it seems to me that the remark in the judgment that through unreasonable actions " the relationship with my wife would be destroyed " advances a consideration which, although of great importance for the emotional life of the persons concerned, could hardly have a legal bearing on the question of my *legal capacity*. The marital partnership between myself and my wife has in any case for years almost completely ceased to exist in consequence of my illness and would, p. 434
particularly if my tutelage were prolonged indefinitely, remain in abeyance until the end of the life of one of the partners. If the remark about the threatening destruction of the relationship with my wife is to make any sense at all, it can only mean that the feelings of respect and love which my wife still harbours for me could thereby be shaken and stifled. Clearly one is dealing with a most delicate matter, which third persons who have never known the intimacy of that marital relationship should judge most carefully and hesitantly. Above all else I must emphasize most decidedly that *a person can be placed under tutelage only in his own interest*, in order to safeguard him from threatening dangers caused by his tendency to unreasonable actions; but a person can never be placed under tutelage in order to safeguard others however closely related from any annoyances, or to maintain them in a certain state of feeling; this may be of importance to their spiritual equilibrium, but does not belong to those affairs of life which are regulated by law. Apart from the vital interests of the person to be placed under tutelage, the care of relatives can only be taken into account in so far (compare the order of the Royal Ministry

of Justice at the beginning of the judgment) as the person to be placed under tutelage is *by law responsible* for such care, that is to say in the circumstances of the present case in so far as it is a matter *of providing legal maintenance.* I would never attempt to avoid this obligation including providing my wife with the necessary means of living apart from me, should circumstances turn out to be such that my wife could not be expected to live with me. If
p. 435 I were really so insensible to my *moral duties* towards my wife as to cast aside every thought for her health, her peace of mind and her natural feelings as a wife, I would give cause for doubt in the *moral worth of my own person, but one could never deduce therefrom grounds for denying my legal capacity.* For if I were really so insensible as not to take the loss of my wife's love as a misfortune, no other disadvantage could possibly arise from the extinction of this love; to employ her love in some manner for my physical or mental well-being, by caring for me physically, tending and nursing me, as well as by exchange of intellectual interests—all this is in any case impossible because of our actual separation. In the face of this my wife's visits and the presents she occasionally gives me hardly count; the latter I would easily be able to buy for myself were I master of my means.

I think I have proved that everything said in the report and in the judgment about the " threatened destruction of the relationship with my wife ", " damage to the marital state ", etc., is irrelevant for the decision of the present case.

In order to appear in a somewhat better light to my Judges than I do from certain statements in the report and in the Court's judgment, I want to add a few more remarks about my relationship to my wife and the inconveniences to my present
p. 436 (and possibly future) environment arising from my so-called attacks of bellowing. All the statements in the report concerning my relationship to my wife, based apparently on discussions between the medical expert and my wife, show *gross misunderstandings;* but I will leave undecided whether my wife has misunderstood me (this could be possible because of the rarity of our meetings), or the medical expert has misunderstood my wife. I have never played with the idea of *divorce* or shown myself indifferent to the future of our marital bond, as one might be led to believe from the expression used in the report that " I at once come out with the hint that my wife could divorce me ". The whole extensive correspondence which I have carried on with my wife for years would prove the true love I feel towards her and

how painful it is for me that she too has been made most unhappy by my illness and the factual dissolution of our marriage, and how much I always take lively interest in her fate. Only in this sense have I discussed the possibility of divorce, mentioning a few times to my wife that *if* it were impossible for her to maintain her previous love and respect for me because of a certain idea, naturally unsympathetic to her, which rules me and causes peculiarities in my behaviour, she had the right according to law to start divorce proceedings because of mental illness persisting longer than three years. I always added that I would regret this very much; nevertheless I remarked to her that in such an eventuality she would naturally have no claim on the interest of my capital nor on the pension to which I am entitled by twenty-eight years in the service of the State. (My wife it is true has money of her own, but the greater part of the interest she draws comes from mine). I p. 437
have at all times had full understanding of the consideration I owe to my wife and have expressed it to her in the usual way. As example and proof I append footnote 76 of Chapter XIII of my Memoirs:

> "I must use particular discretion in contact with my wife, for whom I retain my former love in full. I may at times have failed by being *too frank* in conversation or written communications. It is of course impossible for my wife to understand my trends of thought fully; it must be difficult for her still to retain her previous love and admiration for me, when she hears that I am preoccupied with ideas of possibly being transformed into a woman. I can deplore this, but am unable to change it; even here I must guard against false sentimentality".

I do not know how one came to assume that I would neglect that tact and fine feelings towards my wife for which one otherwise praises me. *Naturally*—and I have acted accordingly up to now—I would spare my wife any painful sight; I showed her my female ornaments only with some reluctance when out of forgivable feminine inquisitiveness she insisted upon it. In the same way I would *naturally* not expect my wife to live with me nor misuse my marital rights to force her in this direction, if experience should prove that living together with me is unbearable for her because of the so-called vociferations or attacks of bellowing. The medical expert therefore misjudges me a little when he speaks of "patho- p. 438
logically increased egoism" in that I "do not give a thought" (!!)

to how much my wife suffers " through my behaviour " and also that I look upon the annoyance to my environment as irrelevant and complain only of my own malaise. Yet the medical expert acknowledges that the vociferations proceed compulsively and automatically against my will.* As far as these are concerned my wife does not suffer at all by them at present because she lives apart from me; if by speaking of " my behaviour " one means my occasional putting on of female ornaments, I have already said above that I would never do so in my wife's presence; but when I am alone I have the most cogent reasons for it. The assertion that I consider the annoyance to my environment as irrelevant and only complain of my own malaise, I deny only—not to be too discursive—by referring to a statement sent to the Director of the Asylum on 16th October 1899, in which I stated:

> " I am still subject to attacks of bellowing which I have repeatedly described to the Director of the Asylum. They occur at different times and occasions in very varying strength and duration, but at times assume such dimensions that I myself feel *I could not show myself on the corridor without molesting*
> p. 439 *the other patients*. Sometimes they even occur in the garden and last almost incessantly during the whole walk, in fact they occur whenever (to which I now add: but only then) I lack the possibility of talking with educated people, etc ".

Besides, the nuisance caused by the bellowing or so-called vociferations is a matter for the *police* only, which, as the judgment itself acknowledges, must remain out of consideration in deciding the legality of my tutelage. Should breaches of the peace occur through my bellowing attacks when I am out of the Asylum which " could not be endured in a house shared with other people " —which unlike the medical expert I do not take for granted and which in any case would have to be proved by experiment—I would be sufficiently sensitive to the impossibility of staying outside a closed institution and would return to it of *my own free will* without there being any necessity for compulsion which could be employed on police grounds.

(B) A second " example " how far my actions are subject to the compulsion of pathological ideas, is supposed to be furnished

* This is not quite correct. As far as the vociferations are articulated words my will naturally plays some part. Only the inarticulate bellowing is really purely compulsive and automatic. I use loud *words* only at certain times because the inarticulate bellowing which would otherwise occur, would be even more disturbing to myself and my environment.

in the judgment I contest by my " Memoirs " and my wish to have them published. Surely in itself it is not unreasonable that a person should wish to bring to the notice of a wider circle the product of his mental labours. Every poetaster who has hammered out a few verses strives to have them printed and everybody thinks this is reasonable, even if the poems are obviously without any poetical value. Similarly my Memoirs might at first appear p. 440
to the reader as muddled, fantastic, and not worth the printer's ink. Nevertheless, it remains precarious to judge in advance whether a mental product is fit for publication or not; not even the authorities in the fields of human knowledge are always capable of such a judgment, much less individual persons: it would not be the first time in history for a new scientific discovery, a new way of looking at the world, a new invention, etc., to be ridiculed by its contemporaries, mocked at and taken as the product of an insane mind, which later had to be granted more or less epoch-making importance. Nevertheless—so the Country Court informs me—my Memoirs are not fit for publication because in them I and my family are compromised in an unheard of manner which would expose me to the danger of criminal proceedings; because I use in them most offensive vulgar words, reveal the most intimate family secrets, and use insulting descriptions for people still living and highly respected, give without modesty an account of the most delicate situations and prove thereby that I have totally lost the capacity to distinguish between the permissible and the impermissible.

In reply I want to say first of all that my intention of publishing my Memoirs is not to be understood in the sense that I will necessarily give them to the printer *in their present form without changes*. I did not write them with the purpose of publishing them. I mentioned this expressly in the " Preface " (which can be read at the beginning of the " Memoirs "). As this Preface contains *in nuce* my (anticipated) reply to the reproaches in the—at the time not even existent—medical report and judgment, I append it here word for word.

> " I started this work without having publication in mind. The idea only occurred to me as I progressed with it; *I did, however, not conceal from myself* doubts which seemed to stand in the way of publication: mainly considerations for certain persons still living. Yet I believe that expert examination of my body and observation of my personal fate during my

lifetime would be of value both for science and the knowledge of religious truths. In the face of such considerations all personal issues must recede ".

This is an indication that I will, in the eventuality of my " Memoirs " being printed, first check the content whether some parts could not be cut out without detracting from the whole, or some expressions rendered more mildly, etc. The possibility of my work actually being printed is by no means as remote as the medical expert assumes. When the latter says in his report (on the penultimate page of my copy) that I was negotiating with a publisher " naturally so far without result ", he did not know that I had two letters in my possession from the publisher (Friedrich Fleischer in Leipzig) of the 5th November and 2nd December 1900, with a fairly definite promise that following my discharge from the Asylum he would be prepared to co-operate in the publication of my " Memoirs ".

Even if my " Memoirs " should be printed in their present form *without any changes*, I would have to deny emphatically that
p. 442 members of my family would thereby in any way be *compromised*. My father's and my brother's memory as well as my wife's honour are as sacred to me as to anyone in similar circumstances who has the reputation of his near relatives at heart. I have not reported the slightest matter which could damage their memory or my wife's name. It is a matter of giving an account of *pathological states* in part most peculiar, which can never be taken as throwing any aspersions on these persons. As far as the danger goes into which I place *myself* by making my " Memoirs " public, " laying myself bare " or compromising myself, I shoulder this risk in full confidence and with complete equanimity. The worst that could happen to me after all, is that one would consider me mentally deranged and *this one does already in any case*. I could therefore hardly lose anything. But I cannot convince myself that there is any fear of people thinking less of me after reading my " Memoirs " attentively. If sexual matters are widely discussed, this is not due to my taste or predilection, but rests entirely on the fact that these matters have played a very large role in the communications of the voices that talk to me, and this again is linked with the fact that voluptuousness is closely related to the state of Blessedness of departed spirits—a fact hitherto unknown to other human beings (compare Chapter XXI of my " Memoirs "). I am sure nobody could say I have shown particular pleasure in vulgarities; on the contrary one cannot miss the moral seriousness which pervades my whole work and

which seeks no other goal but the achievement of truth; no one can p. 443
avoid the impression that wherever it was necessary to be critical of God and divine matters, so to speak, I always anxiously endeavoured to avoid any misunderstanding which could endanger the basis of true religion (compare Chapter V of the Memoirs towards the end, footnote 97 of Chapter XVI of the Memoirs, Postscript V to the Memoirs, etc., etc.). It is true that I used strong language occasionally; but these words did not spring from my own spiritual soil, but are used only as far as I can see, *when I relate* the content of a conversation the voices carry on with me. It is not my fault that these voices often use expressions not fit for drawing rooms; to give a faithful picture I had to render these forms of speech literally. I will give only one example as proof that the "strong language" used by the voices could not have been produced by my own nerves: that particularly offensive word beginning with f. . . . hardly passed my lips ten times in my earlier life whereas in the course of the last few years I have heard it ten thousand times from the voices. How could my nerves unaccustomed to using this word, suddenly without external influence be able to shout or lisp this word at me again and again? Besides, my Memoirs are not written for flappers or High School girls; no understanding person will therefore want to blame me if I have not always hit the form of expression which sensitive school matrons think fit for their charges. A person who wishes to pave a way for a new conception of religion must be able if need be to
use flaming speech such as Jesus Christ used towards the Pharisees p. 444
or Luther towards the Pope and the mighty of the world. The surest proof of "my not compromising myself before other people" in any way, that is to say lose their respect by publishing my Memoirs, is afforded me by the behaviour of the doctors in this Asylum, among them the medical expert himself. There can be no question—and the gentlemen concerned will tacitly agree with this —but that I have been treated very *much more respectfully* in this Asylum since the contents of my Memoirs became known and my intellectual and moral personality appreciated differently than had perhaps been possible before. Similarly I believe I would gain not lose in the moral evaluation of other people.

But it is also said that I "used insulting words about persons still living and highly respected." This can only refer to Professor Flechsig in Leipzig. It is however not true that I used insulting words about him; I request that one point out to me one single passage in my Memoirs where I have used one opprobious word

about Professor Flechsig. It is only correct that I have reported certain events which I must believe were true from the information of the voices that talked to me and which, if they were true and did refer to the *human being* Doctor Flechsig, could be calculated to lower him in public esteem, and if they were untrue would be libellous. The danger of penalty could perhaps arise here. But I am fully alive to this risk and prepared to run it. To clarify my
p. 445 point of view I will quote two of my earlier written elaborations; both date from the time before the judgment, and *before* I was acquainted with the contents of the medical reports. In its entirety the report has only been available to me in the last few weeks (end of May to beginning of July 1901). I sent the following letter to the Director of the Asylum on 4th February 1901:

> "It is known to the Director of the Asylum that I am thinking of publishing my Memoirs and hope to do this after the order placing me under tutelage is rescinded.
>
> For a long time I was in doubt whether publication was permissible. I am fully aware that with respect to certain sections of my Memoirs, Professor Flechsig in Leipzig could feel urged to prosecute me for libel or even demand the withdrawal from circulation of the whole book as constituting a punishable offence (§-40, Str.G.B.). Nevertheless I have at last decided to proceed with publication.
>
> I know I am free from any personal animosity against Professor Flechsig. I have therefore only mentioned such matters concerning him in my Memoirs, which in my opinion are essential for understanding my thesis. I might erase the perhaps somewhat offensive and unessential footnote (erased)
> p. 446 of my Memoirs in case of publication. I hope that Professor Flechsig's scientific interest in the content of my Memoirs will outweigh possible personal susceptibilities. If this should not be the case, the importance I place on the publication of my work, in the hope of thereby enriching science and clarifying religious views, is so great that I would run the risk of prosecution for libel and the threatened financial loss in case of a possible withdrawal of my book from circulation.
>
> I do not make this communication to the Director of the Asylum to obtain an opinion whether a penalty is considered possible, *but only to furnish new proof once again of how carefully I consider the consequences of any of my actions in advance, and so to demonstrate how little one is justified in maintaining that I am incapable of managing my affairs*".

I further added at the end of Postscript VI of my Memoirs the following:

> " In case this book should reach publication, I am well aware that there is one person who could feel hurt by such a publication: it is Professor Flechsig in Leipzig. I have already discussed this in detail in a memorandum of 4th February 1901 to the Director of this Asylum, the wording of which I reproduce here (The above follows here).
>
> I would like to add a few remarks to this.
>
> I naturally have to presume that Professor Flechsig has at p. 447
> least some recollection of the external events connected with my stay in the Nerve Clinic in Leipzig, of which he is Director. On the other hand I dare not state definitely that the supernatural events with which his name is connected and during which his name was *and is still daily given to me* by the voices, ever reached his awareness. It is of course a possibility that in his role as a human being he was and remains removed from these events. The question how it is possible to speak of the soul of a still living person as different from him and existing outside his body naturally remains mysterious. I am absolutely certain that such a soul or at least part of a soul did exist and *still exists* after experiences repeated a thousandfold. I must therefore also acknowledge the *possibility* that everything reported, particularly in the first chapters of my Memoirs in connection with the name Flechsig, is only to be taken as referring to the soul Flechsig as distinct from the living person, the separate existence of which although certain, cannot be explained in a natural way. It follows that I do not in any way wish to attack the honour of the living Professor Flechsig in my intended publication ".

Little remains to be added to the statements repeated above. It
is clearly evident that when I first resolved to publish my Memoirs p. 448
I had the *fullest understanding* of the possible consequences which might follow such a step, *and this appears to me the decisive moment as to whether the question of my legal capacity is to be answered in the affirmative or negative*. Should I wish to add the martyrdom of a threatened penalty to the burden of the untold suffering which has already been mine for a holy purpose, no human being in my opinion would have the right to prevent me. I cannot wish that the knowledge of God which has been revealed to me shall vanish for ever with my death, whereby mankind would lose an oppor-

tunity of attaining truer conceptions about the beyond which may perhaps never occur again. Besides it is an open question whether Professor Flechsig would bring an action, and if he did whether such an action would lead to my punishment. In any case I refuse with due acknowledgment the *protection* planned for me: it would mean, in order to save me from a few months' imprisonment at the most, locking me up in an Asylum *for a lifetime* deprived of freedom of my person and fortune.

I could close the grounds of my appeal with the above; I believe I have refuted all the more important points which were made in the report and in the judgment upholding my tutelage.

But a new moment concerning my health, which arose while I
p. 449 was writing this manuscript, causes me to make an addition, as my future plans cannot remain entirely untouched by it. Until now I lived in the belief that the sleeping drugs provided for me in this Asylum had no effect on my sleep, but that my sleep depended *solely* on the influence of the rays (compare footnote 31 in Chapter V and footnote 45 in Chapter VII of my Memoirs). I only took the sleeping drugs ordered for me because in this as in all other matters I submitted to the doctors' orders. But several nights this month one tried to dispense with sleeping drugs altogether, with the result that during those nights I slept very little if at all. This could have been coincidence as there had previously been nights in which I slept badly. Nevertheless it now seems a possibility or probability that for the time being I cannot do without sleeping drugs. But this would not in the slightest influence my fundamental belief that my person is the object of divine miracles and that my sleep is primarily dependent on the union of all rays. Possibly I can only achieve the *length* of sleep necessary for human beings with the help of medicines. If this is really so, my plans for the future would of necessity have to be somewhat modified. *I do not belong to the class of mental patients who insist constantly and vehemently on their discharge without giving any thought to how their life outside the Asylum would shape both for themselves and their environment.* Further, my stay in this Asylum is at present not so unbearable that I would prefer a
p. 450 lonely life outside the Asylum to the present state of affairs—should it turn out to be impossible to live with my wife. I cannot even be certain whether a hired servant would put up with the attacks of bellowing should they occur frequently. As long as I need

artificial aid to sleep, I am satisfied *to do the correct and sensible thing* and stay under medical supervision; the simplest being to remain in this Asylum where I have now been for seven years. But while I thus give fresh proof of ample and reasonable circumspection, I must insist that my stay in this Asylum is a measure in the interests of my health—irrespective of police considerations—to which I give *my free assent* as a sensible human being capable of looking after his affairs. After all it is a *point of honour*: which person of my high intellectual standing would not feel it an indignity to be treated in legal matters like a child under the age of seven, to be denied every disposition of his fortune even in written form, and, what is more, to be prevented from obtaining information about his financial affairs, etc., etc. Great *practical* significance attaches to the matter over and above this. The need for sleeping drugs might pass sooner or later, the attacks of bellowing now giving rise to police concern, diminish so as to be no longer a serious nuisance **p. 451**
to other people. If such were the case, and I would then suggest a change, perhaps transfer on trial to a private institution, I would as long as I am under tutelage have to fear being sent from pillar to post with my request. The Asylum authorities and my relatives, as also my guardian and the judicial authority—the latter naturally can never be correctly informed about my state—could easily be tempted to shift the responsibility for my release or any change in my circumstances from one to the other. It is therefore of the utmost importance to me to deal in this matter *only* with the Asylum authorities, in whose insight and faithfulness to duty I have complete trust; but whom I cannot spare the burden to act *on their own responsibility* when keeping me against my will in the Asylum, and having this clearly in mind in all their decisions.

I close by repeating the hope that the medical expert will not take any of my statements amiss, as I have no intention whatever of offending him or denying him the high respect which is his due.

Sonnenstein, 23rd July 1901.

Dr. Schreber, *Senatspräsident* (retired).

O.I. 152/00. p. 452

D. *Dr. WEBER'S EXPERT REPORT OF 5TH APRIL 1902*

Sonnenstein, 5th April 1902

To the Superior Country Court,
Civil Division,
Dresden.

To be asked on 14th January 1902 by the Superior Country Court of Dresden, Civil Division, following the evidence of 23rd December 1901, to furnish a further report on the mental state of President Dr. Schreber, is a task little congenial to me. I have been the appellant's doctor for some years, for a long time he was my daily guest at meals, for my part I regard the relations between him and me, if I may say so, as a friendly one, and it is my sincere wish that this man, so sorely tried in the past, will obtain that measure of enjoyment in life to which he thinks he is entitled after so much p. 453
adversity. It has now fallen to me to render a conscientious report about his state as it appears from my observations, and thereby furnish the material which might lead to the confirmation of his tutelage which he is contesting, and the success of which is all-important for his future enjoyment of life. It is always possible that the disclosure of observations made in intimate contact is felt and interpreted as a breach of medical confidence, and although the physician is released from his usual secrecy towards the Court, none the less the free discussion of the patient's morbid symptoms must always remain for the latter a touchy matter, not calculated to make the mutual relationship unconstrained and trusting as it should be. However objective the medical expert attempts to be in his statements, he will never be able to make the mentally ill patient share his opinion in the objectivity of these findings, unless the patient himself were able to judge his condition correctly, whereby he would in fact show that he was *not* ill.

I would therefore have welcomed if another expert had been ordered to give an opinion on this case from the factual evidence provided; in view of my position I have been particularly careful in my earlier reports to keep within my competence as medical expert as I see it. This attitude has been called unjustified by both the appellant and the Crown; all the same I believe I should adhere to this point of view, although in the ordinary clear-cut case the
p. 454 expert himself (and I am no exception) usually draws the conclusions from the established mental illness or mental weakness for the sake of brevity. I refer for instance to Endemann's exposition (Introduction to the Study of the B.S.C., 3rd Edition, p. 147 ff.), and believe I am justified in assuming from the content of the resolution on the evidence that the Court does not find fault with my point of view, as an expert declaration was not demanded from me as to whether the appellant is incapable of looking after his affairs in consequence of his mental illness, but only a comment on and a *supplement* to my previous report. With regard to the request for a supplement, I have somewhat delayed rendering this report in order to be able to take into account events of more recent times when the appellant was able to move about more freely and had command over larger sums of money.

In dealing with the resolution on the evidence I want to start with the question formulated in its third part, because it is a general one and answering it will throw light on some of the questions raised before.

If it is said, perhaps with some exaggeration, that no single leaf of a tree is completely like another, this holds good to a much greater extent for the diseases of the human brain, in so far as it is the substrate of psychic function. It is so very complex an apparatus and developed in so varying degrees, that its disturbances show an infinite variety, the separate abnormalities combine in infinite forms, and no individual case is therefore absolutely like another. This will at once be evident even to the layman, when it is remembered how different the psychic individualities of healthy persons are, how much people vary in promptness and number
p. 455 of associations, in liveliness and depth of feeling, in energy of will and impulses, etc., so that one personality is hardly ever completely like another in all details. If one bears in mind that the original individuality has a marked influence on the form of pathological processes, that pathological ideas in form and content are bound to be of a different character in a person intellectually richly endowed, very knowledgable and ethically prominent,

compared with an individual inferior from the start, poorly developed and mentally dull, and if one further allows that the complicated machinery of psychic life can be disturbed in many different directions, the widest possible variations in the detailed elaboration of the pathological picture must result. But however varied and differently coloured the individual cases of mental illness may be, however characteristic and singular an individual case may appear to careful observation, yet surveying the individual cases one cannot deny that among them certain groupings emerge, certain complexes of pathological manifestations, which in their development, course and outcome, in the involvement of single psychic functions are more or less clearly demarcated from each other; and on the basis of thousands of observations have led to the delineation of a certain number of different disease forms. As colourful and inexhaustible the individual variations of cases of mental illness may be, as constant are the main outlines, and apart from the arabesques of the individual case the basic characteristics of the forms of illness are repeated with almost surprising, monotonous regularity.

Considered from this scientifically established point of view the appellant's mental illness and its peculiarities, far from not being p. 456
known to psychiatry, clearly belong to a well-known and well-characterized form of mental illness, paranoia, and shows all its important distinguishing features. But however common a mental illness paranoia may be, the present case is certainly not a usual commonplace one, just as little as the patient himself is the usual average individual. In paranoia more than in any other form of illness the original personality of the patient is of decisive importance for determining the manifestations of insanity, and as long as secondary dementia (a rare occurrence in paranoia) has not set in, the pathololological products of an intellectually significant man with far-reaching knowledge, lively interest in scientific and philosophical problems, rich in fantasy and of well-trained judgment, will bear the stamp of the original intellectual endowments; but on the whole in the formation and systematization of the delusional ideas, the disease will show the same character as that of another person whose range of ideas does not rise above the most trivial events of daily life.

In my earlier reports I have already described the special features of the mental illness called paranoia, but because of the questions put to me I must repeat them briefly here. Paranoia is a distinctly chronic illness. It mostly develops insidiously but can also start

acutely with the signs of hallucinatory insanity, and after the stormy symptoms have run their course the slowly progressive course starts. It is characteristic of paranoia that delusions develop, frequently in connection with hallucinations and false memories, without the patient's mood being primarily much affected, soon become fixed and are elaborated into a persistent, uncorrected and unassailable delusional system, side by side with
p. 457 presence of mind, unimpaired memory, orderliness and logic of thought. Whether the delusional ideas refer to the condition of the patient's own body (the hypochondriacal form), or to the field of politics, religion, sex, etc., is without great importance for judging the total state. But it is characteristic that the centre of these delusional ideas is always the patient's own person, and that usually ideas of influence, particularly of persecution on the one hand and megalomanic ideas on the other combine, and that mostly—at least for some time—the delusional ideas are limited to a definite group of ideas, while other spheres remain relatively intact. For this reason one used to separate a "partial insanity" and even if this term has now been given up, there is a certain amount of justification for it. It is true that every delusional system must somehow influence all the patient's ideas because its bearer is an 'individual', that is indivisible; this could be proved if we were able to follow in all detail a person's every idea in all its connections. But in fact it is impossible to do this and despite careful observation in not a few cases of paranoia, judgment in some larger complex of ideas, which are only insignificantly and indirectly related to the delusional system, is so little influenced by the latter that for practical purposes it is in some cases nil. It may help to understand this, if I give an example from healthy mental life. It is possible to be in lively scientific contact with another person for a long time, without gaining any insight into his religious convictions, because the latter have no close connection
p. 458 with his scientific views, rather both complexes of ideas lead so to speak a separate existence in his brain. But the time will almost inevitably come when we notice that even the scientific views have been influenced in a significant manner by the religious convictions, which up till then had not come to the fore, perhaps without the person concerned being aware of this influence. The case of the delusional system of a paranoiac is similar: unless specially touched upon it will easily remain hidden from other people, and hardly be noticeable in his ordinary conduct, whereas in reality it forms the substrate of his mental life. It is therefore

neither rare nor remarkable that paranoiacs although perhaps for a long time considered oddities, carry on their business sufficiently well and their professional duties in an orderly manner, can even work scientifically with success, although their mental life is seriously disturbed and they are in the throes of a delusional system which is frequently quite absurd. Such cases are known in large numbers to every psychiatrist of some experience, indeed they illustrate nicely the special features of paranoia. In this always chronic illness the patient may be disturbed by some event in the *modus vivendi* he has maintained towards the outer world, his pathological ideas collide in some way with his environment, he exceeds the limits of what is tolerable in his actions, and thus he is recognized as ill and treated as such. This is common experience; but it can hardly be denied that some cases of paranoia never reach the orbit of medical experience, but remain outside it, recognized perhaps only by their closest associates, and lead the ordinary life of a citizen without any marked disturbance.

Without doubt the appellant's psychosis, in the form it has shown
itself for some years now, belongs to this group of illnesses, although p. 459
it did not, as commonly, start gradually and insidiously, but developed out of an acute stage.

Following the demand of the Appeal Court in its resolution on the evidence, that I deal with the appellant's written communications in the file, I wish to deal briefly with some of the objections the latter raised against my report.

The appellant states (p. 118) that my report is based *a priori* on the tacit supposition that everything he made known about his contact with God and the divine miracles occurring on his body, is based only on pathological imagination. This is not so. Apart from the fact that I do not think I have anywhere used the expression " imagination ", I have in no way assumed *a priori* the pathological nature of these ideas, but rather tried to show from the history of the patient's illness how the appellant first suffered from severe hyperaesthesia, hypersensitivity to light and noise, how to this were added massive hallucinations and particularly disturbances of common sensation which falsified his conception of things, how on the basis of these hallucinations he at first developed fantastic ideas of influence which ruled him to such an extent that he was driven to suicidal attempts and how from these pathological events, at last the system of ideas was formed which the appellant has recounted in such detail and so vividly in his Memoirs, the individual points of which I repeated as far as possible in my earlier

reports. The appellant's legal representative is not quite correct when in his statement he suggests that the medical expert and the Judge saw in his " belief in miracles " and the complex of ideas
p. 460 around them only the basis for the assumption of mental illness, and that this cannot be so, as very many people believe in miracles without anybody thinking of declaring them mentally ill. What is usually called belief in miracles, the naïve theoretical belief intentionally or unintentionally exempted from every criticism, that through His almighty will God sometimes causes events beyond or even against the laws of nature, does not apply in the present case. His ideas, as the appellant himself repeatedly stated and as their content clearly shows, do not emanate from a pious child's belief, but are contrary to his earlier opinions and undoubtedly due to pathological processes of the brain; they are evidenced by disturbances of common sensation and hallucinations and so belong to a category very different from the harmless " belief in miracles ". It cannot be expected that the appellant will gain the insight that these hallucinatory events (in the widest sense the muscular sensations described by the patient belong to them also) are entirely subjective; his expositions on page 164 ff. are aimed particularly at showing that *his* hallucinations are something very special, and at vindicating them by finding a basis in reality for them. But this is bound to be done by every hallucinating person, as otherwise he would not be suffering from real hallucinations. It is their characteristic that they are taken for factual and real and have the same acuity as other sensations. It would be wrong to say that it was *as if* the hallucinating person saw or heard something he does really see and hear, and it would be a waste of time to argue with him about the reality of his impressions. " If what I perceive should
p. 461 be erroneous ", said one patient, " then I must also doubt everything you say to me, in fact I must doubt whether I see you." It would perhaps be going too far to enter further into the subject of hallucinations here, and would serve little purpose in the present matter; it only remains to add briefly that in hallucinations the *inner* abnormal state of excitation of the apperceiving brain apparatus brings to the individual's consciousness what in normal circumstances is only produced by external impressions, that is to say sensations; a process one can also describe by saying that the hallucinating person does not apperceive the world, but himself, i.e. events in his own central nervous system. That hallucinations usually gain much greater power over the total content of patients' consciousness than *real* perceptions is not only due to

their distinctness as sensations, but also to the fact that they fit in with the direction of the dominant complex and grow on the same soil as those perhaps still obscure and unclear trends of thought by which in turn they are mightily fostered and fortified. There can be no doubt that the appellant was and still is hallucinated, and his hallucinations and delusions (subjective pathological interpretation of real events) are not markedly different from those of very many other patients, only they have been shaped according to his individuality. The doubt which he has expressed whether such continuous hallucinations have ever previously been observed is without foundation; they are frequent enough even if rarer than the intermittent cases.

Equally there is no foundation for the statement that " attacks of bellowing " have never been observed before. Among so-called catatonic patients the automatic uttering of inarticulate sounds or endlessly repeated words is not rare, and I have also observed it in paranoiacs. For instance, there was for a number of years among my patients a gentleman of good family, of exceptionally good mental endowment and unusually wide education, who was ruled p. 462
by the delusional idea that people he had known previously, particularly those he thought unfriendly towards him, were locked up in the hollow walls of his house and were from there annoying him by insulting jeering remarks, etc. This paranoid patient, who behaved in an orderly manner, was very entertaining socially, and had quite a successful poetical streak, used to repeat compulsively several times daily for half an hour without interruption very loud inarticulate sounds (" sounds of bellowing ") or abusive language, almost only when he was in his room—he called this " clearing his throat mentally ".

I must further contradict the appellant's repeatedly expressed belief that I have changed my opinion about his condition in the course of time, and as far as one could see would in the future arrive at yet a different opinion about him. It is not my opinion but the condition itself which has gradually changed and gone through markedly different phases. I have already mentioned this in my previous report in detail, and in my opinion comprehensively, and do not think it is necessary to go into the whole process of development of the present state of illness again. Between his earlier state of being occupied by tremendous hypochondriacal delusional ideas, of severe hallucinatory stupor, of markedly negativistic behaviour, characterised by refusal of food and turning away from every contact and occupation, and the present picture of

sensible and sociable approachability, no longer shut off from the demands and interests of the day, there is a vast difference, a difference which is of importance naturally for appraising the total state. How much his condition has changed is also shown by the changes in his hallucinations. Whereas previously in form and content they were of a powerful nature accompanied by lively affect and therefore had a strong, direct influence on him, they have
p. 463 gradually become weaker and at present according to the patient's own graphic account (compare p. 166 ff.) are only a soft lisping noise, a hissing comparable to the sound of sand running out of an hour-glass, while their content also is poorer and more scurrilous, the hallucinated words follow each other more slowly, the "voices" are drowned by an ordinary conversation and, though a nuisance and a burden to the patient, do not influence his feelings and thoughts to any great extent. This is, as I have said before because the acute stage of the psychosis with its vivid changes of feeling passed into a chronic state long ago; out of the stormy turbid flood of the acute stage of the illness the well-known complicated delusional system has crystallized out and become fixed and the patient has come to terms with it in the manner described above, so that to a certain extent it now leads a separate existence in his mental life, and although it represents a very important part of it, being less affect-laden it only acts and reacts little on the rest of his mind, particularly on that part concerned with daily life, and does not influence his actions significantly.

That does not mean that it has no influence at all; in given circumstances it could easily make itself felt in trivial matters and lead to faulty conclusions. I will only touch on one point on which the appellant asks for an expert opinion, namely his peculiar ideas about the male and female body which play a role in his delusional system.

In his opinion the female body in contradistinction to the male has "nerves of voluptuousness" everywhere, particularly on the bosom; he believes he resembles the female type in this and
p. 464 therefore has the corresponding sensations. He cannot be induced to give up this belief, although in actual fact "nerves of voluptuousness" are only present on the genitals, and the female breast owes its form to the development of milk glands and the deposition of fat.

Following these general remarks in answer to the last question in the resolution on the evidence, I now proceed to answer the first and more important question.

It must first be stated that since the previous report was furnished the appellant has been granted gradually increasing freedom of movement in view of his general improvement. Whereas before he was only allowed to go on excursions, visit restaurants and places of public amusement, go shopping, etc., accompanied by an attendant, since the summer of this year he has been allowed out unaccompanied. At that time the appellant's mother and sister took up residence in Wehlen nearby, as planned and arranged by President Schreber himself. For a number of weeks he visited them almost daily, often for the greater part of the day, without an attendant whose presence for obvious reasons would have been disturbing quite apart from the not inconsiderable expense involved. As no untoward incident came to the notice of the Asylum authorities from the omission of this precautionary measure, it was left in abeyance when his relatives departed.

Since then the appellant has been granted absolute freedom of movement outside the Asylum without restriction except for having to conform to the order of the house. He has used it for making almost daily excursions on foot, by ship or railway to visit places p. 465
of interest in the neighbourhood, partly alone, partly in company of one or other patient whom he had invited to join him, sometimes visited concerts, theatres, public shows, etc. He also went repeatedly to Dresden while waiting for the sitting of the Court, visited his wife and did some shopping. At the invitation of his relatives and with the agreement of the Asylum authorities he recently journeyed alone to Leipzig, returning yesterday after an eight days' absence; from his sister's information the visit went off quite well.

One must testify that in the appellant's behaviour on all these occasions there was never anything unreasonable or unfitting. He always discussed frankly and openly his plans, if they were outside his routine, always made certain that the authorities were in agreement before he carried them out, and having obtained permission went ahead after careful planning and consideration of all circumstances, and always returned home from his excursions at the right time. Therefore I believe I am right in assuming that the appellant's conduct in the outside world was never incorrect. One disadvantage of the patient not being accompanied by an attendant from the Asylum was that there were of course no longer reliable reports about his behaviour outside the Asylum. His own accounts cannot be relied upon exclusively in this matter, although he is most truthful and would I believe never

knowingly tell an untruth; but it has often been noticed that he understandably lacks objective judgment of the repercussions and
p. 466 effects of his behaviour. For instance the patient's nightly noisy outbursts not infrequently led to lively complaints by the neighbourhood; when confronted with these he would not believe that he had caused such a disturbance and thought nothing of it. Realizing how noisy the patient is not only in his own room but in the rest of the Asylum and how striking his other peculiarities are, it is difficult to believe that he can *altogether* avoid being conspicuous in other places, and indeed this is not the case.

I have previously described the patient's very striking symptoms even when in company during his daily meals and on other occasions, which any layman would consider pathological: not only the grimacing, screwing up of his eyes, clearing of his throat, the extraordinary position of his head, etc., but still more his occasional almost total distraction and absent-mindedness, so that he does not notice what is going on around him; even recently —*although only once*—he could not restrain himself from letting out the well-known " bellowing sounds " at table, and thereby caused great consternation among the ladies present. At that time he was also so noisy during his wife's visit that she soon had to leave. Eye witnesses further informed me that the appellant became noisy near the Asylum (on the steps) and was gazed at with astonishment in the streets because he was pulling faces. Finally I must not hide the fact that a citizen of Pirna last June wrote protestingly to me about " allowing in public " a patient who behaved like the appellant. This complaint seemed so exaggerated and was denied so convincingly by the patient that I was not
p. 467 inclined to give it much credence; indeed I have heard nothing similar since.

Nevertheless, one cannot doubt that the appellant, unless his total state improves further, will be unable to avoid being a disturbance to his environment after his eventual return home owing to his abnormal compulsive motor impulses in the form of these noisy outbursts. This leads me to say a few more words about the appellant's relation to his wife. It is understandable that he was pained when I referred to his " pathologically increased egoism " in this matter. Nothing was further from my mind with this remark than to disparage his ethical and moral feelings; I am fully aware of their undiminished existence towards his wife as well; the accent is on the word " pathologically " and I only meant the egocentric direction of his thoughts, which occurs in every patient and makes events happening to him the centre of everything, while the effect on other people is underrated because what they suffer at the same time is not appreciated. However that may be, there can be no doubt that in the existing circumstances, unless there is further improvement, the behaviour of the patient is such that marital union could only be resumed with a fair degree of self-denial on the part of his wife, which she might not be able to offer considering her own variable state of health.

Since the appellant has been allowed full freedom of movement outside the Asylum he has also been given a somewhat larger sum (. . . marks monthly) as pocket money in order to cover his excursions and small necessaries. There has been no evidence p. 468 that he squandered this money as a consequence of which it might not have sufficed. Nor was he particularly parsimonious, although he thought carefully before spending money, avoided expensive items and did not buy useless articles (apart, perhaps, from the previously mentioned small trinkets). From his wife's repeated statements I have the impression that in her opinion the patient was spending relatively too much money; but as I do not know details of his financial affairs, I cannot judge whether these remarks were justified; nevertheless I think one will find that he did not spend in excess of his circumstances. In any case the appellant is thoroughly informed about his financial position and at present there is no reason to think he would exceed his means from some pathological motive and, if he had full powers of disposal, that he would squander his fortune.

One cannot say that the appellant does not understand how to look after his health nor that he would damage himself by arbitrary actions. He is clean and looks after his person, eats sufficiently if not to excess, is very moderate in drinking and concerned to maintain his fitness and mobility by means of regular physical exercise. But from his drawn expression it is clear that the frequent, marked sleep disturbances—for which by the way he now only rarely receives drugs—as well as the states of restlessness and agitation occurring by day, have a bad effect on him generally. Only recently was it observed that when he was indisposed he acted very irrationally: he had an attack of indigestion with diarrhoea and p. 469 vomiting, in itself not serious, became greatly excited, saw in it a "divine miracle" and instead of staying in bed and adhering to a strict diet and taking the drugs prescribed, he was driven by his morbid mental processes to doing the very reverse (as far as possible) and so prolonged his indisposition. But as a rule he will not do anything which might influence his health adversely; the above-mentioned episode, however, shows how unaccountable his impulses can be at times through his morbid ideas.

The appellant's oft-repeated firm intention of publishing his "Memoirs" must also be regarded as pathologically determined and lacking sensible consideration. It is unnecessary for me to enter into the details of this manuscript again—it is in the possession of the Appeal Court and its contents will have been carefully examined. Every impartial observer particularly the expert would call this a very interesting presentation of a complicated delusional system, but would regard an unabridged version "impossible" for publication as being both offensive and compromising for the author. But reasoning with him about the propriety of publishing it is hopeless; he sees in it the revelation of a new truth vital for the world and, though he renounces verbal propaganda, he wishes to make known to mankind through the printed word the knowledge granted him of God and the beyond; he is prepared to shoulder all personal unpleasantness that may arise.

p. 470 The Court will know best in how far to judge the foregoing deviations from the normal as a "tendency to unreasonable and wrong action" in the sense of their resolution on the evidence; but it is stressed from the medical side in agreement with the appellant's legal adviser and with himself, that at present the pathological manifestations noticeable *outwardly* concern mostly relatively unimportant fields, exert their disturbing influence more in intimate domestic and social relations, and by their nature bear more on society and welfare-police interests than on the law; the patient's most vital personal interests, his health, fortune and honour, interests which could be safeguarded by the institution of a guardian, do not seem greatly endangered. Only with regard to the last-mentioned can his efforts to get his Memoirs published be regarded as a harmful action.

But the Court also wants to know under [*b*] of the resolution whether in spite of the patient's present favourable behaviour, there are grounds for anxiety in *the nature* of the existing mental illness that the appellant might endanger the above-mentioned and other important interests of life through insensible and injudicious actions, as soon as the freedom of legal action is restored to him. In my earlier report I pointed to the fact that in the nature of so deep-seated an illness as paranoia it is impossible to predict whether and in what direction at a given moment the existing pathological ideas will influence the patient's conduct; I also mentioned that many

paranoiacs with a developed delusional system live in the world
without difficulty, following their profession, until at a given
opportunity they reveal their pathological condition by contrary
actions; I have given above an example of how much the p. 471
appellant can be disturbed by external events and forced to inappropriate action through his pathological revelations, and therefore I
have only to repeat that even now it is not impossible that the
appellant could be influenced in his actions by pathological processes.
When the appellant states (pp. 118 and 119) that the insight gained
into the true nature of divine affairs, the certainty that he is dealing
with God and divine miracles, have become the centre of his whole
life, that God still reveals Himself to him daily and hourly in His
miracles and in His speech, that his constant cheerfulness of mood,
his benevolence towards people little worthy of it, etc. rest on this,
then it is not likely that this mighty current of thoughts and
feelings would never under any circumstances influence his actions,
particularly as even at present some of his actions are caused against
his will directly by "miracles." The appellant's assurances "that
he does not permit his delusions to influence his affairs" can hardly
alter this, as on the one hand he need not become aware of such
influences and on the other the pathological processes may gain so
much in strength that resistance becomes impossible. No assurance
can therefore be given in face of the nature of the illness that
important life interests of the patient might not be endangered
were he freed from his tutelage. Two other points are important
medically. Firstly, it is doubtful whether mere *apprehension* for the
future, the *possibility* of endangering himself severely, is sufficient
grounds for the assumption that he is incapable of looking after
his affairs. Secondly, the danger for the future is now not great,
because the sphere of the appellant's delusional ideas has gradually p. 472
become more sharply demarcated from the rest of his ideas, and has
for some time led a relatively separate existence. Experience so far
shows that his judgment and treatment of a number of important
life interests were not significantly influenced by these complexes
of delusional ideas, but have been carried out faultlessly. Present
conditions do not entitle one to expect any great change in
the appellant's mental state, e.g. deterioration, in the foreseeable
future. Apprehension for the future, therefore, need not weigh
as heavily to-day as previously in judging the over-all situation.

(signed.) Dr. Weber.

E. *JUDGMENT OF THE ROYAL SUPERIOR COUNTRY COURT DRESDEN* p. 473

of 14th July 1902.

O.I. 152/01. No. 22

Pronounced
14th July 1902
Signed: Dr. Förster,
Clerk to the Court.

Day of Exhibition
14th July 1902
Signed: Diethe,
Clerk to the Court.

F. XI 6894/02

IN THE NAME OF THE KING

In the case of

Daniel Paul Schreber, Doctor of Law, *Senatspräsident*, retired, formerly residing in Dresden, now in the Country Asylum Sonnenstein,

Plaintiff and Appellant

(Solicitor: Windisch)

Versus

the Public Prosecutor at the Royal Country Court, Dresden, p. 474
now Public Prosecutor at the Royal Superior Country Court, Dresden, Defendant and Respondent,
re: contesting the order placing plaintiff under tutelage,
the Royal Superior Country Court of Saxony, with Judge Hardraht, President of the Senate of the Court, together with Counsellors of the Superior Court Vogel, Dr. Steinmetz, Nicolai, Dr. Paul,
find:

Appeal of plaintiff is allowed, and the judgment of the Seventh Civil Chamber of the District Court, Dresden of 13th April 1901 confirming the order of the Lower Court,

Dresden, of 13th March 1900 placing plaintiff under tutelage is *rescinded*.

Plaintiff is allowed costs of the proceedings including those of the Court of Appeal.

p. 475

FACTS OF THE CASE

(Pleadings and Evidence.)

Plaintiff was *placed under tutelage* as an insane person at the instance of the Royal Prosecuting Authority by an order of the District Court at Dresden of 13th March 1900. The District Judge declared that he was convinced by virtue of Dr. Weber's expert report in whose care plaintiff had been since 1894, and by the impressions he personally gained by interrogating the patient, that plaintiff was deprived of the use of his reason and therefore incapable of managing his affairs. He held that Dr. Schreber was dominated by delusions, that he considered himself chosen to redeem the world and to restore to it the lost state of Blessedness. This however he could only do by first being transformed from a man into a woman. In this sexual transformation the patient imagined himself the object of continuous divine miracles, and believed he could hear the birds and the winds talking to him, which fortified him in his belief in miracles.

A person influenced by such delusions and hallucinations is no longer master of his own free will. He is subject to external influences independent of his own will, against which he is powerless and which render him incapable of managing his actions and affairs according to practical and reasonable deliberation.

Plaintiff in due course *contested* the order placing him under tutelage by bringing a legal action for suspension of the order. He denies that he is in any way prevented from managing his affairs by the mental illness (paranoia) diagnosed by the medical expert:
p. 476 factual evidence of this assumption had not been produced by the District Court. It is merely a *petitio principii* when it is stated that: a person under the influence of delusions and hallucinations is not master of his own free will. What to the Court may appear as delusions has nothing whatever to do with the question of his legal capacity; in any case his illness is not of a kind to make him incapable of judging correctly those matters of social behaviour which in law are "his affairs", even if one understands "affairs" in the broadest sense, that is to say including everything concerning:

life, health, freedom, honour, family, fortune. In all these matters the clarity of his judgment was not clouded by his illness.

Nobody would be able to say of him that he does not bestow the necessary care upon his body and *health*. Although he admitted *suicidal ideas* in the first years of his illness, he says they disappeared long ago with the continual improvement in his condition. That he sets much store by his *personal freedom* and his *honour* was proved by his endeavour to free himself from the shackles of tutelage; his sense of manly honour was hurt by being treated in law as an infant. He is on the best terms with his wife and his *family* and also has their interests at heart. Finally he is completely capable of managing his *financial affairs* himself. He feels he is as safe as every other person against being taken advantage of in business dealings. Even the District Court in the order placing him under tutelage held that he is still capable of presiding over a panel of Judges, of deciding the most intricate cases and delivering most difficult counsel's opinions with striking juristical reasoning. If this is the case it is difficult to understand why he should not be capable of dealing with the simple legal acts p. 477
involved in looking after his own well ordered finances.

The Country Court ordered a delegated judge to interrogate plaintiff personally, and the Director of the Country Asylum, Sonnenstein, Dr. Weber, to give a further report on his mental state with special reference to: whether the nature of plaintiff's illness and the medical observations made on him in the last few years up to the present time, give grounds for the assumption that plaintiff in case the order for his tutelage were rescinded, would endanger his life, his health, his property or any other interests of life by unreasonable actions. The result of the Judge's personal interrogation of plaintiff is laid down on page 38 ff. of the protocol, while the medical expert Dr. Weber has rendered the requested report in a detailed written document of 28th November 1900 (pp. 44 to 53). With it the medical expert handed to the Court Dr. Schreber's manuscript in 23 copy-books under the title "Memoirs of my Nervous Illness" dealing with his religious views and the history of his illness.

The Country Court in its judgment of 13th April 1901 dismissed Dr. Schreber's action. It agreed with Dr. Weber's expert opinion that plaintiff's high intelligence and his capacity of thinking according to formal logic might not be markedly clouded by his mental illness; nevertheless there was danger of unreasonable action. As perusal of the "Memoirs" proves and the medical expert

Dr. Weber confirms, plaintiff suffers to a considerable extent from hallucinations and delusions, which centre on his relation to God and his exceptional position in the universe. This delusional
p. 478 system dominates his whole feeling and thinking, it influences his conception of the world and his judgment of men and things. Under such circumstances it is quite incalculable what plaintiff's decisions might be if freedom of action were restored to him; whether they would be taken according to the sphere of ideas which remained comparatively untouched by his madness, or under compulsion of his morbid psychic processes. In two matters the detrimental effect of Dr. Schreber's delusional ideas on his whole outlook, is particularly clear: in his relation to his wife who suffers much from his delusion of being unmanned, and to whom, when she tries to object to his ideas, he always readily suggests that she could divorce him. Further, plaintiff has the urgent desire to make his " Memoirs " known to the public in print, and strives to have the order of tutelage rescinded mainly to be able to conclude a valid contract for publishing his manuscript. Actually the " Memoirs " are quite unfit for publication; plaintiff would thereby compromise his family and himself in an unheard-of fashion, might even expose himself to the danger of criminal prosecution. That plaintiff cannot recognize this himself proves to what extent, in consequence of his pathologically altered conception of the world, the proper appreciation of the actual circumstances of life, the capacity of distinguishing between the permitted and the impermissible, have been lost.

Plaintiff appealed against the Country Court's judgment and repeated his request for rescission of the Order placing him under the care of a guardian, while the Public Prosecutor asked for dismissal of the appeal. The contested judgment referred to in
p. 479 its entirety, besides all documents cited in it, Dr. Schreber's personal written communication to the Court and to the Asylum authorities, as well as the content of the tutelage file of the District Court CJI 64/99, were read out in Court. The reading of Schreber's " Memoirs " was restricted to Chapters I, II, XVIII, XIX, as agreed between both parties.

Plaintiff appeared personally at the hearings before the Court of Appeal and frequently pleaded himself beside his legal representative. He presented from his own pen a number of rejoinders contradicting the conclusions of the First Instance and Dr. Weber's expert opinion on which it was based, and discussed thoroughly his opposite opinion in factual and legal respects. Plaintiff stressed that the formal treatment which he personally gave to his case should be taken into consideration by the Judges in deciding the question of his legal capacity. A person who is capable of dealing with so involved a legal matter in self-composed representations with circumspection and expert knowledge, and is tactful and discreet where other people's opinions are concerned, should be trusted to be capable also of managing the simpler and less important matters of ordinary life in a competent way.

The following of plaintiff's pleadings are to be stressed:

I

p. 480

First, plaintiff denies that in the District Court he admitted being or having been mentally ill. He only concedes that his nervous system has for years been in a morbid state; but his mind, that is to say the working together of the sum total of his intellectual powers, is as clear and healthy as any person's. When the medical expert suggests that he is suffering from a form of insanity (paranoia), in that he declares *a priori* everything as morbid imaginings that plaintiff reported in his "Memoirs" about the intimate communication between himself and God and about divine miracles, he goes in the face of truth. He naturally knows the medical expert could do no other than apply to his (Dr. Schreber's) case the standards of common scientific experience, and he does not in the least want to chide him because of this approach. Dr. Weber stands with his feet firmly planted in rationalism, which denies out of hand the possibility of supernatural happenings.

In opposition to him plaintiff champions fundamentally the contrary point of view: the *certainty of his knowledge of God* and the absolute conviction that he is dealing with God and divine miracles *tower for him above all human science*. It has become and must remain for him the centre of his whole life, because God still reveals Himself anew to him daily and hourly in His miracles and in His language. His steady serenity of spirit rests on this; it remains with him despite all the adversities of life and can be p. 481 observed by everyone who meets him; from it also springs the calm, kindly feeling which he entertains even towards those who in earlier years unwittingly hurt him, and this explains the great stress he lays on the publication of his "Memoirs". He does not wish to make propaganda for his belief in miracles, much less would he want to sacrifice one penny for it. His only reason in wishing to publish his "Memoirs" is to raise doubt whether it is possible that after all his " delusional system ", as one sees fit to call it, has a basis in truth and he has really been granted a glance behind that dark veil which otherwise hides the beyond from the eyes of man. He is convinced that after the publication of his book the scientific world will take a serious interest in his person. Far from wishing to play the prophet of a new religion he looks upon himself solely as an object of scientific observation. Whatever one may think of his belief in miracles, no one is entitled to see in it a mental defect which makes plaintiff require State care. One does not usually and without further reason declare the adherents of spiritualism mentally ill and put them under a guardian, although their way of looking at things supernaturally is also neither shared nor comprehended by the vast majority of their fellow men.

II

Even supposing that psychiatrically speaking he had to be counted mentally ill, it would have to be proved that *in consequence* he is *incapable* of managing his affairs.

p. 482 The expert refused to express a definite opinion on this last point. He only stated that it was *unpredictable* whether and in how far plaintiff might be induced to act unreasonably, if his freedom of action were restored to him. With such general forms of speech and vague fears the matter is not settled. Rather it would have to be proved on the basis of facts and actual experiences particularly those of the last few years, that and in what direction he has a tendency to act unreasonably because of his " delusions and hallucinations ".

He admits that there is less chance of making such observations on a person detained in an Asylum than on a person at large. Strictly speaking, the medical expert Dr. Weber only came to know plaintiff more closely since Easter 1900 when he was permitted to share meals regularly at the family table. This has changed considerably in the meantime. Since the previous report was furnished, more than a year has passed during which he has been granted considerable freedom of movement by the authorities of the Asylum. He has undertaken numerous greater and smaller excursions, visited places of public amusement, shops, churches, theatres and concerts, in the last six months without being accompanied by an attendant, and was provided with a certain amount of money. He declares that nobody will ever have noticed the least sign of

faulty conduct on these occasions. It never occurred to him to molest other people by making known his delusions. He believes for instance to be justified in maintaining that the ladies of the family table of the Director of the Asylum would not have the faintest idea of his delusions, unless informed of them some other way.
It is true that at times he mentioned them to his wife, but this is p. 483
adequately explained by the close bond that exists between them.

The only way in which his behaviour to the outside world is influenced to a certain extent by his " delusional ideas " and which could perhaps make him appear unreasonable in the eyes of other people, is the circumstance also stressed by the expert Dr. Weber, that he sometimes decks himself out with some feminine ornaments (ribbons, trumpery necklaces and suchlike). This he admits might appear silly to many people, but states that he has good reasons for it. He thereby usually achieves considerable amelioration of the states of bellowing which would otherwise be extremely troublesome to him and his environment. At worst it is only a whim, absolutely harmless and not in any way detrimental either to himself or others.

The financial aspect does not enter into consideration; the whole lot cost him hardly more than a few marks.

III

The medical expert stressed in his report:

> " The most important point for judging the patient's capacity for appropriate action is the fact that everything which to objective observation appears as delusions and hallucinations is for him unalterable truth and *adequate motive for action* ".

He unreservedly admits the first part of this, but must counter the second with an unconditional " No ". The religious conceptions he cherishes could never lead him to unreasonable action in
practical life. They are completely without influence on his p. 484
capacity to manage his own affairs and care for his interests. He cannot understand how Dr. Weber arrived at the contrary opinion. He certainly has not given any grounds for it in his actions up till now. He does not dream of bringing pecuniary sacrifices to further his belief or to have the presence of " nerves of voluptuousness " in him confirmed. The certainty of his knowledge of

God is so great and unshakable, that he is indifferent to what other people think about the truth or probability of his ideas.

He wishes to be trusted in his assurances about his future behaviour, because he has never given any cause to doubt the inviolability of his love of truth. The expert's apprehensions that it was " entirely incalculable " to what extent plaintiff could be led to unreasonable action by his delusions are therefore unfounded. The Country Court itself considers this apprehension justified chiefly in two points: firstly in respect to the matrimonial relation to his wife which could be destroyed by rescinding the tutelage order, and secondly in view of his plan to publish his " Memoirs ", as he would thereby compromise himself and even run the risk of a penalty. But neither of these considerations suffices to uphold his tutelage.

(a) The *matrimonial bond* between himself and his wife has in consequence of his illness for years been as good as non-existent and would remain in abeyance, if his tutelage were continued in the future, perhaps even to the end of the life of either spouse. It is possible that the return to his family for which he strives might entail inconveniences for his wife. But this does not come
p. 485 into consideration because a person can be placed under tutelage only in his own interests, in order to safeguard him from the threatening dangers of his unreasonable actions, but never to protect other persons, however closely related, from unpleasantness. Of course he has legal liabilities to his wife in that he has to provide adequate maintenance for her. He would never shrink from fulfilling this legal obligation; rather he would at all times be prepared to provide his wife with sufficient means to live apart from him, in case after his return from the Asylum circumstances should arise in which she could not reasonably be expected to live with him.

The expert's remark that, when his wife argues about his belief in miracles he is quick to indicate that she could divorce him, apparently rests on a misunderstanding. He has never toyed with the idea of divorce nor shown indifference to the continuance of the marital bond. The whole extensive correspondence he maintained with his wife for years proves how heartfelt his love for her still is and how it pains him that she too has been made so deeply unhappy by his illness. Accordingly he discussed the possibility of divorce only by mentioning a few times that if his disturbing states of bellowing should make life with him intolerable, or should it be impossible for her to continue loving and respecting him because of certain other peculiarities arising from his belief in miracles, she had the legal right to divorce him.

(b) The second example of to what extent he acts under the compulsion of his pathological ideas was seen by the District Court p. 486 in the content of the " Memoirs " and his wish to see them published.

He never concealed from himself and in fact expressed in the Preface to the " Memoirs " that there are certain objections to their publication. Should they reach the printer, he would continue to keep in mind erasing certain passages and toning down certain expressions beforehand. He does not intend publishing them in their present form. He only submitted the manuscript for inspection to the publishers in Leipzig with whom he entered into negotiations about the publication of the " Memoirs ".

Even if the manuscript remained completely unaltered he wishes to protest strongly that he would thereby " compromise " any member of his family, as the District Court seems to assume. There can be no question of this. The " Memoirs " do not contain the least that might be construed as damaging to the reputation of his father, his brother or his wife. Plaintiff accepts fully any risk of compromising himself in publishing his " Memoirs ". The worst that could befall him is that one would consider him mentally deranged and this one does in any case. Actually he believes that there is no danger that anybody who reads his " Memoirs " carefully would think less of him afterwards than before. At all times his only aim has been to discover the truth. It is true as the contested judgment criticizes in his manuscript, that he occasionally uses offensive strong language. But these expressions do not originate from him, but occur only where he relates the content of the conversations the voices held with him. It was not his fault that these voices frequently used expres- p. 487 sions not fit for drawing rooms. Besides, his " Memoirs " were not written for flappers or High School girls. Admittedly there is one person who might feel hurt by the publication of the " Memoirs " and who might possibly bring a libel action against him; it is Professor Flechsig in Leipzig. Even, here, however plaintiff only related events about him which from information received from the voices talking to him he had to believe were true. He is certain that Flechsig will forgive him, and he had even thought of sending him a copy of the " Memoirs " because he believed that Flechsig would take a scientific interest in the problems discussed. It was far from him to attack Flechsig's personal honour. But should, despite his expectations, the publication of the manuscript lead to his being punished for libel, he was prepared for the sake of the cause to accept this new martyrdom also, and no one in his opinion had the right to prevent him from doing so.

The Public Prosecutor considers the continuance of the tutelage legally necessary and dictated by plaintiff's own interests; he holds there is not the slightest doubt that Dr. Schreber suffers from paranoia judging from his pleadings before the Court of Appeal. It is equally beyond doubt that in consequence he is not in a position to manage his own affairs reasonably, although the medical expert wishing to limit his competence, did not express a sufficiently definite opinion on this point. As Dr. Weber rightly says psychic processes are an organic unity and it is impossible that those areas of mental life not immediately filled with delusional ideas would remain entirely untouched by them; one should not be misled by
p. 488 plaintiff's verbal and written statements giving in part the impression of clarity.

There is no need to detail individual facts to show plaintiff's incapacity to manage his own affairs. Such facts exist. For instance plaintiff is obviously incapable of judging how much longer he will have to remain in the Asylum. If his tutelage were rescinded he would sooner or later certainly endeavour to be discharged from the Asylum. In one of his letters to the lawyer Dr. Thürmer, his Counsel in the District Court (pp. 68, 74 of the file), he wrote:

> "He knows exactly and better than any doctor what is good for him physically and mentally, as it is a matter of defending himself against the harmful effects of divine miracles".

One may see from this that plaintiff has no real insight into his illness and that he will not listen to advice. In addition he is visited by hallucinations which according to Dr. Weber's evidence preoccupy him in the middle of a conversation and disturb his concentration. It is evident that this might be disastrous when he is dealing with money matters. It is not so simple to administer his and his wife's estate. According to the last inventory made by the President of the District Court Schmidt in Leipzig in his capacity as guardian (p. 177 of the tutelage file) it consists in part of real estate and in a share of a copyright. Dr. Schreber's behaviour towards his wife also gives rise to well-founded doubts whether

he would be capable of freeing himself from the influence of his delusional ideas in his dispositions for her. Despite all assurances p. 489
to the contrary given by plaintiff in this respect, one must also fear that in pursuing the idea of a divine mission he might be led to expenses which he would not incur as a man acting of his own free will. How much Dr. Schreber's whole way of thinking is faulty is shown not least by his persistent and firm intention of publishing his " Memoirs ".

Plaintiff denies all these allegations. He states that the experience gained since Dr. Weber's last report of 28th November 1900, has proved that despite all alleged delusions and hallucinations he is perfectly capable of conducting reasonably his business and other affairs alone and in accordance with his legal interests. He is convinced that in the face of these new experiences Dr. Weber himself would no longer wish to maintain his statements in an earlier report about plaintiff's incapacity to manage his affairs.

It is correct that he strives to achieve his release from the Asylum in the not too distant future. He expects no further improvement in his health by continuing his stay at Sonnenstein. But a little delay may yet be necessary. He agrees that it might be sensible to remain in the Asylum as long as his states of bellowing persist, although he has observed that the bellowing occurred only while he was in the Asylum but almost never outside, when travelling, etc. But these " vociferations " have nothing to do with his capacity or otherwise of managing his affairs. They are only a welfare and police matter which in certain circumstances might give the Asylum authorities—in their capacity as organs of the security police—the right to keep him in the Asylum against p. 490
his will. He wishes to repeat however that no force would be necessary in this direction, as he would not oppose remaining in the Asylum while disturbances could be feared from frequent attacks of bellowing.

The Court of Appeal in its resolution on the evidence of 30th December 1901 asked Dr. Weber to furnish a supplement to his first report clarifying three matters under *a*, *b*, *c* of the resolution, and particularly requested information about the experiences made since November 1900 respecting plaintiff's capacity to move freely outside the Asylum and manage his affairs. Dr. Weber rendered the report (p. 203 ff.) in writing under oath, and supplemented it with a postscript (p. 231) prompted by some of Dr. Schreber's (p. 223 ff.) arguments against the factual basis of his report. Both reports were read in Court.

Plaintiff believes that the statements of the later report can be interpreted as more favourable to him. He is satisfied that the medical expert is now *in doubt* as to whether continuation of his tutelage is imperative. In point of fact in the last two years not a single instance of unreasonable action could be proved against him. Even the occasional disturbing bellowing sounds which stilll seem to cause the medical expert some apprehension, but which outside the Asylum never amount to a serious annoyance and breach of the peace, have lately decreased. During his week's stay in
p. 491 Leipzig they never once occurred as his relatives would confirm. As the bellowing is caused automatically, that is to say independently of his will, it could not possibly be considered a sign of a tendency to unreasonable behaviour.

The medical expert is wrong in stating that he acted unreasonably in a recent illness (diarrhoea and vomiting) by refusing the medicines ordered for him. He closely followed medical instructions (proof: attendant Müller), and it cannot be said that he fails to appreciate the value of medicines, even despises them. The reverse is seen to be true from the fact that he did not refuse to take sleeping drugs for his insomnia.

Besides, he has diligently sought every opportunity lately of conversing with other people including strangers while on his walks, excursions, and journeys. He wished to refer to their evidence. Of the great many people concerned he wished to name as witnesses for the time being only the following: his brother-in-law, the merchant Karl Jung in Leipzig and his wife, his eldest sister; his brother-in-law, the Country Court Judge Krause in Chemnitz and his wife, his youngest sister; his guardian, President of the District Court Schmidt in Leipzig and his wife; the physician Dr. Nakonz; the lawyer Dr. Schill; Dr. Hennig; the publisher Nauhardt, the possible publisher of his "Memoirs", all in Leipzig; finally the retired President of the Court Thierbach in Dresden and Majors Meissner and Sander in Pirna. They would all confirm that during their meetings with him they received the impression of
p. 492 a completely reasonable person capable of every demand of social and business life, in whom they as laymen did not notice the least sign of a mental illness, let alone one making him incapable of managing his affairs.

More recently a very important fact was added for judging his legal capacity. In order to make the Asylum authorities take a more definite stand regarding the question of his tutelage, he tried to sound them whether there was any objection to his possible discharge from the Asylum in the near future. He did not mean immediate discharge from one day to the next. The precarious health of his wife, with whom he wishes to live together again and the choice of a home suitable for her as well as himself, would require careful consideration and preparations which would take time. He also assumes that the Asylum authorities would wish to consult his guardian and perhaps even his wife before his discharge and above all would wish to ensure that living arrangements had been made. He therefore formulated his question in a letter to Dr. Weber of 29th May 1902 in the following way:

> " Whether, the present state of affairs prevailing and provided no objection were raised by the guardian or judicial authority against discharge, and provided his wife were not averse to having him or some other residence were found, the Asylum authorities would consider *granting* his wish to be *discharged* in due course taking into consideration only welfare police matters ".

Dr. Weber answered on 30th May 1902 (p. 252b/253 in the file) p. 493
as follows:

> " The Asylum authorities would at present *not* place an obstacle in the way of your discharge with the provisos mentioned in your letter and as long as there is no deterioration in your condition.
>
> For the Asylum authorities, apart from possible medical advice, the decisive moment when considering discharge or a trial leave period, is only the possible ' danger ' which the patient's illness may bring to himself or others. Such does not exist in the present case . . . etc."

The *Public Prosecutor* acknowledges the letters exchanged between plaintiff and Dr. Weber. Nevertheless, he opposes rescinding the tutelage, because despite all plaintiff's protestations to the contrary, the fear cannot be denied that he may be driven to foolish and unreasonable actions under the compulsion of his delusional insanity. For instance plaintiff would certainly have to bring considerable financial sacrifice in order to carry through his planned publication of the " Memoirs ", as an ordinary contract with a publisher is most unlikely to be concluded.

Plaintiff counters the last point as follows:

> " The publication of the ' Memoirs ' is planned, according to preliminary agreement with the publisher Nauhardt in

Leipzig, in the form of a contract on the basis of a commission, the same form of publication in which his father's 'Medical Indoor Gymnastics' appeared. The financial risk he runs is restricted to the production costs of the book, a sum of ......
p. 494 marks. Such an expenditure is small in relation to his total means which may be estimated at ...... marks. For the rest he wishes to repeat his previous assurance that he would not make propaganda for his belief in miracles and that it would not occur to him to sacrifice one penny of his capital for it."

GROUNDS OF THE JUDGMENT

The Court is in no doubt that the appellant is insane. One would not wish to argue with him whether in fact he suffers from a mental illness known as paranoia. He lacks insight into the pathological nature of the inspirations and ideas which move him. What to objective observation is hallucination and delusion is for him irrefutable certainty. Even now he holds fast to the conviction that God manifests Himself to him directly and continuously performs His miracles on him. This conviction, as he says himself, towers high above all human insight and science.

But it is not sufficient grounds for placing plaintiff under tutelage that his mental processes are pathologically disturbed. The Civil Code demands under §6 No. 1 apart from the existence of a mental illness that the patient in consequence thereof is *incapable of managing his affairs*. Not every mental abnormality therefore leads necessarily to a negation of legal capacity. Placing under tutelage is justified only when mental illness is so severe that it prevents
p. 495 the patient from managing *all* affairs like a child under the age of seven. If the patient is not completely deprived of the capacity of acting sensibly and reasonably, but is only restricted through mental illness in appreciating special matters or a certain range of his affairs, this can in certain circumstances cause him to be made a ward of the Court (§ 1910, section 2 of the Civil Code), but never to be placed under tutelage.

"Affairs" referred to by the law in §6, No. 1, is not to be understood only as pecuniary affairs as the District Court rightly assumed.

The concept embraces the entirety of all circumstances of life, the ordered regulation of which is of interest to the law: protection of the person to be placed under tutelage, of his life and health, no less than the care of his relatives and his estate. Tutelage is primarily a protective measure. It is designed to assist him, who in consequence of being without insight is incapable of protecting himself, from being taken advantage of, and against exploitation by others. The State's duty to the patient extends as far as the patient's need of protection. But the precautionary measure of tutelage offered by law to the patient to save him in civil life from dangers arising out of his lack of will-power, must in fact be adequate and effective. Placing under tutelage is only permissible if such dangers to the person concerned are present which can be successfully countered by abjudication of his legal capacity (§104^3 of the Civil Code) and by appointing a guardian for the general care of his personal and pecuniary affairs (§1896). (Compare memorandum to the draft of the Civil Code, p. 2.).

In this sense is appellant in need of such protection or is he p. **496**
capable of managing his affairs himself?

The medical expert Dr. Weber gives no definite answer to this question in his two reports. He does not answer it with a direct yes or no. The decision is clearly difficult for him. Whereas in the usual clear-cut cases of mental illness he generally does not hesitate to draw the legal consequences from a proved mental illness (p. 203b) himself for the sake of brevity, he declines to do so in the present case. He limits himself to delineating the picture of plaintiff's mental illness and to assembling the actual instances in which the patient's disturbed mental life presents itself conspicuously, leaving it to the Judge to decide for himself from his reports whether plaintiff is to be considered capable of safeguarding his life interests in civil affairs.

One cannot raise any objection to the medical expert's attitude. It is in fact not within the province of the medical expert to decide the practical legal aspect of the ascertained mental illness of a person, nor its influence on his legal capacity. To form an opinion on this question is solely the responsibility of the Judge.

Because the medical expert calls the illness which is manifested by plaintiff's delusions *paranoia*, one might be tempted to regard the question *sub judice* as thereby already decided. Thus Endemann in his textbook (§31, p. 136, No. 8, p. 137, 3rd Edition) states *simply* that every person suffering from paranoia can be placed under tutelage; he is satisfied that the *nature* of this mental illness is in itself sufficient proof that the person suffering from it is p. **497**
incapable of weighing reasonably the consequences of his actions.

This goes too far. As the medical expert Dr. Weber, an acknowledged authority in the science of psychiatry, correctly emphasizes, there are numerous paranoiacs who, despite severe mental derangement and although their thinking sometimes moves in the confines of the most absurd delusional ideas, are hardly recognized as sick by their environment, carry on their daily business correctly and in general fulfil the duties of their profession adequately. One might consider them peculiar, call them whimsical and think that they have fixed ideas, but as a rule one does not think of placing them under tutelage. The progress of recent legislation lies precisely in the fact that it is now possible to leave such more or less harmless persons in possession of their legal capacity of free disposition necessary to their progress in life, despite their ascertained mental derangement. Even though such persons are influenced by compulsive ideas which make them appear irresponsible in those fields of mental life directly affected they have not *altogether* lost the faculty of acting reasonably. In those fields of mental activity removed from their delusional ideas or less exposed to them, they are mostly capable of carrying out their professional duties in a manner which gives rise to no objection.

Compare Krafft-Ebing, Doubtful Mental States, p. 8; also Samter, in Gruchots *Beiträgen*, June 1901, p. 3.

According to Dr. Weber's report (p. 206) to *this group of illnesses belongs plaintiff's psychosis* in the form it has taken in the last four years after the transition from the stage of acute insanity to the chronic illness. It is true plaintiff's way of looking at the world is falsified
p. 498 by the idea ruling him about his extraordinary position towards God, and Dr. Schreber suffers much from hallucinations. He acknowledges that the centre of his life is his conviction that he is the continual object of the divine power of miracles. But only *one single field* of plaintiff's mental life is affected, the field of religion. What in our views is connected with divine matters and our belief about the relation of man to God, plaintiff will never be able to judge correctly, because he lacks insight into the pathological nature of his mode of thinking. But it does not necessarily follow that his judgment in all other fields of mental life must be equally pathologically altered. A person's religious feelings may have many and important points of contact with other fields of his mental life; nevertheless one cannot maintain that all these need be equally affected. The religious conviction which fills the believer and often enough is the centre of life of the mentally

healthy, does not enter into all aspects of life; Dr. Weber points out convincingly how a person can be in close scientific contact with another for a long time without gaining any idea of his religious convictions; these usually have no very close connection with his scientific views, both complexes of ideas leading up to a point a *separate existence* in his brain.

The case of the *paranoiac's* delusional system is similar according to the medical expert's statement (p. 205b). The Prosecuting Authority is therefore not correct when it holds against plaintiff, following Endemann's expositions, that because he is under the influence of delusional ideas his whole thinking therefore rests p. 499
eo ipso on a false basis, and that in consequence all his acts of will must be pathologically influenced; as mental life is a unity, pathological fields of thought must of necessity spread to parts apparently healthy and little touched by the delusional system.

It would appear that this notion of the unity of all psychic events is reflected in the scientific views of modern psychiatry. The medical expert Dr. Weber in his report also makes it his starting point (pp. 447, 205). Nevertheless its immediate importance is only theoretical. Opposite views used to be held; one unhesitatingly recognized "partial insanity" and that this concept is still somewhat justified even today, is seen in Dr. Weber's report (p. 205b). Whatever one's scientific or theoretical views about this question, the Judge ordering tutelage has to consider the fact proved by experience, that the influence of delusional ideas ruling a paranoiac does not affect equally all fields of his *ordinary civil life*. Frequently there is present only a "partial insanity", the pathological ideas withdraw to a certain circumscribed field and within these limits maintain a kind of "separate existence", while other fields of life remain comparatively untouched and do not show any signs of mental derangement in the patient (p. 205).

Certainly, one cannot deny the possibility of a partial disturbance spreading to a person's total mental function. This is a theoretical possibility in every form of mental abnormality. Dr. Weber perhaps wished to express this and nothing but this, when he declared in his first report (p. 53) that it was unpredictable how at p. 500
any given moment plaintiff might decide, should his legal capacity be restored; whether according to the dictates of his relatively healthy ideas or under the compulsion of the pathological belief in miracles which fills him.

This alone however does not suffice for placing him under tutelage. As plaintiff rightly argues, one cannot deprive him of his legal capacity on the mere *suspicion* that his delusional ideas might lead him to unreasonable action in this or that field. According to law it is necessary to *establish positively* that in consequence of mental illness he is incapable of managing his affairs (§6[1] of the Civil Code). The burden of proof lies with him who requests an order placing a person under tutelage. If proof cannot be furnished against plaintiff and if official inquiries according to §653 C.P.O., into the mental state of the patient have also not led to any definite result, then the order of tutelage cannot be maintained.

It is a debatable point what demands such proof should fulfil. One certainly cannot go as far as plaintiff who wishes to allow a patient to be placed under tutelage only when the danger of his acting unreasonably is based on certainty. On the other hand one must not be satisfied with mere doubts. The doubts must at least be tangible and have, through facts or otherwise, become probabilities.

The showing of proof is therefore shifted to that field which alone can offer a conclusive answer to the question to be decided, namely the field of *factual experiences*.

p. 501 In order to place a person under tutelage it must be ascertained to what extent a patient's delusions influence his actions and omissions in social life. Is the person to beplaced under tutelage still capable of meeting the demands of practical life despite his clouded mind, or are his senses so disturbed that his judgment for the reality of things and their sensible comprehension has been lost? This can only be decided with certainty on the basis of experience. The patient must actually have been exposed to the demands of life and have had to deal with affairs of legal consequence. Observations made on him in such circumstances would be the best test for establishing the correctness of his statement that though ill, he is nevertheless able of managing his affairs sensibly and in accordance with his interests like any other reasonable human being. The *nature* of his mental illness does not afford a reliable clue for the medical specialist. It only admits of suppositions. As already stated the presence of paranoia does not exclude the continuance of complete legal capacity.

In this opinion the Court is in agreement with the medical expert. Even in his first report of 28th November 1900 Dr. Weber expressed regret that plaintiff had till then been rather restricted in acting independently in the ordering of his affairs outside the walls of the Asylum, so that the matter had not been put to proper test (p. 45). He therefore limited himself mainly to giving a picture of the illness as it presented at the time to the eye of the expert observer.

This situation has improved in the meantime. Since the first report the patient has been permitted greater freedom of movement. He has been allowed contact with the most varied circles of p. 502 the outside world. He has had the opportunity of showing, in dealing with his relatives and others, to what extent his delusional ideas rule his general thinking and feeling and to what extent they influence his relation to his fellow men. The Court of Appeal now has much more factual material for its judgment than the lower Court had at the time. The observations which have been made in this matter are altogether *favourable* to plaintiff.

One observation was forced on the Judges of the Court of Appeal in their dealings with plaintiff during the proceedings; it was that Dr. Schreber's intellectual powers and the clarity of his thinking had *in no way* suffered by his illness. The way he personally took up the fight against the tutelage under which he was placed and how he carried it through according to plan, the acuity of the logical and juristical operations developed by him, the reasonableness with which he conducted himself, and last but not least the refined measured attitude he showed when in opposition to the medical expert and the Prosecutor—all this affords indisputable proof that in *this* field plaintiff has no need of protection by a guardian; rather in conducting his case he was able to preserve his interests to the full and independently, better indeed than anybody else could have done it in his place.

Too great a weight must, however, not be placed on this side of plaintiff's mental life. The capacity to think logically and correctly appears, as Dr. Weber remarks (p. 50b), well developed in paranoiacs; it is not an infallible sign of the patient's equal capacity to judge correctly matters of life that lie outside pure thinking. In this sphere the complementary experiences are important p. 503 which the medical expert Dr. Weber has had the opportunity of collecting about the patient's behaviour in his relation to the outside world during the last eighteen months, and on which he reported in his second report of 5th April 1902.

In his first report Dr. Weber, despite little opportunity of collecting observations on Dr. Schreber's social behaviour, had to acknowledge that the pathological sphere of his mind was already fairly sharply demarcated from the rest, and had to add that plaintiff's judgment in matters and affairs far removed from his firmly established delusional system was usually correct (pp. 47, 50b); in his second report he repeated this with great emphasis.

The picture of the illness itself has not changed. In the main it is the same as when he was placed under tutelage. Only more material based on observation is available, giving the medical expert the opportunity of supplementing his previous opinion which was based on fairly limited factual material, and where necessary of correcting it. There can therefore be no hesitation in applying the results reached by the medical expert only in his later report, and using them in retrospect directly for judging plaintiff's mental state at the time when he was placed under tutelage.

Dr. Weber is now convinced that plaintiff's delusional ideas lead a relatively *separate existence* in his mental life and that outside the religious field which they mainly dominate they affect other fields particularly of daily life *hardly* at all; and that hallucinations from which plaintiff continues to suffer, do not now influence his
p. 504 feeling and thinking to *any significant degree*. Such pathological manifestations as do appear are noticeable outwardly mostly in comparatively *unimportant* fields only. Especially the *more important* life interests have withdrawn from their domination and are appreciated in a manner *beyond reproach* (pp. 208 a/b, 211b, 212b).

In order to furnish further grounds for his opinion the medical expert mentions a number of actual events *in part observed* by himself, *in part* reported to him by reliable observers; all these have also strengthened the Appeal Court in its conviction that the danger of plaintiff's wrong and inappropriate action in affairs of legal consequence appears almost nil, in any case not so imminent as to justify the upholding of his tutelage.

For a few years appellant has eaten daily as a guest at the family table of the Director of the Asylum without causing any annoyance to the others present. On the contrary Dr. Weber, who looks upon his relation to plaintiff as a friendly one, extols the patient's delicate tact and forbearance which prevented him from molesting the company at table with his miraculous ideas (p. 50b). Dr. Schreber believes he can be certain that other persons at table, particularly the ladies, have never noticed even a trace of his mental illness. In view of Dr. Weber's statements about patient's conduct one can give the latter credence.

The appellant's movements outside the Asylum also have not given rise to any trouble worth mentioning. While Dr. Schreber until the summer of 1900* was only allowed outside the Asylum accompanied by an attendant, he has since then been allowed unlimited freedom of movement unaccompanied outside the Asylum. He has used it to make almost daily excursions on foot, by ship or railway, to visit all noteworthy parts of the environment of Pirna, partly alone, partly in company and also at times to frequent concerts, theatres, public performances, etc. He has repeatedly been to Dresden to keep appointments at Court, to visit his wife or do some shopping, and lately at the invitation of his relatives and with the agreement of the Asylum authorities he even undertook a journey to Leipzig on his own, from which he returned after a week's absence and which according to his sister's report went off quite well. p. 505

Dr. Weber confirms that plaintiff never carried out *any unreasonable or incorrect action*, always discussed *openly* and *without keeping anything back* those of his plans and intentions which fell outside his normal daily activities, and before carrying them through made sure he had the sanction of the Asylum authorities; when carrying them out he *always acted cautiously and sensibly, taking into consideration all the circumstances*. Dr. Weber thinks he is equally justified in believing that *no great annoyances* were *ever* caused by plaintiff in his contact with the outside world (p. 290a/b).

With the 50 marks a month pocket money which plaintiff has received for about a year to meet the expenses of his excursions and smaller necessaries, he has dealt in an *orderly* fashion and in the manner of a careful head of a family. It never came to notice that he squandered the money and therefore ran short. Neither did one have the impression of particular parsimony. Rather one noticed that he considered every expenditure well beforehand, avoided expensive things, and did not buy anything useless (apart from the small feminine trinkets).

In short, in the whole of plaintiff's behaviour during his contact p. 506 with the world outside the Asylum, there has until now *not been a single fact* which could give well-founded grounds for anxiety, that the patient would allow himself to be led astray under the compulsion of his delusional system, or impair his legal interests through wrong actions if freedom of action were restored to him. Practical experience has shown that plaintiff's insane belief in miracles although forming the basis of his mental life does not dominate

*Wrong: until the summer of 1900 I was *not* allowed out *at all*, and without being accompanied by an attendant only since the autumn of 1901.

him so exclusively that he is deprived of the capacity of quiet and sensible consideration of other affairs of life. It is a fact then, that no important legal interest would be jeopardized were plaintiff to have full legal capacity restored to him.

It is impossible that plaintiff would endanger his *life*, just as little as he is a danger to the lives of others. His tutelage cannot therefore be upheld as a necessary precaution to protect the patient's environment. It is admitted that disturbances are caused by the " bellowing attacks " which at times plague plaintiff and which could be very molesting to his environment, although he states that outside the Asylum he is almost completely free of them. In any case the so-called automatic and compulsive vociferations occurring against the patient's will have no bearing on the question of his tutelage. They might necessitate police intervention should the peace of the neighbourhood be disturbed, but they cannot justify maintaining his tutelage especially as tutelage is not an effectual measure against them.

Also irrelevant is the Prosecutor's statement that during the bellowing attacks and at those moments when the patient's thoughts
p. 507 are deflected by hallucinations, his freedom of will appears completely suspended. This may be so. But no immediate danger would thereby arise for plaintiff; it is obviously a matter of rapidly passing disturbances of consciousness lasting a few moments during which transactions of legal consequence are in any case precluded.

There is also no danger to plaintiff's *health* according to Dr. Weber's report. In general he knows well how to look after himself and is careful not to damage himself by wilful actions (p. 211). In this respect also there is no need for protection by a guardian.

It is true the medical expert mentions in his second report of 5th April 1902 one episode, when under the influence of his mental disturbance, plaintiff is said to have acted inappropriately in respect of the treatment of a short illness (diarrhoea and vomiting). He places little importance on this episode, and agrees retrospectively with plaintiff's remonstrance that the latter finally did acquiesce in the measures ordered by the doctors (p. 231 a/b). It is certainly not correct to say that plaintiff because of his belief in miracles despises medicines in general. Plaintiff appropriately points to his having in earlier years almost daily and of his own free will taken artificial sleeping drugs (pp. 226, 231b). Even if it were the case, placing him under tutelage would not remedy it. The patient's dislike of doctor and pharmacy, which actually does not exist, would neither be conquered by recognizing his legal capacity nor by placing him under tutelage.

It would give rise to more serious concern, if plaintiff's illness required for its improvement a prolonged stay in the Asylum, and his mental derangement prevented him from realizing this, p. 508 and if he were fighting for his tutelage to be rescinded only to enforce his discharge from the Asylum after being freed from the surveillance of a guardian. According to official information which the Asylum authorities of Sonnenstein only recently gave plaintiff in answer to his question of 29th May of this year (pp. 252/253), there is now no need for apprehension. Dr. Weber agrees in principle with plaintiff's discharge from the Asylum, with certain self-explanatory precautions. He expressly declares that he does not consider the patient "dangerous" to himself or others and furthermore has no hesitation in returning plaintiff to free congress with human society. This negatives the need for the care of a guardian with respect to the patient's health. Should the Judge nevertheless wish to affirm the necessity of tutelage from this point of view he would thereby place himself in opposition to the authoritative judgment of the medical expert and of the Asylum authorities.

There is also no need to fear that the patient might endanger his *monetary affairs* through wrong and unreasonable actions.

As the medical expert states, Dr. Schreber is fully informed about the state of his finances. The trial in latter years of letting him act financially on his own by giving him pocket money has worked out very well; plaintiff has shown himself in every way careful and economical. There is no reason to think he would squander his fortune, if unrestricted power over it were restored to him. Dr. Weber who knows plaintiff best and is most able to judge the influence of his delusional ideas, in any case gives the p. 509 assurance that he has *no reason* to think that *through pathological motives* he would exceed the limits of his resources and squander his fortune (p. 211).

The apprehension expressed by the lower Court that plaintiff might be induced to offer awards for scientific investigation under the compulsion of his wondrous ideas and in order to make propaganda for them, was from the outset not very serious. One has never noticed a tendency in plaintiff to spend money for the sake of his belief in miracles. The Court of Appeal has therefore no reason to mistrust plaintiff, particularly as the medical expert concurs in this opinion, when the former affirms he does not intend making sacrifices for the advancement of his belief in miracles and that it never entered his head to spend one penny for this purpose.

Of course one cannot exclude the possibility that plaintiff despite his assurances *might* at a given moment unconsciously be influenced in his financial dispositions by the fantastic ideas which dominate him. The possibility of such an influence exists in every mental abnormality even if it has not assumed the form of established insanity. It is, however, a matter of consideration for law and legal order only when such a possibility has become a real *danger*. There is nothing like that in this case. Only in one single instance has a direct influence of plaintiff's religious delusions on the disposition of his fortune been proved. To this Dr. Schreber himself drew attention. It concerns his attraction to all kinds of small ornaments with which like a woman he occasionally decorates
p. 510 his breast which he believes is changing into a woman's bosom. To spend money on such nonsensical stuff would never occur to him if he were mentally completely normal. But it is a matter of such insignificant sums that they could not play any part in the difficult decision as to whether or not he is legally capable of managing his affairs. Even if one totally disregarded the patient's statements that these decorations are a kind of mental medication which help to calm his attacks of nervous excitation, one could at worst only consider them a whim. Besides, much larger sums of money are spent on such whims by otherwise healthy people.

It is beyond dispute that plaintiff is completely capable of using his reasoning faculties to administer his and his wife's finances. These are not so intricate as the Prosecutor maintains, even regarding the individual items which according to the inventory on p. 175 ff. of the judicial guardian's files make up the fortune of the married couple Schreber. Plaintiff has only recently brought clear proof of his competence in this direction, in that he dealt with the extraordinarily difficult question of making further use of his father's book "Medical Indoor Gymnastics" after its publisher had gone into liquidation; he showed such acuity, clarity and circumspection in a report which he wrote at the request of his family, that they had no scruples whatever in following his suggestions. This is according to trustworthy information from his brother-in-law Jung, the merchant in Leipzig (pp. 41/43 of the file of the tutelage proceedings). This circumstance not only proves Dr. Schreber's technical ability of managing such matters, but proves at the same time that he does not lack inclination or interest to devote to the affairs of his fortune the necessary businesslike attention. p. 511

It is said Dr. Schreber's relationship to his *family* is threatened, *the marital bond with his wife* in danger of being destroyed. This also cannot be conceded.

As plaintiff rightly stresses, marital union with his wife has been almost completely in abeyance for years owing to his mental illness and the necessity created by it of living apart from her. How then could this relationship be worsened if freedom to decide over his person were now returned to plaintiff? Dr. Schreber has the sincere wish to resume domestic union with his wife and to live in the seclusion of a quiet country seat for the rest of his days, as soon as his discharge from the Asylum is granted. He therefore strives on his part to *improve* existing marital relations. Whether this can be achieved in reality is of course a different matter. The miraculous ideas which dominate plaintiff's mental life and which probably will become a much greater nuisance to his wife in intimate contact with him than to outsiders further removed, make it appear doubtful whether the married couple's living together will work in the long run. One would have to try and see.

But however this may work out has no influence on the decision whether his tutelage is to be upheld. Even on this point one must agree with plaintiff that consideration of other persons' well-being, even of nearest relatives cannot be taken into account. Placing under tutelage is primarily for the well-being of the person concerned. It is inadmissible in the interest of others.

Compare §2 of the Ministry of Justice's regulations for placing a person under tutelage because of mental illness, etc., 23rd December 1899. p. 512

Moreover Dr. Schreber is well aware, as can be seen from his statements in the procedings, of the moral duties which he owes to his wife in these difficult circumstances. His mind is not disturbed to such an extent as to make him blind to the degree of self-denial which may be demanded of his wife when living together with him. He will make no unfair demands on her if life together is impossible; also he would grant her everything to which she is legally entitled. He rejects altogether the suggestion that he might neglect his legal duties as regards her maintenance or that he would dispose of his fortune to her disadvantage out of resentment towards her. He states that in any case a joint will of the year 1886 exists which precludes such dispositions. Further, however careful one must be in trusting the assurances of mentally ill persons, plaintiff's great moral seriousness and candour of character, not lessened by illness, also stressed by Dr. Weber and evidenced in all his declarations in Court, disperse all doubt in their trustworthiness.

Thus the medical expert's earlier remark that Dr. Schreber in his relation to his wife is quick to speak of divorce, if she does not willingly agree with his delusions, loses in importance. Apparently this report is based on Dr. Schreber's wife's statements and rests on misunderstandings. Plaintiff has clarified this matter in statements which make his behaviour towards his wife free from any objection; these explanations are not contradicted in Dr. Weber's
p. 513 second report after he had seen them.

It only remains that plaintiff might compromise himself and his family by his intended publication of the "Memoirs" and even place himself in conflict with the criminal law.

No reasonable person would wish to deny serious scruples about publishing the manuscript. Not even Dr. Schreber could ignore them. If nevertheless he urgently insists on publication this is not proof of his deficient capacity of anticipating the results of his actions, but only proof of the strength of his belief in the truth of the revelations which have been granted him by God:

> "I cannot wish"—he remarks in his own words—"that the knowledge of God which has been revealed to me should sink into oblivion with my death and an opportunity be lost to mankind of achieving more correct ideas about the beyond which might never occur again".

The appellant knows that this might have unpleasant consequences for him. But he is justified in denying the accusation of the Lower Court that he had written anything in the "Memoirs" damaging to the honour of his family. It is a fact that nothing of the kind can be found in the manuscript. One also cannot maintain that the contents of the "Memoirs" are such as to compromise plaintiff himself. The manuscript is the product of a morbid imagination and nobody reading it would for a moment lose the feeling that its author is mentally deranged. But this could not possibly lower the patient in the respect of his fellow men, particularly as no one can miss the seriousness of purpose and striving after truth which
p. 514 fill every chapter. As Dr. Schreber remarks correctly, the worst that could happen to him would be that one consider him

mad, and this one does in any case. One cannot be offended by the strong language in the book. It is not plaintiff's; he only repeats what the voices of spirits spoke into him in earlier years when he was most severely hallucinated.

This must be kept in mind when one tries to find the correct standard for judging the defamation which Professor Flechsig suffers in the " Memoirs ", as he is accused of soul-murder and worse. Even here plaintiff is not in any way talking for himself or acting on his own behalf, but only reporting what the voices of miraculous spirits told him, with whom in his opinion he was in communication. He certainly had no intention of attacking Professor Flechsig nor of wittingly insulting his honour while writing the "Memoirs". The danger of being sued by Flechsig for libel is not very great, particularly as certain alterations are to be made in the manuscript before it is printed. Punishment appears in any case out of the question because plaintiff is protected in all eventualities by §51 of the Criminal Code. Even should plaintiff expose himself to the risk of criminal conviction by it, this would not suffice as a reason for denying his legal capacity. Placing under tutelage cannot be used as a means of preventing a person with a mental defect but *otherwise* capable of managing his affairs, from undertaking *one single* wrong action or to save him from the possible adverse effects of such an action. The same applies to the Prosecutor's view of the disadvantages of the contract which plaintiff would p. 515
be forced to conclude with the publishers of the " Memoirs ". Firstly, it is by no means certain that the conclusion of the contract with the publisher on a commission basis must involve financial loss for plaintiff, though it is probable enough. But one must remember that the business risk which plaintiff runs is really not very considerable in comparison with the rest of his fortune. To save him from such a risk is not the task of tutelage. Plaintiff knows full well that the publication of the " Memoirs " could become a financial burden; in this matter also he does *not* require legal *protection* such as tutelage would afford him.

The Court of Appeal has therefore arrived at the conviction that plaintiff is capable of dealing with the demands of life in all its spheres here discussed—these are the most important ones, the orderly regulation of which is the object of the Law. There is no evidence and it cannot be regarded as ascertained that he is incapable of managing his affairs owing to his delusional ideas. Therefore in considering the Appeal which has been lodged this must lead to the tutelage inflicted on plaintiff being rescinded without entering into new evidence by witnesses offered by him (§672 C.P.O.).

The decision on costs rests on §673 C.P.O.

Signed: Hardraht, Vogel, Dr. Steinmetz, Nicolai, Dr. Paul.

Dresden, 26th July 1902.

(L.S.) Heinker, Clerk to the Royal Superior Country Court of Saxony.

p. 516 No notice of appeal has been received at the Imperial German High Court in the above action within the required period ended on 1st September 1902.

Leipzig, 3rd September 1902.

(L.S.) Schubotz, Secretariat VI of the Imperial German High Court.

VI.Z.1520/02.

The above judgment became valid on 1st September 1902 as hereby witnessed.

Dresden, 17th September 1902.

(L.S.) Müller, Clerk to the Royal Superior Country Court of Saxony.

NOTES*

In these Notes we have limited ourselves to giving reasons for our translation of various difficult and important terms in Schreber's text. We have only commented on the text so far as it was necessary to explain the translation. We have not attempted a detailed commentary on the clinical insight which Schreber's Memoirs furnish on so many aspects of mental illness. Such an endeavour would mean almost writing a textbook of psychiatry.

Schreber page

Fleeting-improvised-men: *flüchtig hingemachte Männer.* These were not beings produced by sexual reproduction, but souls put down temporarily in human form directly by divine miracle. The word *hingemachte* indicates they are not complete beings, but improvised, and has an anal implication as *hinmachen* can also mean to defecate; *flüchtig* (suggesting an element of punning with Flechsig) refers both to their being fleetingly-improvised and that their existence was transitory or fleeting; *Männer* because they appeared in human shape. Their special purpose is explained later (S. 54): they maintain and provide with the necessities of life the sole survivor selected to renew mankind after world catastrophes, until his offspring are sufficiently numerous to maintain themselves. Then they vanish. Their appearance therefore proved to Schreber that mankind had perished. In the English translation of Freud's (1911) paper the fleeting-improvised-men are translated as " miracled men, cursory contraptions ". p. 4 footnote 1

The sun plays an important part in Schreber's story. Because its gender is female in German we refer to the sun as she throughout the Memoirs. p. 8

Quotation from Schiller's " Ode to Joy ", from which Schreber quotes again later (S. 281). p. 8 footnote 3

To form a nerve-contact: *Nervenanhang nehmen.* This neologism, meaning to attach to, or be in contact with nerves, is used by Schreber as a concrete expression for a supernatural, mystical union with God, Who is taken to be the sum total of all nerves, or with nerves in the p. 11

* Page numbers given as p. . . . and (S. . . .) refer to the original pagination of Schreber's Memoirs, which runs alongside the translation.

sense of souls, the remnants of departed human beings. Schreber could not explain how Flechsig's and other souls of still living persons could be in nerve-contact with him without having departed. In footnote 5 (S. 11) which he added in 1902 when he had improved greatly, he reverts to the original abstract, i.e. psychological meaning of attraction: "Attractive is that which interests". During his illness he considered it concretely as a mechanical attachment.

p. 12 Blessedness: *Seligkeit.* Grimm's *Wörterbuch* gives several meanings: (1) Eternal joy and security in communion with God, used in relation to life after death; (2) In more modern use, other than in a religious sense, to emphasize excessive and greatest happiness. Schreber combines both senses in his use of the word. A further complication is that Blessedness is "closely related to voluptuousness" (S. 281), even identical with it (S. 359), which is "uninterrupted enjoyment coupled with the contemplation of God". This is the state in which souls (departed human beings) live in heaven after having undergone a gradual process of purification, and await reincarnation.

p. 12 Forecourts of heaven: *Vorhöfe des Himmels.* This refers to the hierarchy in God's realms detailed in footnote 19 (S. 29). During the process of purification souls were stripped of their wordly memories and identities, and so gradually became pure, until finally reunited with the totality of all nerves, that is, God. The erstwhile human souls who accumulate in the forecourts of heaven are those who have become blessed and have some supernatural power but are not yet absolutely purified. Above the forecourts of heaven were the anterior realms of God, and still higher (and hence behind them) the posterior realms of God which were subject to a "peculiar dualism," consisting of Ormuzd and Ariman. Schreber was much influenced by the dualism of the Persian religion. Both Ariman and Ormuzd are concerned with creation in the Persian religion. For Schreber, Ormuzd was in favour of his being unmanned (changed into a woman) but Ariman had the power of reversing this miracle when necessary.

p. 13 Basic language: *Grundsprache.* The word *Grund* is the English "ground", referring to the ground, basis or fundament of all things; hence *Grundsprache*, basic language, for God's language. It also has the meaning of below, in German as well as in English, and is used in this sense in relation to a devil as *Grundteufel* (S. 14). We preferred the word ' basic ', because it seems to render the meaning in a somewhat more current form.

" Your Majesty's obedient servant ": " *Ew. Majestät* ". This is an p. 14
untranslatable pun: *Ew.* being the customary abbreviation for *Eure Majestät*. Schreber puns on *Ew.* as short for *Ewigkeit*, meaning eternity.

Tested souls: *geprüfte Seelen*. This might have been translated as p. 14
qualified, examined or approved, but we chose tested because it renders the punning contained in *geprüfte* in the sense of " severely tested ". Hence the " euphemisms " of the basic language by which the meaning of words used to be reversed. Tested souls were those still undergoing the process of purification, and hence still impure but already endowed with some supernatural power.

Zoroaster rays. Light phenomena play a part in the Persian p. 20
religion; later in the book Schreber refers to spectacles of great footnote
splendour produced by rays. 13

Soul murder. This is the most obscure issue in the Memoirs and p. 22
also the most important one. It caused the crisis in God's realms, in other words his illness (see Memoirs, Table of Contents, Chapter II). It is mentioned in his " Open Letter to Professor Flechsig ", where he describes the phenomenon in a more abstract sense as any influence or ascendancy one person can gain over another, as for instance in hypnosis, or achieve some advantage at another person's expense such as prolongation of his own life. In this way the Schrebers may have been denied offspring or choice of profession such as that of nerve specialist (S. 26-27). In connection with Schreber's references to soul murder and soul theft, it must be remembered that his " philosophy " was based on the dualism of soul and body; the soul, the life substance, is part of God and put into a human body at conception or birth and drawn up to Him again after death. Soul = breath = spirit = nerves = rays = God: it is the life substance in circulation. Schreber regarded the soul as separate and detachable from the body. When the soul leaves the body permanently and returns to God, the person dies; illness, particularly nervous illness, is caused when the soul leaves the body temporarily, or is under another's influence. The theme of soul murder or soul theft is widespread in religions and folklore. Schreber refers to the part it plays in Goethe's Faust, Weber's

Freischütz and Byron's Manfred (S. 20, 22), the theme of which is a mythical contact with the beyond, and the meaning and fate of man's soul, i.e. of life.

p. 24 Because Schreber here refers to members of his family living in the eighteenth century, we have given details of some of his illustrious ancestors in the Introduction.

The soul of Daniel Fürchtegott Flechsig vanished years ago (flitted away): *Die Seele Daniel Fürchtegott Flechsig ist schon seit Jahren verschwunden (hat sich verflüchtigt)*.

p. 25 Contact with divine nerves: *ein göttlicher Nervenanhang*, was granted to a person who specialized in nervous illnesses (*eine Person . . . , die sich mit Ausübung der Nervenheilkunde befasste*). Asylums for the mentally ill were therefore called in the basic language "God's Nerve Institutes": *Die Heilanstalten für Geisteskranke hiessen daher in der Grundsprache "Nervenanstalten Gottes"*. We have commented on this passage in the Discussion.

p. 33 Chapter III was deleted from the Memoirs before publication; but the Judges of the Appeal Court who had the complete Memoirs before them, stated that there was nothing particularly damaging or offensive in them.

p. 38 Interferences: *Störungen*. These play a large part later in the Memoirs. They are explained by Schreber as events caused on him or his surroundings in order to interfere with or impede the development of soul-voluptuousness in his body, and so stop his transformation into a woman.

p. 45 Seer of spirits: *Geisterseher*. Schreber explains that a seer of spirits is in contact with spirits or blessed souls of departed human beings (S. 77).

p. 46 Nerve-language: *Nervensprache*. This refers to an altered awareness of his own thoughts and mental processes, perhaps best described as an awareness of unconscious mental processes.

p. 47 Compulsive thinking: *Denkzwang*.

p. 49 Schreber's preoccupation with Catholicism and conversion may have some basis in the actual situation in Saxony, ninety-five per cent of the population being Protestant, but the Royal House Catholic.

Corps Saxonia—Students' Club with distinctive colours and badges, which encouraged duelling. p. 50

Drinking member: *Konkneipant.* Old member of a Corps who is allowed to take part in evenings devoted to drinking and revelry. p. 50

Member of a Students' Union: *Burschenschaftler.* Members of a Students' Union professing national and liberal principles. p. 50

Unmanning: *Entmannung.* The authorized translation of Freud (1911) uses the term "emasculation". We have chosen "unmanning" because its primary meaning is "to remove from the category of men", which is what Schreber intended. Only its fourth definition in the Oxford English Dictionary is given as castration. Emasculation, on the other hand, has castration as its primary meaning, i.e. rendering sterile. From the pages immediately following, as well as from Schreber's further text, it is quite obvious that he meant transformation by an evolutionary process into a reproductive woman which was to render him fertile. Schreber himself stresses this by usually putting "change into a woman" in brackets after the word "unmanning". (See also Discussion). p. 51

The theme of change of sex is as widespread in early myths and religions as it is in psychiatry (Feuchtersleben, 1845; Griesinger, 1861; Bleuler, 1911; Macalpine and Hunter, 1954 b). The Indogermanic deities from which the Persian religion derived were bisexual. The fundamental story behind all religions, that of sun-gods and creators in the sky, shows frequent changes of sex: the earliest God was the Great Mother. The sexual, phallic element was only added much later to this "heliolithic" complex of ideas centring around the origin of life, creation and procreation (Smith, 1929). In Genesis the first being produced Eve from his rib. Schreber believed this original state could occur again following world catastrophes, which necessitated creation of mankind anew after its destruction. This is "the fountainhead and parent story" of all myths and religion (Smith, 1919). The sole survivor procreated single-handed until the sexes were established again, and in sufficient numbers to reproduce themselves. Hippocrates (quoted by Feuchtersleben. 1845) relates that the

Scythians were subject to a "sacred disease", also described by Herodotus, which caused men to turn into women. Schreber states that he suffered from the plague, which the souls considered "a disease of nerves and hence a 'holy disease'" (S. 93).

p. 56 Policy of half measures ("*half-heartedness*"): *Politik der Halbheit* ("*Halbschürigkeit*").

p. 56 Simply "forsaken", in other words left to rot: *einfach "liegen gelassen", also wohl der Verwesung anheimgegeben.*

pp. 57–60 These pages give an interesting insight into suicidal attempts on the basis of delusions. They also show the close connection between suicidal ideas and suspicions or delusions of being killed, which in turn may lead to outbreaks of violent behaviour, as in Schreber's case.

p. 62 Order of the World: *Weltordnung.* In the authorized translation of Freud (1911), this is rendered as "order of things".

p. 70 End of the world: *Weltuntergang.*

p. 83 Impure souls: *unreine Seelen.*

p. 86 The cursed play-with-human-beings: *die verfluchte Menschenspielerei.*

p. 93 "Searing" and "blessing" rays: "*Sehrende*" *und* "*Segnende*" *Strahlen.*

Concerning the plague, see Note to p. 51, on "sacred disease".

p. 94 The idea to "forsake me", that is to abandon me: *Die Vorstellung mich "liegen zu lassen", d.h. zu verlassen.* Schreber expresses his fear that God might withdraw from him before impregnation had occurred, that he would thus be excluded from the cycle of life, and his body used "for sexual purposes only".

p. 94 Nerves of voluptuousness (female nerves): *Wollust-(weibliche) Nerven.* Schreber explains that the nerves of voluptuousness, also called female nerves, are found all over the female body, particularly under the skin of the breasts, whereas in the male body only around the genital organ. That, as he believed, nerves of voluptuousness were palpable all over his own body was evidence for Schreber that his body was being transformed into a female body. The development of these female nerves of voluptuousness increased his power of attraction on divine nerves (rays): therefore the greater the development of voluptuousness in his body, the more ready his body to receive and indeed force divine impregnation, which could be accomplished by attracting all divine rays. Soul-voluptuousness, *Seelenwollust*, is the permanent state of enjoyment in which souls exist, which is their permanent expectation of creating and being reborn. According to Grimm, the word Wollust originally did not contain a deprecatory element, nor was it used with reference to sex. Even now it is used independently of sex, in its original general sense, as in *Wollust des Lebens*, *Wollust der Freiheit* (literally, voluptuousness of life, voluptuousness of freedom). See also Note to p. 12. Schreber combines both senses, as can be seen clearly from pp. 281, 282.

Nerve of determination: *Bestimmungsnerv*. p. 95

Wandering clocks: *Wandeluhren*. Schreber's meaning is not clear: *Wandel* could also mean changing, that is changes in the souls of departed heretics contained in these clocks. p. 96

Schreber's descriptions of his surroundings in Pierson's Asylum (the "Devil's Kitchen") and his acute observation of other patients, throw an interesting light on how much patients observe, even when grossly alienated, and how much they may be influenced by their surroundings. pp. 102–107

With regard to the Determining: *Rücksichtlich des Bestimmenden*. p. 106 footnote 54

Magazine of rays: *Strahlenmagazin*. p. 114

Moonshine Blessedness: *Mondscheinseligkeit*, a neologism referring to the female state of Blessedness, of which Schreber says there are two kinds: a flatter and a more robust one. The former may be regarded as Child-Blessedness, *Kinderseligkeit*. This also is a neologism and could mean both the Blessedness of a child, and the blessed state of being with child. As it applies only to the female state of Blessedness, and as the moon is possibly an allusion to menses, it probably indicates a state of being with child. Further p. 114

weight is given to this interpretation by the subsequent associations of creating " a new human world (" new human beings out of Schreber's spirit ") ". This is followed (S. 115) by his having the soul of the " Apostle (National Saint) " in his abdomen.

p. 115 National Saint: *Nationalheiliger*, is probably borrowed from the Persian religion in which Zoroaster is the national hero as well as the prophet. Incidentally, in the Persian religion Zoroaster was going to bear a son after three thousand years, who was to awaken the dead and create a new and immortal world.

p. 116 Law for the restoration of the rays: *Strahlenerneuerungsgesetz*.

p. 120 Scoundrels: *Hundejungen*, literally dogs-chaps; Could also mean kennel-boy, referring to the souls having to perform some menial task as part of purification. (See footnote 56).

p. 121 " To remove themselves ": *sich wegzusetzen*.

p. 122 An attempt has been made to keep something of the naive ballad form of the original. The refrain " God's still and silent peace " is *der stille Gottesfriede*.

p. 125 Tying-to-rays: *Anbinden an Strahlen*.

p. 125 Tying-to-celestial-bodies: *Anbinden an Erden*.

p. 126 The writing-down-system: *das Aufschreibesystem*.

p. 127 " Miss Schreber " may be a pun and mean " miss Schreber ", which in German as in English means to omit. Schreber might be implying that he was missed out from having offspring. It can also mean in English as in German " bad or wrong " as in mis-shapen, i.e. a freak.

p. 128 footnote 62 The notion of " representing ": *der Begriff des " Darstellens "*.

p. 128 footnote 62 At every " sight " (twinkle of an eye): *in jedem " Gesichte " (Augenblicke)*. This phrase recurs repeatedly and is a pun: *Gesicht*, meaning both sight, that which is seen, and face. *Augenblick*, literally glance of the eyes, also means moment, momentary, immediately or now.

" We have already got this ", *scil.* written down: " *Das haben* p. 132
wir schon " (*gesprochen;* " *Hammirschon* ") *scil. aufgschrieben.* We have omitted the words in brackets (spoken: " *Hammirschon* ") because they merely represent the sound of the words when they are spoken rapidly.

Learnt by rote: *auswendig gelernt.* p. 137 footnote 64

The " cursed creation of a false feeling ": *die* " *verfluchte Stimmungs-* p. 144
mache ".

The mood-falsifying-miracle: *das Stimmungsfälschungswunder.* p. 145

The compression-of-the-chest-miracle: *Engbrüstigkeitswunder.* p. 151

Schreber here explains his reasons for refusing food; Dr. Weber p. 151
in his report stated that for a long time Schreber also refused meat footnote 69
altogether (S. 381).

Dangerous obstruction of my gut: *Darmverschlingung.* p. 153 footnote 72

Soul-conception: *Seelenauffassung*, the soul's way of looking at p. 164
things.

The pages that follow contain an interesting description of compulsive rumination on the theme of male and female.

The not-thinking-of-anything-thought: *der Nichtsdenkungsgedanke.* p. 169

I did not encourage the miracle (" pacify it " was the expression in p. 171
the basic language): *dass ich das Wunder nicht begünstigt habe* (" *begütigt habe* ", *wie der grundsprachlich Ausdruck lautete*). The clang association of the original cannot be rendered in English.

The round wing of the Asylum: see legend to Plates II, III, and p. 175
IV of Sonnenstein Asylum.

Spirited woman: *Geistreiches Weib.* Literally: a woman full of p. 178
spirits.

p. 193 So-what-party: *Je nun Partei.*

p. 196 Schreber mentions that he had to shave off his moustache; this was the first outward sign of transvestitism (August 1896).

p. 197 footnote 83 Many in One and One in Many: *Vielheit in der Einheit oder Einheit in der Vielheit.*

p. 205 The bellowing-miracle: *das Brüllwunder.*

p. 210 Similarity of sounds: *Gleichklang der Laute.* Schreber describes the alliteration, ' clang association ', and hence punning so frequently found in schizophrenics.

p. 228 ff. Schreber describes the common phenomenon of obsessional rumination. These pages seem to confirm Freud's observation that in the last analysis all obsessive questioning and doubting originate from the first question " Where do I come from ". As Schreber puts it naively " Between divine creation . . . and the individual processes of life there are innumerable intermediate links, which are eminently interesting to work out " (S. 230).

p. 232 To picture: *Zeichnen;* also to draw.

p. 241 Spontaneous creation: *Urzeugung.* This he exemplifies on insects (S. 242). For this reason we mentioned his famous great-uncle's study on newly discovered insects in the Introduction.

p. 254 Schreber makes clear that his being in contact with, and wishing to attract all rays expresses his hope for offspring. He says " the *capacity* to transform themselves into *animals* of all kinds, ultimately even into a human being, is the *latent potential* of divine rays: they can create these creatures out of themselves "; and on p. 250: " The frightening miracles are perhaps to be regarded as the very first beginnings of divine creation, which in certain circumstances could be further condensed to fleeting-improvised men and from there lead up to the creation of real human beings or other permanent beings ".

p. 255 See plate V.

p. 262 ff. An extremely interesting description of ideas of reference.

Note that Schreber does not identify with Jesus Christ as Freud thought, but only compares the magnitude of his sufferings with the martyrdom of Christ. p. 293

The automatic-remembering-thought: *der unwillkürliche Erinnerungsgedanke*. p. 311

Essentially without thoughts: *die Hauptgedankenlosigkeit.* p. 325

FOOTNOTES

Footnote 28 is missing. Schreber refers to it on pp. 67, 69, and 75. It was not printed because it contained a reference to the reigning King (S. 67).
There are footnotes 93 and 93B, but no footnote 94.
Footnotes 24 and 91 were not printed because they referred to Flechsig (S. 341, 445–6).
There are two footnotes 74.

LEGAL TERMS

Str.G.B. *Strafgesetzbuch:* Criminal Code.
C.P.O. *Civil-Prozess-Ordnung:* Code of civil procedure.
B.-G.-B. *Bürgerliches Gesetzbuch:* Common Law Code.
Str.-Pr.-O. *Straf-Prozess-Ordnung:* Code of Criminal Procedure.
G.u.V.Bl. *Gesetz und Verordnungsblatt:* Gazette in which new laws and orders are published.
District Court: *Amtsgericht.*
Country Court: *Landesgericht.*
Superior Country Court (Court of Appeal): *Oberlandesgericht.*

TRANSLATORS' ANALYSIS OF THE CASE*

I. INTRODUCTION

Freud (1911) formulated his views on the relationship of paranoia to homosexuality in his paper "Psychoanalytic Notes Upon an Autobiographical Account of a Case of Paranoia (Dementia Paranoides)".† He described his analysis as "only a fragment of a larger whole" (F. 466) and said "how much more material remains to be gathered from the symbolic content of the fantasies and delusions of this gifted paranoiac" (F. 467). He recommended that the original be read "at least once" prior to his analysis of it (F. 389).

Yet no attempt seems to have been made to exploit the original material further. Particular difficulties, it is true, stand in the way of studying Schreber's autobiography: the book is almost unobtainable, the only edition is said to have been bought up and destroyed by his family, and it has not before been translated. Further, some passages from Schreber's Memoirs "appear in the English translation of Freud's text in such a manner that not only is their meaning lost, but sometimes actually reversed" (Niederland, 1951). Niederland also refers to passages which are "completely incomprehensible in the English version", criticisms which cannot be too strongly emphasized.

Perhaps the decisive reason, however, is that the taboo of a 'classic' was immediately attached to Freud's paper, setting it above critical scrutiny.

Review of Literature

For the purpose of reviewing briefly the literature it is convenient to remember that Freud's paper is divided into three parts: 1, Case History; 2, Attempts at Interpretation; 3, On the Mechanism of Paranoia.

* Reprinted, with additions, from The Psychoanalytic Quarterly, 1953, **22**, 328.

† Quotations from Freud's paper are given as (F. ...), Freud quoting Schreber as (FS. ...), and quotations from Schreber's Memoirs as (S. ...), referring to the original page numbers which run alongside the text.

1. *Case History.* Use has not been made of any of Schreber's material other than that extracted by Freud. Baumeyer (1951) reported that Schreber had a further psychotic breakdown in 1907, which lasted to his death in 1911. This we have not been able to verify.

2. *Attempts at Interpretation.* Katan (1949, 1950, 1952, 1953) forced the whole psychosis into a struggle against masturbation and homosexuality, the dangers of which "forced him to sever his ties with reality"; the sun and the stars "represent the male genitals of God". He merely enlarges on Freud's thesis of the origin of the illness in unconscious homosexuality. Niederland (*loc. cit.*), supporting Freud's analysis and searching for common precipitating factors in Schreber's first and second illnesses, laid stress on the fact that in 1884 Schreber was a candidate for the *Reichstag*, and in 1893 had just taken office as *Senatspräsident*. He assumes that in each case "under the impact of a threatening reality which imperiously demanded of him an active masculine role, his latent passive feminine tendencies broke into consciousness and he fell ill".

3. *On the Mechanism of Paranoia.* The bulk of the literature is concerned with confirming the mechanism of projection in paranoia and with the importance of unconscious homosexuality in "neurotic" symptom formation, as in jealousy, alcoholism, drug addiction, etc. The earliest and most important evidence is by Ferenczi (1911), followed by Tausk (1919) and Nunberg (1920, 1921); Fenichel (1945) lists later relevant publications. Many papers of course contain incidental allusions. A confirmatory case was reported by Freud himself (1923) under the title of "A Neurosis of Demoniacal Possession in the Seventeenth Century".*

No open criticism of Freud's interpretation is to be found in psychoanalytic literature: "Perhaps no psychoanalytic theory of a psychosis rests on firmer foundations or has been less frequently attacked" (Knight, *loc. cit.*), "in spite of obvious logical fallacies" (Menninger, *loc. cit.*). However, careful reading shows that doubts as to whether repressed homosexuality alone can explain paranoia must have exercised Ferenczi's (*loc. cit.*) mind when he wrote "in paranoia it is mainly a question of recathexis with unsublimated libido of homosexual love objects which the ego wards off by

* We reinvestigated the original manuscript and paintings on which Freud's (1923) study was based, and showed that the same criticism applied as to his Schreber study, in that undue stress was placed on libidinal homosexual drives (Macalpine and Hunter, 1954 b). The original manuscript and paintings are reproduced in a separate volume (Macalpine and Hunter, 1955).

projection. This statement, however, leads us to the bigger problem of 'choice of neurosis', i.e. under what conditions does infantile bisexuality, ambisexuality, lead respectively to normal heterosexuality, to homosexual perversion, or to paranoia". A similar note of reservation can be detected in Nunberg (1938): "The question why it is that, out of the same fundamental situation, a paranoia develops in one instance and in another does not, must remain unanswered for the present". Glover (1932) found that "Schreber was described mainly in terms of libidinal conflict and related to repression of the inverted oedipus situation", and noted the lack of reference to pregenital aspects.

It is surprising that not even the changes in the libido theory, namely the introduction of the death instinct, and the changes in the concept of transference (Macalpine, 1950)—for instance the recognition of negative transference—led to any re-evaluation; particularly as Schreber was interpreted by Freud solely on the basis of libidinal transference from father, to his physician Flechsig, to God. Menninger (*loc. cit.*) stressed the importance of "the destructive tendencies and the impulses of hate . . . mingled with homosexual attraction". Knight (*loc. cit.*) attempted to revise Freud's theory of paranoid symptom formation in the light of the changes in the theory of instincts, because he felt that it "leaves something to be desired in the way of completeness", and discussed the problems raised by psychotherapeutic failure. Klein (1946), stressing aggressive (death) instincts, saw in Schreber's delusions "anxieties and fantasies about inner destruction and ego disintegration". His ideas of the end of the world are interpreted as projections of his own aggressive impulses: "the 'world catastrophe' fantasy . . . implies a preponderance of the destructive impulse over the libido" (Klein, *loc. cit.*).

All confirmatory studies of Freud's paper, as well as those which attempt to bring the paper into line with the libido-death theory of instincts, are however, based exclusively on manipulating those parts of Schreber's Memoirs which Freud had extracted in order to prove his point. This may explain why, despite obvious weaknesses and discrepancies, no fundamentally different interpretation of the whole of Schreber's illness and the dynamics of the case had been attempted.

It is not intended to go into details of the criticisms with which Freud's paper was received in psychiatric circles. But mention should be made of the review by Bleuler (1912), one of Freud's friendliest critics: "This publication bears the hallmark of an important contribution by the very fact that it provides food for further thought, questioning and research", though "difficulties arise by trying to separate Schreber's illness from schizophrenia ... Paranoid and schizophrenic symptoms not only coexist in one patient, they also seem to merge and indeed appear to be two aspects of the same process". He felt that "not even in Schreber's case itself does it seem proved that the denial of homosexuality is the factor which produced the illness, although it plays a large part in the symptomatology of the case". This sentence also sums up our findings.

Summary of Literature

Freud's views on Schreber's illness stand unquestioned, no new material has been added nor different interpretations advanced. Subsequent literature is almost unanimously confirmatory; such reservations as can be detected are only implied. This is all the more surprising in view of the many changes in psychoanalytic theory and practice and in the concept of transference since 1911, and the extension of interest in the psychoses.

Freud's Analysis

Freud believed "that the exciting cause" of Schreber's psychosis "was the appearance in him of a feminine (that is, passive homosexual) wish-fantasy, which took as its object the figure of his physician ... The patient's friendly feeling towards his physician may very well have been due to a process of 'transference', by means of which an emotional cathexis became transposed from some person who was important to him on to the physician who was in reality indifferent to him: the patient having been reminded by the physician of his brother or of his father (F. 431). The feminine fantasy, which aroused such violent opposition in the patient, thus had its root in a longing, intensified to an erotic pitch, for his father and brother (F. 435). Thus in the case of Schreber we find ourselves once again upon the familiar ground of the father-complex (F. 440). The object ... was probably from the very first his physician, Flechsig" (F. 426), as he had been under his care nine years before: "Perhaps that illness had left behind in him a feeling of affectionate dependence upon his physician, which had now, for some unknown reason, become intensified to the pitch of an erotic desire (F. 426). An intense resistance to this fantasy arose on the part of Schreber's personality, and the ensuing defensive struggle, which might perhaps just as well have assumed some other shape, took on, for reasons unknown to us, that of a delusion of persecution. The person he longed for now became his persecutor, and the content of his wish-fantasy became the content of his persecution" (F. 431–432), because it implied degradation and castration: hence "it was impossible for Schreber to become reconciled to playing the part of a female prostitute towards his physician" (F. 432). Flechsig was then replaced by "the superior figure of God (F. 432). He took up a feminine attitude towards God; he felt that he was God's wife (F. 413). This seems at first . . . a sign of aggravation of the conflict, an intensification of the unbearable persecution, but . . . soon . . . becomes the solution . . . Schreber could not reconcile himself to playing the part of a female prostitute towards his physician but the task of providing God with the voluptuous sensations that he required called up no such resistance on the part of his ego. Emasculation was now no longer a disgrace, it became 'consonant with the order of things', it took its place in a great cosmic chain of events, and was instrumental in the re-creation of humanity after its extinction. 'A new race of men, born from the spirit of Schreber', would, so he thought, revere as their ancestor this man who believed himself the victim of persecution. By this means an outlet was provided which would satisfy both of the contending forces. His ego found compensation in his megalomania, while his feminine wish-fantasy gained its ascendancy and became acceptable. The struggle and the illness could cease. The patient's sense of reality, however, which had in the meantime become stronger, compelled him to postpone the solution from the present to the remote future, and to content himself with what might be described as an asymptotic wish-fulfilment" (F. 432). His delusional self-aggrandizement is interpreted as caused by the flooding of his ego with narcissistic libido, consequent upon the abandonment of object love (reality); and his delusions as attempts at restitution, "reconstruction" (F. 457) and regaining his homosexual love objects at a safe distance from the ego. "For we learn that the idea of being transformed into a woman (that is, of being emasculated) was the primary delusion, that he began by regarding that act as a piece of persecution and a serious injury, and that it only became related to his playing the part of Redeemer in a secondary way. There can be no doubt, moreover, that originally he believed that the emasculation was to be effected for the purpose of sexual abuse and not so as to serve some higher design. To express the matter in more formal language, a sexual delusion of persecution was later on converted, in the patient's mind, into a religious delusion of grandeur. The part of persecutor was first assigned to Professor Flechsig, the physician in whose charge he was; subsequently, however, the place was occupied by God himself (F. 397–398). He then arrived at the firm conviction that it was God Himself who, for His own satisfaction, was demanding femaleness from him (F. 415) and looked upon his transformation into a woman as a disgrace with which he was threatened from a hostile source (F. 414). But the first author of all these acts of persecution was Flechsig, and he remains their instigator throughout the whole course of the illness (F. 421) . . . Flechsig . . . remained the first seducer, to whose influence God had yielded (F. 422) . . . In general, however, the illness is looked upon as a struggle between the man Schreber and God, in which victory lies with the man, weak though he is, because the order of things is on his side" (F.409).

Certain weaknesses are obvious in Freud's analysis, many of which he pointed out himself.

1. Freud sought to establish the mechanism of paranoia on Schreber's case. But Schreber, as Freud himself said, was not suffering from pure paranoia, but "a mixed state" of schizophrenia plus paranoia, for which Freud suggested the term paraphrenia. He saw no incompatibility in both being present in one patient as they merely represent different points of fixation according to the libido theory. Contrary to present-day psychiatric opinion, he felt it to be essential that "paranoia should be maintained as an independent clinical type, however frequently the picture it presents may be complicated by the presence of schizophrenic features . . . It would be distinguished from dementia praecox by having its dispositional point of fixation differently located and by having a different mechanism for the return of the repressed" (F. 463). But Freud also stated "it is not at all likely that homosexual impulses which are so frequently (perhaps invariably) to be found in paranoia, play an equally important part in the aetiology of that far more comprehensive disorder, dementia praecox" (F. 464). It would appear that in Freud's opinion Schreber was suffering from both paranoia and dementia praecox. The homosexual factor alone cannot then afford the whole explanation of the case.

These remarks may appear petty and of no great consequence. On the contrary, they light up sharply the difference in approach, sometimes the gulf, which exists between clinical psychiatry and psychoanalysis. The psychiatrist primarily focuses his interest on the clinical picture, the signs, symptoms and course of mental illness, and tries to separate clinical entities. The psychoanalyst centres his interest on the mechanisms involved in symptom-formation with little respect for the whole disease picture and no aversion to 'double pathology'; he speaks of psychopathological states. Such mechanisms are then taken for the disease proper and give their names to it (cf. Paranoia in Introduction). This emphasis on and sometimes exclusive preoccupation with mental mechanisms, irrespective of clinical distinctions, has been pressed furthest in Klein's 'psychotic positions' which are even claimed to be part of normal development.

2. Freud applied to Schreber's illness the criteria of a neurosis in the classical psychoanalytic sense, and discussed it on the basis of libidinal conflict: Schreber is said to have fallen victim to "an outburst of homosexual libido" (F. 426) which his personality repudiated, his delusions (symptoms) constituting a compromise. Thus the wish-fulfilment, enjoying intercourse like a woman, is said to have "gained its ascendancy" (F. 432) although Schreber to the day of his discharge from hospital continued only to hope that in "the remote future ... his transformation into a woman would come about" (F. 432). To the unbiased reader this appears a bare minimum of gratification: "if, in this process, a little sensual pleasure falls to my share, I feel justified in accepting it as some slight compensation for the inordinate suffering and privation that has been mine for so many past years" (FS. 415).

Furthermore Schreber's illness is explained by Freud on a genital level only, centring on the inverted oedipus situation. Hence when Schreber speaks of "new life springing from his lap" and "feeling the quickening of a human embryo in his body", Freud uses this procreation fantasy as proof of passive homosexual wishes, and as arising in consequence of, or merely incidental to such wishes; in all cases derived secondarily.*

Freud (1923) summarizing his views on Schreber made this point clear beyond any doubt: "Amongst all the observations concerning the mental life of children which psycho-analysis has made, there is hardly one which sounds so repugnant and incredible to the normal adult as the boy's feminine attitude to the father and the fantasy of pregnancy derived from it. Only since Daniel

* It may appear as if we were neglecting the pregenital stages of development postulated in psychoanalysis. But even if these are taken into account, the core of mental illness, "the infantile nuclear complex" lies in "the familiar ground of the father-complex" (F. 440).

Paul Schreber . . . published the history of his psychotic illness and almost complete recovery, have we been able to speak of such things unconcernedly and with no need to apologize. We learn from this invaluable book that . . . the President became absolutely convinced that God—who incidentally had many of the characteristics of his father . . . had formed the decision to castrate him . . . In his revolt against this decision on the part of God . . . he fell ill with symptoms of paranoia . . . ".

3. While stressing that the precipitating factors can only be surmised in the absence of sufficient material in the Memoirs, Freud in support of his thesis speculates on what some of them may have been.

(*a*) Schreber had " no son to console him for the loss of his father and brother—to drain off his unsatisfied homosexual affections " (F. 442). This does not seem a satisfactory explanation, applying as it does to so many people similarly situated who never fall ill. In fact the reverse might be argued, namely that Schreber's homosexuality was neither aroused nor revived by the very fact that he had no son.

(*b*) Freud felt he " must not omit to draw attention to a somatic factor which may very well have been relevant . . . Dr. Schreber was fifty-one years of age, and he had therefore reached a time of life which is of critical importance in sexual development . . . for men as well as women are subject to a ' climacteric ' " (F. 430). The influence of a ' somatic ' male climacteric seems to the writers uncertain and not backed by the findings of modern endocrinological research. Moreover, even if it were accepted as a factor, it could have served as a precipitating factor only in his second illness in 1893, and not in his first in 1884.

(*c*) Extending Freud's argument, and starting from an upsurge of passive homosexual feelings as if it were an established fact, Niederland (1951) assumes that a common precipitating factor for Schreber's two illnesses can be found in ' masculine responsibility ': which he could not face in his first illness in standing for Parliament, and in the second in his new office as *Senatspräsident*. This implies that he had had no such masculine responsibility before, whereas it is very much more likely that he was promoted to high legal office for the very reason that he carried responsibility so well.

4. If " the basis of Schreber's illness was an outburst of homosexual feeling (F. 425) . . . of a feminine (that is, a passive homosexual) wish-fantasy, which took as its object the figure of his physician " (F. 431), to whom Freud postulated Schreber longed to return in his second illness, this cannot apply to the first. Freud himself says that a knowledge of the causes of the first illness " is no doubt indispensable for properly elucidating the second " (F. 425). Schreber also knew that both were intimately connected. On several occasions prior to the outbreak of his second illness he had anxiety dreams that his former illness had returned: " Naturally I was as unhappy about this in the dream as I felt happy on waking that it had only been a dream " (S. 36). Freud interpreted that this may have " simply expressed some such longing as: 'I wish I could see Flechsig again!' " (F. 425).

If it can be substantiated that Schreber had another acute episode in 1907, further doubt must arise in the validity of these precipitating factors, as none of them could apply.

If the homosexual significance of these precipitating factors is unconvincing, they can no longer be used to support Freud's theory that an upsurge of homosexuality was the cause of Schreber's illness.

5. One of the main pivots of Freud's analysis is that Schreber could not accept his homosexual wishes for Flechsig and therefore turned his love into hate, and later transferred his feelings for Flechsig to God, thus making God the loved, hated and feared male love object. We will discuss later the sequence of events in the Memoirs which shows that this is not what actually happened according to Schreber's own account. Freud claimed repeatedly in definite terms that Schreber identified God and the sun, and that " the sun, therefore, is nothing but another sublimated symbol for the father " (F. 439), a point much belaboured by Katan (*loc. cit.*). Freud even adds a postcript to his paper adducing new mythological evidence in support of his view that " the patient's peculiar relation to the sun (F. 467) . . . expressing his filial relation . . . has confirmed us once again in our view that the sun is a symbol of the father " (F. 469).

Yet Freud himself quotes Schreber's physician's report that one of Schreber's stereotyped utterances during his early catatonic phase was his shouting for hours " The sun is a whore " (FS. 438). Freud also quotes Schreber speaking of the monstrosity of God allowing " himself to be f . . . . d " (FS. 408). That both these quotations are given in footnotes by Freud throws light on his conviction that God and the sun were "nothing but" father symbols for Schreber; he ignores their obvious female significance, and gives them in illustration only of this other facet of the boy's libidinal attachment and submission to the father: the son's rebellious, derisive and belittling attitude toward him (F. 435–437).

But it is evident that Schreber clearly considered the sun both male and female, ambisexual, a point also made by Abraham (1913): "this bisexuality of the sun appears in Schreber's case too . . . there can be no doubt of the female character of the sun symbol". Further, Schreber refers to the sun as "the eye of God" (S. 10), an ambisexual symbol according to Abraham (*loc. cit.*), who quotes Rank and other authors in support. This is in agreement also with mythological evidence (Perry, 1923) and further borne out by the different gender of the sun in different languages; in Schreber's the sun is feminine.

We lay great stress upon this point because, if the sun was not a father symbol for Schreber, Freud's theoretical deductions only partially cover the facts. The passive homosexual wish-fantasy, ultimately derived from his infantile relation to his father and evidenced in his relation to the sun, could not afford the whole explanation, but would throw light only on one aspect, however important, of his psychosis and the content of his delusions.

All the evidence goes to show that the sun, far from representing only the father, mirrored Schreber's own ambisexuality, being both male and female. In other words Schreber was confused about his own sex and procreative possibilities. For Schreber the sun was the concrete expression of God's miraculous powers of creation; "the sun is not really a power in itself and separate from God, in a certain sense she is even identified with God, in other words she is the instrument nearest to earth of God's power of miracles" (S. 247; 8, 9).

When Freud assumed the sun to be a father symbol and God equivalent to an earthly father, he failed to see that Schreber was preoccupied with the origin and giving of life, i.e. creation and procreation in the primitive, presexual sense which precedes knowledge of sexual reproduction both in the history of the individual and of mankind. This group of ideas in fact forms the basis of all primitive religions (Perry, 1923) which arose in answer to the question 'where do I come from' and 'whence life'. These "prephallic" (Smith, 1929) speculations gave rise to the belief in sun gods in the sky who hold the life-substance—the soul—which they send down at every birth and draw up again at every death.

Free- and high-flying birds were believed to act as carriers of this soul substance in their flight between heaven and earth.* Because they were mere carriers of souls of erstwhile human beings (S. 248) the free-flying birds only spoke to Schreber in phrases learnt by rote (S. 215). Birds incapable of flight such as a canary in its cage, ducks, geese and hens in the yard of the Asylum, never spoke to Schreber (S. 214).

Because Freud missed that Schreber's psychosis was concerned with the origin of life in this, its original, most primitive sense, he thought that the talking birds " must be young girls. In a carping mood people often compare them to geese, ungallantly accuse them of having ' the brains of a bird ' " (F. 418).

Schreber's theme of soul murder which must have been committed on him by someone, of which Freud could make nothing, now becomes clear. It runs through the whole of the Memoirs as the cause of the crisis in God's realms, in other words of Schreber's illness. It is the most obscure issue in the book, perhaps evidence that it was the centre of his psychosis. Schreber could only explain it as somebody taking possession of another's soul, his life substance, to prolong his life, to gain a kind of immortality, or for some other advantage (S. 22, 23). In this way soul murder or theft of soul substance meant denying the Schreber family, i.e. himself, offspring (S. 26, 27), because the life substance which God gives to all human beings to perpetuate themselves was taken away. In this way Schreber, being without children, was excluded from the eternal cycle of Life. This also explains his conflict with God and his ' end of the world ' fantasy, because new life had to be put into him again to restore his soul and so allow him to procreate. Hence also his delusion that he was immortal: a person without a soul, i.e. life substance, cannot die. His quest for life and immortality in its mystical and mythological meaning reminded Schreber of Goethe's Faust, Weber's Freischütz and Byron's Manfred (S. 22).

The nexus of ideas of sun and sky gods (originally the Great Mother with subsequent repeated changes of sex), the holders and givers of life and life substance or soul, the destruction of mankind followed by a succession of new creations, the origin of mankind from stones, the preservation of the body after death to allow the soul to return (cf. Schreber's diatribe on cremation (S. 344–348)), together make up the "heliolithic culture".† To it belongs

* Compare the Holy Ghost in the shape of a Dove.

† " Heliolithic ", from Greek, meaning sun-stone (cf. Sonnenstein and Schreber's reference to Deucalion and Pyrrha).

also the strange custom of the *Couvade* (Smith, 1929; Dawson, 1929): " when the women are delivered, the men lie-in . . . , keep their bed, and are attended as if under real sickness " (Lettsom, 1778). In this widespread custom, primitive prephallic procreation fantasies in the male are expressed in physical symptoms (hypochondriasis) without prior upsurge of homosexual libido. A clinical example is furnished by patients with intractible pruritus ani (Macalpine, 1953), which was found to be due to reactivation of unconscious, intestinal, procreation fantasies.

6. Such physical (somatic) hallucinations figure prominently in Schreber's Memoirs; descriptions of " his physical tortures " play as large a part as his delusional deliberations, and indeed merge with them. But Freud pays little attention to them in his analysis. He mentions " the enormous number of delusional ideas of a hypochondriacal nature which the patient developed ", but interprets them only as coinciding " word for word with the hypochondriacal fears of onanists " (F. 441). Yet Freud seems to have been aware of deficiencies in his estimation of these somatic hallucinations: " I must not omit to remark at this point that I shall not consider any theory of paranoia trustworthy unless it covers also the *hypochondriacal* symptoms by which that disorder is almost invariably accompanied " (F. 441). Freud's disregard of them in his evaluation of the case is all the more surprising as Schreber's first illness in 1884 was an " attack of severe hypochondria . . . 'without the occurrence of any incidents bordering upon the sphere of the supernatural' " (FS. 390), marked by insomnia, depression, preoccupation with loss of weight and other " hypochondriacal ideas " (S. 35).

Freud assessed the physical symptoms as organ pleasure, as masturbatory equivalents or expressions of guilt and anxiety over masturbation, particularly the fear of castration. Other authors have followed Freud with the result that psychoanalysis has little else to say about hypochondriacal symptoms and their significance; commonly they are treated with less interest, respect and understanding than mental symptoms (Macalpine, 1954). Yet most psychiatric patients present with complaints referred to their body, which are often investigated and treated by physicians and surgeons as if they were due to organic disease.

One historical reason, as mentioned in the Introduction, is that hypochondriasis was classed as an actual neurosis by Freud (1895), of which he stated: " The problems of the actual neuroses, in which the symptoms probably arise through direct toxic injury, offer no point of attack for psychoanalysis; it can supply little towards elucidation of them and must leave this task to biological and medical research"; and "The symptoms of an actual neurosis have no 'meaning', no signification in the mind" (Freud, 1917). Jones (1951) regretted that Freud could not be persuaded to take up the problem of the actual neuroses again from where he had left it in 1895. As it stands today the concept is unacceptable and useless, the theory of damming up of libido in one organ has not led to deeper insight but merely to a barrage of terms such as organ-neurosis, pregenital conversion, and erotization of organs. The toxic effect of undischarged libido is an outmoded concept, however hard it seems to die.

Because we believe that Schreber's hypochondriacal symptoms express primitive, pregenital procreation fantasies in the form of body hallucinations, we searched the psychoanalytic literature on pregnancy fantasies. We ourselves prefer the term procreation fantasies to stress the absence of mature sex drives, whether homo- or heterosexual.

Literature on Pregnancy Fantasies

It is surprising that so little interest has been shown in pregnancy fantasies as Freud held that the child assumes first that everybody is like itself, and that when it discovers that this is not so, it wishes to have what it has not got. Thus the girl's penis envy fills psychoanalytic literature to overflow, while the boy's envy of child-bearing receives almost no attention. Glover (1946) notes "... although less attention is paid to the fact, it is undeniable that the boy's unconscious disappointment at being unable to emulate his mother's feat of baby-production is as deep as the corresponding jealousy of the girl that she does not possess male organs..." Jones (1942) finds "mutual envy between the sexes is common in early childhood ... the male one, envy of the female capacity to give birth to children, is less recognized than its counterpart".

In "A Neurosis of Demoniacal Possession", a case similar in many smaller details and, like Schreber's, subject to confusion between neurosis and psychosis, Freud (1923) spoke expressly of pregnancy fantasies which the painter must have had since the figure nine recurs significantly in his pacts with the devil, and states: "What he is struggling against is the feminine attitude to the father, which culminates in the fantasy of bearing him a child ". And again: " The feminine attitude to the father became repressed as soon as the boy realized that his rivalry with the woman for the father's love implies the loss of his own male genital, that is to say, implies castration ". Like Schreber he had somatic symptoms which Freud makes no attempt to detail or interpret; he " experienced all manner of things: also convulsive seizures accompanied by extremely painful sensations; on one occasion paralysis of the lower limbs occurred; and so on " (Freud, 1923).

It is remarkable that Freud does not even consider pre-genital fantasies. Only two years before he wrote his study of Schreber's Memoirs he had found that infantile sex theories assume " . . . that babies come out of the anus; the second theory which follows logically from the first is that men can have babies just as well as women " (Freud, 1909). Freud (1908), discussing the infantile " cloacal theory " of baby making, " the child being voided like a stool ", says that the child does not accept the fact that woman alone has the painful privilege of giving birth to babies: " If babies are born through the anus then a man can give birth just as well as a woman. A boy can therefore fancy that he too has children of his own without our needing to accuse him of feminine inclinations ". Rank (1909, 1912), from his anthropological studies, confirmed that procreation fantasies in children precede the knowledge of sexual differences, and that infantile birth theories are by no means linked to the female, so that both boys and girls are supposed to bear children.

Binswanger (1911) analyzed a " hysterical phobia " in a girl and found it due to reawakening of archaic, intestinal pregnancy fantasies, following appendicectomy; conception was thought to be caused by eating certain foods.

Nunberg (1920) says of a catatonic schizophrenic : " The process ran its course in two series: in a somatic series aimed at attaining organ pleasure, and in a psychic series directed toward the recovery of the lost objects ". The material, like Schreber's, is essentially concerned with transitivism, impregnation, self-impregnation, birth, rebirth, immortality, the propagation of mankind, and death. The patient himself " thought eternal life would result from my making these motions ", and Nunberg says " it is a birth fantasy tied up with the process of defecation ". Yet he concluded that " the attack represents a perfect wish-fulfilment and gives full assent to all perversions . . . the patient's whole endeavour is aimed at ridding himself of unpleasure and at gaining pleasure through stimulation of the erotogenic zones or organs . . . " In the period of hypochondriasis preceding the illness, "the connection of the body sensations with sexual processes is obvious ". "A desire to be transformed into a woman and to propagate himself" is taken as "the psychic expression of the sexuality while it was still genital; it is therefore comprehensible that the accompanying sensations bear this character ".

Eisler (1921) concludes that his patient indulged in "a passive homosexual wish-fantasy . . . the neurosis mobilized a multitude of anal-erotic memory traces ", and "a memory . . . of childbirth observed in childhood led to identification with the suffering woman thought of as being tortured in childbirth ". The patient longed for a child and his marriage was childless. He was referred for treatment solely on account of somatic symptoms which included "a boring pain in the left side 'as if a solid object were trying to emerge' ". An X-ray examination was found to have had the unconscious significance of impregnation. Eisler speaks of the *fruit-pip* complex to illustrate patients' preoccupation with the contents of faeces and their carrying new life.

Boehm (1930) coined the term "parturition envy ". Whether envy of the vagina in men has the same close relationship to narcissism as penis envy in women, or is based mainly on a passive homosexual attitude to the father, "cannot be decided ".

Brunswick (1940) in an "exhaustive discussion of the pre-oedipal phase of both boy and girl" written in "collaboration with Freud ", stressed that "the original, asexual, 'harmless' wish for a baby arises very early, is based wholly on the primitive identification of the child of either sex with the active mother . . . is neither active nor passive . . . Contrary to our earlier ideas, the penis wish is not exchanged for a baby wish which . . . has indeed long preceded it ".

Jacobson (1950) speaks of "unconscious feminine wishes to grow children " and of "narcissistic components in a man's longing for children which are apt to revive again his infantile frustrated feminine reproductive wishes ". She gives details of a case who, from early childhood, had suffered from "psychosomatic symptoms (mainly gastrointestinal) and mild hypochondriacal fears ". These fantasies are interpreted entirely as originating on the genital level. Hence such contradictory conceptions as the "pregnant, i.e. castrated, mother ", and the "phallic—equated with pregnant—mother ".

Freeman (1951) could not find a clear relation between unconscious pregnancy fantasies and his patients' passive homosexual impulses, but could not divorce himself from the theory of instincts and therefore concluded that " aggressive and sexual drives were stimulated by the (wife's) pregnancy ".

Evans (1951) described a case of simulated pregnancy in a male, diagnosed as " anxiety hysteria ". His symptoms were all somatic: abdominal pain, diarrhoea, nervous cough, etc. The patient described himself as " a middle sex . . . Attention should be drawn to the particular intensity of his fear of castration . . . it was as if he understood that to be loved as a woman by the father, he must submit to castration and his simulated pregnancy proved on analysis to be an attempt to pay that price ".

Summary of Literature on Pregnancy Fantasies

The literature on pregnancy fantasies is extremely scant and shows several weaknesses.

1. Pregnancy fantasies in men are mostly considered as arising in consequence of, or as a cover for, passive homosexual wishes. Apart from many other criticisms this view is open to, it also presupposes that the boy's mind is sufficiently structured and mature not only to recognize the existence of two sexes and their respective roles in procreation, but also that he is aware that pregnancy follows sexual intercourse, a fact not appreciated in some primitive tribes even today (Mead, 1949; Smith, 1919).

2. That pathogenic pregnancy fantasies are almost exclusively reported in men shows that they are tacitly paralleled to mature, genital, uterine pregnancies, and this may explain why in women they have attracted so little attention. It would appear that in women such archaic pregnancy fantasies are supposed to be precursors of " normal " childbearing. This is however not always so, as shown for instance, by cases of pseudocyesis, by no means always " hysterical " (Bivin and Klinger, 1937). The frequency of anal birth fantasies in psychotic women also shows how pathogenic such primitive procreation fantasies are in females.

3. " Harmless ", presexual pregnancy fantasies preceding genitality are given due weight only by Freud (1908)—but not in Schreber's case—and by Brunswick (*loc. cit.*). Both are theoretical contributions which do not seem to have found their way into clinical practice. Considerable weight attaches to Brunswick's remarks that the wish for a baby long precedes the wish for a penis, because the generally accepted and freely quoted faeces-penis-child equation

tends to perpetuate the genital aspect of pregnancy fantasies, to the neglect of these much earlier and more primitive, presexual procreation fantasies.

4. Because such fantasies are assumed to be sexual (phallic), i.e. genital, most cases reported are labelled " hysterical ". Hence the stress placed on castration fears or wishes, and on the libidinal and later aggressive aspects of the inverted oedipus situation. Detailed reading of the case reports makes it very doubtful whether the diagnosis of hysteria was adequate, whether used to describe the whole picture or only one isolated symptom in an otherwise differently diagnosed case. The term " hysteria " is freely and indiscriminately used, and Kraepelin's (1913) criticism still holds good: " Quite frequently cases of dementia praecox are misdiagnosed as hysteria ". It is doubtful whether hysteria or anxiety hysteria is an adequate diagnosis today, other than as a non-specific assessment of temperament and omnibus label for milder cases of mental disturbance.

5. Lack of understanding and confusion appear to hinge around neglect of hypochondriacal symptoms, their mechanism and diagnostic significance, in favour of the more dramatic, more easily understood, and perhaps less disturbing psychic symptoms (Macalpine, 1954). It is noteworthy that all cases of pregnancy fantasies quoted in the literature had somatic symptoms predominantly; however, they are not accorded any significance and are therefore scattered at random through the case histories.

II. SCHREBER'S MATERIAL

The difficulty which Schreber experienced of making the material clear, if only to a limited extent: " things are dealt with which cannot be expressed in human language; they exceed human understanding " (S. 2), is equally great when attempting to give a *résumé* and analysis. Concreteness of schizophrenic expression, mixture of primary and secondary processes, neologisms and puns, tortuous associations and somatic language, difficulties of translation, comparison with Freud's analysis, all complicate the presentation.

Outline of the Psychosis

Schreber fell ill when a wish-fantasy that he could, would or should have children became pathogenic. Simultaneously he became doubtful of his own sex. His Memoirs might bear the subtitle ' Whence Life? '; reproduction and the origin of life are considered from all aspects: biological, embryological, geological, mythological, theological, astronomical, literary, and supernatural. His extensive and detailed knowledge of these subjects shows the unconscious determination of his interests before he became ill. His psychosis was a quest to procreate; speculations became reality and were jumbled up in a cycle which embraced birth, life, death, rebirth, resurrection, life after death, transmigration of souls. All centred around the fundamental issue of creation and his own creative potentialities.

His Introduction affords insight and an overall view: " the concept of eternity is beyond man's grasp. Man cannot really understand that something can exist which has neither beginning nor end, and that there can be a cause which cannot itself be traced to a previous cause . . . If God created the world, how then did God Himself come to be? This question will for ever remain unanswered. The same applies to the concept of divine creation. Man can always only imagine that new matter is created through the influence of forces on matter already in existence, and yet I believe—and I hope to prove in what follows by means of definite examples—that divine creation is a creation out of the void. The Christian teaching that Jesus Christ was the son of God can be meant only in a mystical sense which but approximates the human sense of these words, because nobody would maintain that God as a being endowed with human sexual organs, had intercourse with the woman from whose womb Jesus Christ came forth (S. 3). I am able to give . . . a . . . detailed explanation of . . . how such things can come about through divine miracles. Something like the conception of Jesus Christ by an Immaculate Virgin . . . happened in my own body. Twice at different times (while I was still in Flechsig's Asylum) I had a female genital organ, although a poorly developed one, and in my body felt quickening like the first signs of life of a human embryo: by a divine miracle . . . fertilization had occurred " (S. 4; FS. 413).

Schreber pursued the quest ' how can I a man be in the process of having or actually have children? '. To live through the various possibilities was his psychosis: as a man, by being changed into a woman, parthenogenetically, by divine impregnation and self-impregnation. He speaks of " parentless generation, spontaneous generation " (S. 2–3, 241, 251). That these speculations refer to himself can be seen when he recounts " the innumerable visions I had in connection with the idea that the world had perished . . . partly of a gruesome nature, partly of an indescribable sublimity" (S. 73), when "I recapitulated . . . the whole history of mankind or of the earth in reverse order" (S. 74).

The different stages of his procreation fantasies, although here presented separately, are interwoven and run together through the maze of the Memoirs. There are three principal themes: procreation, change of sex, relation to God.

Procreation as Man

After "a series of single acts of creation, in general advancing from lower to higher forms of organic life (S. 253) God exercised His power of miracles on our earth . . . only until the ultimate aim of His creation was attained with the creation of the human being. From then on He left the created organic world as it were to itself, and interfered directly by miracle only very rarely if at all in very exceptional cases . . . He Himself retired to an enormous distance (S. 251–252). Every single species was able to preserve itself by being provided with the conditions under which it could live, by their capacity to reproduce themselves and by the continued warmth of the sun" and the "many lower animal forms which serve as nourishment or for other purposes (S. 256, 10). Regular contact between God and human souls occurred in the Order of the World only after death" (S. 12). In the transmigration of souls (S. 15) God approached "corpses in order to draw their nerves . . . out of their bodies and up to Himself" (S. 12). This is the eternal cycle of life, in which God is the sum total of all souls which He sends down to be reincarnated at every birth and draws up to Himself again after every death, when they have to undergo a process of purification (S. 6–15). In this cycle the words soul, nerves, rays have the same meaning (S. 8).

Therefore God could not help Schreber to be fruitful unless a "world catastrophe" necessitated re-creation of the species (S. 10, 52, 53, 240, 252, 289). "In such an event, in order to maintain the species, one single human being was spared—perhaps the relatively most moral": one is "automatically reminded of the legends of Noah, Deucalion and Pyrrha, etc." (S. 53).*

Schreber stressed in many places that he was such a moral man

* The myth of Deucalion and Pyrrha is presexual in character. Deucalion built a wooden chest in which he and his wife Pyrrha were saved from a deluge sent by Zeus. After floating for nine days, they were instructed to renew the human race destroyed by the deluge, by veiling their faces and throwing behind them the bones of their mother. They interpreted this as meaning the stones of the earth. Those thrown by Deucalion became men, those by Pyrrha women.

(S. 292, 427). Into the ancient myth of world catastrophes and new creations (S. 52, 53, 240) he introduced one new feature: besides the universal stories of devastating plagues (S. 74, 91, 92), earthquakes, floods, ice age, immorality (S. 52, 60), the destruction of mankind could be caused by " an increase in nervousness ". That he himself protested at length that he suffered from a nervous and not a mental illness (S. 268, 404–451), also shown by the title of the Memoirs, is further evidence that the ' end of the world ' fantasy centred round him and was set in motion by his desire to bear children: " . . . through my case . . . the earth has once again become the permanent scene of divine miracles " (S. 259).

Schreber lived through the fantasy that the world had come to an end, mankind perished, people around him seemed to be directly created by God in transitory form, " fleeting-improvised-men ". There is an anal implication in the original of " fleeting-improvised-men "—as pointed out by Niederland (*loc. cit.*)—consonant with Schreber's preoccupation with defecation. In the long passage quoted by Freud (FS. 406–408) it is Schreber who speaks of " the symbolic meaning of the act of evacuation . . . in a certain sense the final act " (FS. 406–407), obviously alluding to anal birth fantasies. Schreber's complaint that God does not understand living human beings or the living human organism, being only accustomed to dealing with corpses, is therefore not the son's rebellion against God the father, but refers specifically to Schreber's failure to produce a child by anal birth, because God did not or could not intervene to make him fruitful by divine miracle. Secondly, the punning of Flechsig and *flüchtig* (fleeting) (S. 24) shows that Flechsig's soul had supernatural powers to fill Schreber's body with " little Flechsigs " It goes without saying that this also was asexual procreation, souls are *ipso facto* sexless, because they lose their identity in the process of purification (S. 18).

Schreber could further procreate asexually as a man if he were to die and be born again. Thus he thought himself dead (S. 73), read an announcement of his own death, significantly at Easter (S. 81), and speculated on being buried alive (S. 59, 92). This was not his only intrauterine fantasy. The close connection between sleep, death, birth, and rebirth, particularly in the transmigration of souls, explains his concern with ideas of death (S. 40, 43, 44), and suicide by hanging (S. 41), starvation (S. 57–58) and poisoning (S. 59, 380). These most primitive procreation fantasies coincided with the worst tortures of his catatonic and most alienated phase.

Procreation as Woman

The phase of procreation as a man merged with, and was eventually superseded by fantasies of divine impregnation like the Virgin Mary (S. 4) and Rhea Sylvia (S. 53). He "had to be unmanned (changed into a woman) to bear children" (S. 53, 54). This was in consonance with the Order of the World, a prerequisite and essential (S. 55, 177): "unmanning with simultaneous fertilization by divine rays would have led to my recovery" (S. 139). Once reconciled to the necessity of changing into a woman he improved and indeed left hospital with this idea still florid. The reproductive aspect of the change into a woman is emphasized by Schreber's fantasies centring on breasts and buttocks. "Twice at different times . . . I had a female genital organ, although a poorly developed one, and in my body felt quickening like the first signs of life of a human embryo" (S. 4, footnote 1).

As divine impregnation did not materialize, Schreber felt that it was prevented and even reversed in its purity of purpose in accordance with the Order of the World, by impure rays emanating from Flechsig (S. 54, 139), whom he had endowed with godlike powers (S. 49, 56, 109-111), since Flechsig had promised to "deliver" him of his illness at the first interview (S. 39) If not accompanied by fertilization, unmanning was contrary to the Order of the World (S. 56, 127, 139); here Schreber's homosexual temptations made him fear that his body might be changed into a female body for sexual purposes and abuse only.

Freud singled out this one aspect to explain the whole illness in terms of homosexual conflict, laying great stress on one night of six emissions (F. 429) which occurred several months after admission. Freud assigned to Flechsig the part of "instigator" (F. 421) and "first seducer" (F. 422). Because Schreber "was anxious not to insult the 'man Flechsig' . . . it is nowhere expressly stated that the transformation into a woman was to be carried out for the benefit of Flechsig". It must, however, have been Flechsig, because "no other individual is ever named . . . who could be put in Flechsig's place" (F. 427).

The change into a woman was not castration as a punishment for forbidden homosexual wishes, nor was it a means of achieving such wishes. Rather its purpose was to permit procreation. He "had to be unmanned (transformed into a woman) to be able to bear children. This process of unmanning consisted in the (external) male genitals (scrotum and penis) being retracted into the body and the internal sexual organs being at the same time transformed into the corresponding female sexual organs " (S. 53). Far from meaning castration, i.e. sterilization, " unmanning " meant changing into a woman in order to be fertile. Schreber described how " my body seemed to have got smaller by six to eight centimetres, thereby approximating the size of a female body " (S. 149). The most consistent changes concerned " breasts and buttocks (S. 176). . . . my nipples remain small as in the male sex . . . notwithstanding I venture to assert flatly that anybody who sees me standing in front of a mirror with the top half of my body naked would get the undoubted *impression of a female trunk*—especially when the illusion is strengthened by some feminine adornments " (S. 280). The whole of the female body is covered with nerves of voluptuousness, particularly the mammae: " I can *feel* certain string- or cord-like structures under my skin ; these are particularly marked on my chest where the woman's bosom is . . . and have the peculiarity that one can feel them ending in nodular thickenings " (S. 277).

These nodular tissues are the nerves of voluptuousness (S. 278) with which God's rays or nerves have filled him (S. 87, 279). They are the " female nerves " (S. 94) in which lies " the nature of divine creation " (S. 8, 151, 254, 259). Voluptuousness therefore is readiness to conceive and be pregnant (S. 94, 281) and part of the state of Blessedness (S. 281, FS. 410). Souls, being in a continual state of expectancy to be reborn, are in a perpetual state of " voluptuous enjoyment or Blessedness . . . as an end in itself " (S. 281–282); hence " soul-voluptuousness " (S. 129) and " the close relationship which exists between voluptuousness and everlasting Blessedness " (S. 281). " The new life to come is the state of Blessedness " (S. 12). It is given " to *human beings . . . solely as a means for the preservation of the species* " (S. 281–282).

In this way the words voluptuousness, soul-voluptuousness, transmigration of souls, the state of Blessedness, blessed, blessing, nerves, souls, rays, and talking birds, all refer to creation, procreation, birth, rebirth, and eternal life as a continuation of life after death. In all ' soul ' is used in its original primitive meaning of " the life substance " (Smith, 1919). Freud disregarded the concreteness of schizophrenic thought and expression when he took voluptuousness literally only to mean mature sexual lust.

Ambisexuality

" Transformation into a woman " therefore refers to being a male with female reproductive features, a double-sexed creature well known in mythology (Smith, 1919). " In the absurd relationship between God and myself I have to find a fitting middle course " (S. 283, 284). It follows that Schreber was throughout basically uncertain about his sexual identity: " I must point out that when I speak of my duty to cultivate voluptuousness, I *never mean any sexual desires towards other human beings (females), least of all sexual intercourse*, but that I have to imagine myself as man and woman in one person having intercourse with myself, or somehow have to achieve with myself a certain sexual excitement —which perhaps under other circumstances may be considered immoral—but which has nothing whatever to do with any idea of masturbation or anything like it " (S. 282, 285).

He also " repeatedly had the nerves belonging to my wife's soul in my body " (S. 121-122).

Beginning of Illness

Preoccupation with the homosexual " neurotic " aspect, and overemphasis on frank delusions and hallucinations centring on the outside world—that is alienation—as hallmarks of psychosis are responsible for the neglect of the prodromal phenomena of psychosis which marked the beginning of Schreber's illness.

Schreber's first delusion developed during the weeks of insomnia which followed his taking up office as Presiding Judge on 1st October 1893. " In an almost sleepless night . . . an extraordinary event occurred . . . a recurrent crackling noise in the wall of our bedroom became noticeable . . . naturally we thought of a mouse, although this was very extraordinary . . . in a solidly built house . . . but having heard similar noises innumerable times since then and still hearing them every day . . . I have come to recognize them as undoubted divine miracles " (S. 37, 38). The child symbolism is obvious : *parturiunt montes* . . .*

" On the 8th or 9th of November " Schreber took sick-leave to consult Flechsig who " gave me hope of delivering me of the whole illness through one prolific sleep to last from three o'clock in the afternoon to the following day . . . Naturally I did not get to bed (in my mother's house) as early as three o'clock . . . but it was delayed till the ninth hour (possibly according to some secret instruction which my wife had received) " (S. 39). This was his second delusion and in it the figure nine appears twice. That the figure nine is not a coincidence the following data show:

* " The soul-substance can assume the form of a mouse " (Perry, 1918).

1. His first illness started in the autumn of 1884; he entered Flechsig's Clinic in December and had recovered sufficiently to leave in June 1885. The illness therefore lasted about nine months.

2. His second illness started in October 1893—nine years after the outbreak of the first.

3. It lasted nine years from 1893 until 1902, when his tutelage was rescinded.

4. Schreber was transferred from Flechsig's Clinic to Sonnenstein Asylum on 29th June, 1894. Nine months after the first consultation with Flechsig, "during the first weeks of my stay at Sonnenstein . . . certain important changes took place with the sun" (S. 135).

5. The figure nine appears repeatedly in the book in numerical combinations: for instance he speaks five times of 4-5, 40-50, 4th and 5th (S. 104-107); two further instances follow.

The night after seeing Flechsig "was almost sleepless", and he had to be prevented from suicide by his wife. "Next morning my nerves were badly shattered; the blood had gone from my extremities and to the heart" (S. 40). He was admitted to Flechsig's Clinic "and put to bed which I did not leave for four or five days . . . my illness grew rapidly . . . I was concerned only with ideas of death" (S. 40). "About the 4th or 5th night after my admission I was pulled out of bed . . . and taken to a cell fitted out for dements (maniacs) . . . I was delirious . . . and tried to hang myself . . . I was completely ruled by the idea that there was nothing left for a human being for whom sleep could no longer be procured . . . but to take his life (S. 41) . . . My will to live was completely broken; I could see nothing in the future but suicide" (S. 43, 44).

Acute Stage

On admission "he mentioned mostly hypochondriacal ideas, complained that he was suffering from softening of the brain, would soon die, etc." (S. 380). Although "ideas of persecution" and "visual and auditory hallucinations . . . soon appeared in the disease picture", it was not until four months after admission that "the first signs of communication with supernatural powers appeared, particularly that of nerve-contact which Professor Flechsig kept up with me, in such a way that he spoke to my nerves without being present in person" (S. 44). Schreber felt that his wife's absence for four days, and a night of six emissions were "decisive for my mental collapse" (S. 44).

Freud interpreted this "by assuming that they (the emissions) were accompanied by homosexual fantasies which remained unconscious . . . the mere presence of his wife must have acted as a protection against the attractive power of the men about him" (F. 429). It is difficult to accept this interpretation from Schreber's own attitude to, and description of the rough and ready attendants around him. It seems to us that the presence of his wife may have helped him to maintain the distinction between male and female and keep at bay uncertainty about his sex. In her absence total identification with the reproductive woman took place: "In my opinion . . . a human being ("seer of spirits") must under certain circumstances be "unmanned" (transformed into a woman) once he has entered into indissoluble contact with divine nerves (rays)" (S. 45, 77). A hint to this sentence lies in "certain circumstances", a possible allusion to pregnancy. Contact with divine rays meant contact with divine creative power, i.e. impregnation (S. 256). In other words the idea of "unmanning" is derived from his procreation fantasies and the change into a woman was a means to them.

He continued to deteriorate and was catatonic when transferred to Sonnenstein in June 1894. There, nine months after the beginning of his illness, terrifying and threatening miracles occurred; a second, smaller sun appeared in heaven (S. 135, 71), "it was a holy time" (S. 63, 77). "Holy time" may be a reference to Christmas, the time of the birth of God's son.

Hypochondriacal Delusions

In the acute stage of his illness Schreber lived through a fantasy of giving birth, which can be interpreted from his account. Proof is afforded by examination of his hypochondriacal delusions, which clearly express ideas of change of sex and giving life. That they were most severe during his first year at Sonnenstein (S. 148) may be in part due to the Asylum's name*: the sun as giver of life, and the stone as symbol of the child (cf. Schreber's reference to Deucalion).

"But in the first year of my stay at Sonnenstein, the miracles were of such a threatening nature that I thought I had to fear almost incessantly for my life, my health, or my reason . . . I could fill a

* It will be remembered that Schreber was mystified by his transfer (S. 117).

whole book with them alone (S. 148). This will naturally sound extremely strange to all other human beings . . . But in reply I can only give the assurance that hardly any memory from my life is more certain than the miracles recounted in this chapter. What can be more definite for a human being than what he has lived through and felt on his own body ? (S. 150). Most nearly in consonance with the Order of the World were those miracles which were somehow connected with a process of unmanning " (S. 149). These were the changes into a reproductive woman, the " milder " ones which we have described earlier.

More serious and multifarious were the miracles directed against his internal organs (S. 149). They were " very painful (S. 149) . . . hardly a single limb or organ in my body escaped being temporarily damaged by miracles " (S. 148). They give expression to Schreber feeling new life in all parts of his body and in all sorts of ways. We append a selection without comment, except to point out that some are exact replicas of well-known birth legends, e.g. smashing of ribs (Adam), splitting of head (Zeus), plurality of heads (Janus, the double or four-headed, *fons et origo* of all things, who presided over all beginnings of birth, enterprise and the year).

He had a different heart ; tuberculosis of the lungs, a worm in them, " either an animal-like being or a soul-like creature" (S. 150); his diaphragm was raised up to his neck ; stabbing pains were felt in the chest ; his ribs were repeatedly smashed, but always reformed (S. 151). " One of the most horrifying miracles " consisted of compression of his chest, " so that I could hardly breathe " (S. 151). His stomach was exchanged for another, at times he had to live without one and " food and drink taken simply poured into the abdominal cavity and into the thighs " (S. 151, 152). The abdomen was filled, leading to sudden attacks of diarrhoea (S. 313) ; he suffered from " dangerous obstruction " of his gut ; the lower abdomen went rotten and the smell escaped from his mouth (S. 153, 154).

Many and the most threatening miracles were directed against his head and spine (S. 154) : the skull was sawn to pieces, pulled apart, squeezed together, thinned, and perforated. Holes were bored into it through which threads were pulled, which performed circular movements inside, nerves were pulled out, the shape of the head was changed so that it became elongated and pear-shaped and a central cleft (fontanel) appeared (S. 159). A new membrane covered the brain ; " even now I suffer from uninterrupted headaches . . . hardly comparable to ordinary headaches (S. 270). There was a time when souls in nerve-contact with me talked of a plurality of heads (that is several individuals in one and the same skull) which they encountered in me, and from which they shrank in alarm crying 'for heaven's sake—that is a human being with several heads' (S. 73). The rays (nerves) of the upper God . . . often appear in my head *in the image of a human being* . . . the capacity to be transformed into human shape or to become a human being is an innate potentiality of divine rays" (S. 255–256).

He also had Flechsig's soul in his body, in the shape of "a fairly bulky ball . . . impossible to digest . . . Moved by a kind of sympathetic feeling" he let it escape from his mouth (S. 83). Little men in his feet pumped out his spinal cord which left his mouth "in the form of little clouds" (S. 154). He had severe toothaches (S. 196, 270), pains at the bottom of the spine, paralyses and cramps in the lower back (S. 160, 270); sudden attacks of hunger, nerve pains, severe sciatica, transient paralyses, boring pains in the bones, especially the thighs, and swelling of the feet. Many miracles concerned his eyes (S. 157, 158, 270).

In summary, the deepest layer of his procreation fantasies and his greatest suffering lay in his body hallucinations and delusions (hypochondriasis). These also form the connecting link between his first and second illnesses. They are therefore complementary to and of the same significance as the psychic symptoms. The patient himself showed that he knew this when he spoke of "All the attacks made over the years, on my life, my bodily integrity, my manliness and my reason . . ." (S. 119, 127, 140, 148).

III. CONCLUSIONS

We have interpreted Schreber's psychosis as a reactivation of unconscious, archaic procreation fantasies concerning life, death, immortality, rebirth, creation, including self-impregnation, and accompanied by absolute ambisexuality expressed in doubt and uncertainty about his sex. Homosexual anxieties were secondary to the primary fantasy of having to be transformed into a woman to be able to procreate. These fantasies are best described as somatic hallucinations and hypochondriacal delusions. They led to Schreber's system centring on creation and the origin of life, whether by God or the sun, sexually or parthenogenetically.

Transference

Freud described Schreber's relation to Flechsig as libidinal "transference . . . the patient having been reminded of his brother or father" (F. 431) which "after a lapse of eight years" caused his "severe mental disorder" (F. 430). This "hypothesis" (F. 430) naturally leaves out of account the negative transference not recognized by Freud in 1911. What is more important, it disregards the psychotic aspect of Schreber's "transference".

At the first interview, before hospitalization became unavoidable, Flechsig unwittingly played into Schreber's already active delusions about procreation; he "gave me hope of delivering me of the whole illness through one prolific sleep" (S. 39). Sleep meant to Schreber the time of supernatural happenings: of dreams (S. 11, 47); of connection with divine rays, called nerve-contact (S. 141, 185, 199); of divine impregnation (S. 11, 26, 142, 144, 340); and of unmanning (S. 40, 53). Sleep was also like death (S. 7, 141–142) and rebirth of the soul (S. 7). All this gives meaning to the "torturing bout of sleeplessness" (F. 391), which ushered in his psychosis and took him to Flechsig. On hearing Flechsig's promise he immediately formed a psychotic transference: Flechsig was going to deliver or impregnate him, or both. This idea was facilitated because "the human soul is contained in the nerves of the body" (S. 6), and "God is only nerve" (S. 8). Therefore Professor Flechsig, a nerve specialist, could be expected to have special, even supernatural powers, because he dealt with nervous diseases (S. 25) "and had contact with divine nerves" (S. 25). Hence "Asylums for the mentally ill were called in the basic language God's Nerve-Institutes" (S. 25). Endowed with this divine power as head of the "Nerve-Institute", Flechsig was supernatural and partly a soul (S. vii-xii, 56–57) in direct contact with God (S. 82, 111). Herein lies the easy passage from Flechsig to God (S. 49, 95) and "God Flechsig" (S. 82). Had Freud been aware that Schreber though not overtly alienated was already psychotic at the time of his first interview with Flechsig (S. 36–39), he would not have considered Schreber's transference exclusively libidinal and neurotic.

Freud's analysis was based on Schreber being homosexually attracted to Flechsig. He could not accept this urge and therefore turned his love feelings into being persecuted by Flechsig. Later he transferred his love from Flechsig to God, that is back to the father figure towards whom his homosexual wish originated as a boy. "Schreber could not reconcile himself to playing the part of a female prostitute towards his physician ; but the task of providing God with the voluptuous sensations that he required called up no such resistance on the part of his ego " (F. 432). Freud assumed that only in "November 1895 . . . the connection was established between the emasculation fantasy and the Redeemer idea and the way thus paved for his becoming reconciled to the former" (F. 400). But Schreber at the beginning of his Memoirs states that " twice at different times (while I was still at Flechsig's Asylum) I had a female genital organ . . . and in my body felt quickening like the first signs of life of a human embryo. By divine miracles God's nerves corresponding to male seed had been thrown into my body; in other words fertilization had occurred " (S. 4). This was at least 18 months before the time specified by Freud, that is November 1895, as Schreber left Flechsig's Clinic in June 1894. In fact Schreber was in contact with God and had his first divine revelations in March 1894 (S. 257, footnote 103). Flechsig therefore played a secondary role in Schreber's psychosis from the beginning, and was only woven into his budding delusional system later. The evidence of the Memoirs clearly contradicts Freud's construction that homosexual feelings towards Flechsig were transferred to God, and so became acceptable to Schreber.

What then was Schreber's grievance against Flechsig? Flechsig's soul, and later after his transfer to Pierson's Asylum the senior attendant von W.'s soul (S. 112), assumed the right of disposal over Schreber's body as " tested souls ", that is to say as souls not yet purified : this " profoundly influenced my relation with God and therefore my personal fate " (S. 16). Purely concretely Schreber may be alluding to the actual fact that Flechsig had personally brought him into his Clinic and indeed had him removed to a padded cell; and of course both Flechsig and the senior attendant of Pierson's Asylum had actual power over him. Schreber saying that Flechsig remained the first instigator of the plot against him, may therefore be interpreted as meaning that Flechsig declared him mad and hence " deprived him of his reason " by denying him the reality of his delusions and hallucinations, and in this way committed " soul murder " on him. Schreber also regarded Flechsig as the person who prevented his being unmanned in order to bear children (S. 54), which was the same as soul murder (S. 61).

Homosexuality

Freud felt " justified in maintaining the view that the basis of Schreber's illness was an outburst of homosexual feeling " (F. 429), and the illness the " ensuing defensive struggle " (F. 431) against " castration " and " emasculation ". Hence Freud's central emphasis on castration fears and wishes, because " the idea of being transformed into a woman (of being emasculated) was the primary delusion " (F. 397), and " voices which the patient heard never treated his transformation into a woman as anything but a sexual disgrace " (F. 399). This is correct only for " mocking hypocritical " voices (S. 177) and in so far as it covers Schreber's fears that his turning into a woman might be used for sexual purposes by himself or others, but leaves out of account the reproductive aspect of the change, the deeper and more pathogenic issue. It played a subordinate role to the primary delusion of being transformed into a reproductive woman. " Unmanning " was not castration, implying sterilization, but feminization, implying fertilization. It could even be reversed at any time : " the rays of the upper God (Ormuzd) have the power of restoring manliness when necessary " (S. 54).

Freud misunderstood " contrary to the Order of the World " to refer to " castration ". Schreber himself considered " unmanning " " contrary to the Order of the World " only if it meant lust without procreation. " But now I could see beyond doubt that the Order of the World imperiously demanded my unmanning, whether I personally liked it or not, and that therefore it was *common sense* that nothing was left to me but reconcile myself to the thought of being transformed into a woman. Nothing could of course be envisaged as a further consequence of unmanning but fertilization by divine rays for the purpose of creating new human beings " (S. 177). Schreber makes this point clear in many other passages, as for instance : "All attempts . . . at unmanning me for purposes *contrary to the Order of the World* (that is for the sexual satisfaction of a human being) . . . have failed . . . To be unmanned could have served a different purpose . . . in *consonance* with the Order of the World and this was not only within the bounds of possibility, but may indeed even have provided the likely solution of the conflict " (S. 61, footnote 34 ; also S. 45, 51, 53,54, 55, 124, 127, 128, 139, 289, 337). Schreber, regarding his " unmanning " as an evolutionary possibility, thought " this future transformation into a woman might take decades if not centuries " (S. 387) for its completion, so that " It is probable that to the end of my days there will be strong indications of femaleness, but that I shall die as a man " (S. 289).

Schreber's psychosis is not explicable as an outburst of homosexual libido unacceptable to his personality and repudiated by his ego, nor was his remaining delusion of turning into a woman at the close of his illness an " asymptotic wish-fulfilment " of homosexual drives (F. 432) ; it was by no means the only remnant of his psychosis, as his " Open Letter to Professor Flechsig " (S. vii–xii) evidences.

Relation to God

Freud saw in Schreber's relation to God a revival of the Oedipus situation, i.e. the relation to his father, a physician. It is " singular and full of internal contradictions (F. 401), the strangest mixture of blasphemous criticism and mutinous subordination . . . and of reverent devotion (F. 435–437, 408–409). Through the whole of Schreber's book . . . runs the bitter complaint that God does not understand living men . . . God was only accustomed to intercourse with corpses (F. 402, 405). Could more bitter scorn be shown for a physician such as this than by declaring that he understands nothing about living men and only knows how to deal with corpses ? " (F. 437). But Schreber did not personify God in this way ; for Schreber God was the mysterious, omnipotent power responsible for all creation. God was not just one person, a father figure : " He is One in Many, and Many in One " (S. 197, footnote 83). He is " the sum total of all nerves, of all souls of departed human beings ", in fact the Life Substance.

Schreber did not deride God. He was in conflict with Him. As Schreber explains, God, after one act of creation, delegated His creative powers to man and woman to reproduce themselves. He confined Himself to drawing up to heaven the spirits and souls of the dead, where they again become part of Him after purification and await reincarnation when a child is born. In this " transmigration of souls " God no longer intervenes in the reproduction of mankind on earth except by a miracle. Thus God dealt only with the souls of the dead which ascended after death, but not with living people. This is the Order of the World. The conflict into which Schreber came with God and, through Him, God with His created world, was that Schreber was barren. Thus arose the " circumstances contrary to the Order of the World ". Although God must have given him the wish, because he had left mankind to reproduce itself, He could not intervene to make Schreber fruitful—a flaw in His wisdom and eventually a danger to His creation and so to His own existence (S. 10, 11, 30, 52, 53, 240, 250, 344–348).

The element of megalomania, " the aggrandizement of the ego " (F. 459) as compensation for homosexual wishes, becomes less striking when Schreber's singular position is seen to result from his procreation fantasies ; a point which emerges clearly from Freud's own presentation (FS. 395–396). " The state of Blessedness " is the state of perpetual readiness of souls to be reborn (S. 12) and of continued existence after death (S. 344). " Voluptuousness," far from being only sensual voluptuousness, is closely allied to " Blessedness " (S. 281) ; it serves reproduction.

Mythology and Megalomania

Freud, discussing Schreber's " mission to redeem the world " (F. 395), says this " is a fantasy . . . familiar to us through the frequency with which it forms the nucleus of religious paranoia " ; but in Schreber's case " the additional factor, which makes the redemption dependent upon the patient's being previously transformed into a woman, is unusual and in itself bewildering, since it shows such a wide divergence from the historical myth " (F. 397).

This, however, is only apparently so. The Redeemer idea springs from man's quest to beget eternal life, immortality (S. 31), and represents ideas of rebirth, " except a man be born of water and the Spirit . . . " It is a variant of the " fountainhead and parent story " (Smith, 1919) of the destruction of mankind followed by a succession of new creations, which is man's primitive, presexual attempt at explaining creation (the origin) and procreation (the continuation) of life. All these aspects are discussed by Schreber.

During the florid catatonic phase Schreber experienced bodily procreation in its widest aspects (religious, mythological, evolutionary), which he took to mean that the end of the world had come. The ' psychotic ' idea of feeling new life in his body (S. 4, 82, 115, 116) became conscious in the guise of being chosen to renew mankind. Far from seeing " the end of . . . his subjective world . . . since he has withdrawn his love from it " (F. 456–457, 460), the delusion of world catastrophe necessitated and fulfilled his bringing forth new life (S. 114). The men around him were " fleeting-improvised-men ", not because of " the loss of his libidinal interest " (F. 462) in them, but because only if mankind had perished could Schreber's procreation wishes be fulfilled as " sole survivor to renew mankind " (S. 53, 71, 99, 119, 289) in accordance with biblical and mythological precedent. This also is the reason why he became the centre of attraction of all rays

(S. 87, 262, 265, 322): only through him could souls be reborn. Hence God was inseparably tied to Schreber: rays must create and unless or until they had created something in him, they could not get away.

The idea of male unisexual procreation hidden behind "the Redeemer fantasy" (F. 397) marked the worst phase of his illness, "tremendous hypochondriacal delusional ideas, severe hallucinatory stupor" (S. 462). This fantasy gradually merged with and was later replaced by "something like the conception of Jesus Christ by an Immaculate Virgin" (S. 4). He slowly acquiesced to being turned into a woman in order to bear children (S. 61, 178, 289; FS. 400), and from then on awaited divine impregnation. For a woman it was in consonance with the Order of the World to bear children. This was "the reconciliation" and with it he began to improve. "I would like to meet the man who, faced with the choice of either being a demented human being in male habitus, or a spirited woman, would not prefer the latter" (S. 178).

Freud explained that when Schreber was "reconciled to playing the part of a female prostitute . . . the solution of the conflict . . . the replacement of Flechsig by the superior figure of God . . . called up no such resistance on the part of his ego" (F. 432, 415, 420; FS. 400). In fact "the task of providing God himself with the voluptuous sensations that he required" (F. 432) was *die Wollust pflegen*, an obsolete expression used in Genesis XVIII, 12, when Sarah, old and barren, is promised a child by the Lord and says, *Nun ich alt bin soll ich noch Wollust pflegen*? (Now I am old, am I still to cultivate voluptuousness?). By "cultivating voluptuousness" Schreber meant keeping himself in readiness to receive divine impregnation as a woman by attracting all "rays" (S. 178–179, 281–282, 285). To keep God in contact with his nerves was to ensure that He would complete the change and not "withdraw to an immense distance" until divine impregnation was accomplished.

Schreber's transformation into a woman is thus seen to be in perfect agreement with a variety of mythological and religious beliefs.

Ambisexuality

The sun as creator and promoter of life shares with God the centre of Schreber's delusions. He projects the double nature of his procreative possibilities on to the sun which fertilizes, gives life, brings forth and maintains life, and keeps away death. These functions are synonymous and interchangeable in the primary process of the unconscious, as well as in early religions and among primitive peoples today (Freud, 1900; Rank, 1909; Smith, 1919). But as Freud saw only the male symbolism of the father in the sun, so he interpreted only the homosexual aspects of Schreber's illness.

The maleness and femaleness of the sun mirror Schreber's confusion about his own sex. At one stage even Flechsig was destined to appear as a charwoman (S. 108) and von W.'s soul was almost always the receptive and Schreber's the giving part (S. 192); in another place he records how his mind was exercised as to whether furniture (S. 165) and articles of clothing (S. 166–167) belonged to the male or female sex. His basic bisexuality had developed into a true manifest ambisexuality, male and female potentials being equally matched. He was as much both as he was neither. Thus he says "that I have to imagine myself as man and woman in one person having intercourse with myself" (S. 282) and "playing the woman's part in sexual embrace with myself" (S. 285). These ideas culminated in fantasies of self-impregnation.

In this fundamental doubt Schreber exhibits a common characteristic of schizophrenics. Usually, however, this balanced imbalance of sex has to be deduced from psychotic expression and is not freely accessible. The insight afforded by Schreber on this point gives to his Memoirs their unique value.

It would appear that even in hospitalized psychotics, fantasies of birth and rebirth more easily become conscious and are more easily verbalized in female than in male patients; in the latter, as in Schreber, they often remain confined to hypochondriacal delusions. Appreciation of them seems incompatible even with psychotic mental life.

How disruptive procreation fantasies are can also be seen from the fact that they are rarely uncovered even in lengthy psychoanalyses, whereas the homosexual aspect is always reported.

Precipitating Factors

Schreber's marriage was childless. Freud mentions this "frustration" and says, "Dr. Schreber may have formed a fantasy that if he had been a woman he would have managed the business of having children more successfully"; but adds, "and he may thus have found his way back into the feminine attitude toward his father, which he had exhibited in the earliest years of his childhood" (F. 443). Schreber himself singles out this disappointment:

" After recovering from my first illness I spent eight years with my wife, on the whole quite happy ones, rich also in outward honours and marred only from time to time by the repeated disappointment of our hope of being blessed with children " (S. 36). It is obvious that he alludes to miscarriages or stillbirths. To us it seems legitimate to assess these misfortunes as precipitants of both illnesses, because they reactivated unconscious procreation wishes. With the end of his wife's reproductive period approaching, his disappointment must have become increasingly severe and hence pathogenic.

Promotion to presidency of a court of five judges, most of them up to twenty years older (S. 37), may have made Schreber as a father figure among 'fathers', feel the lack of children more keenly.

" Change of Life "

Freud believed somatic climacteric factors operative in Schreber, a dubious point. But the approaching 'change of life' in Schreber's wife may have given additional impetus to unconscious fantasies culminating in ideas of 'change of sex'. Loss of ability to bear children means loss of a female sexual characteristic; hence 'change of life' in women comes to mean 'change of sex'. This may throw light on the frequency of mental illness at the menopause, and following operations such as hysterectomy. In fact the very expression 'change of life' implies unconscious appreciation of 'change of sex'. Life and sex can be used synonymously, as when an impotent patient complains that 'there is no life' in him. The assumption of a 'change of sex' in women can be extended to men; we have repeatedly found such a belief.

Hence the climacteric in its psychic significance may well have played a part, giving added impetus to Schreber's unconscious uncertainty about his own sex and the possibility of change.

Course of Illness

Schreber went into his psychosis the same way as he came out of it. Shortly before it developed with the break-through of fantasies of being impregnated and with child, of giving birth and being reborn, he felt it would be nice to be a woman having intercourse. He emerged believing he was turning into a woman. To facilitate this he wore " sundry feminine adornments, such as ribbons, trumpery necklaces, and the like" (FS. 400–401). In passing it is of interest that feminine adornments, in particular necklaces, have their origin in the primitive presexual belief in the cowrie shell as giver of life and fertility (Smith, 1919).

Freud argued that because this belief was "the earliest germ of his delusional system . . . also . . . the one part of it that survived his recovery and was afterwards able to retain a place in his practical life" (F. 400), was proof of his thesis that the libidinal homosexual aspect of changing into a woman was the cause of Schreber's illness. But its occurrence both at the beginning and at the end shows that it was not the "salient feature" (F. 400), as it cannot account for the intervening years of his psychosis, including two of catatonic stupor with outbursts of violence spent in the padded cell, the years of "tremendous hypochondriacal delusions, of severe hallucinatory stupor" (S. 462). Had the homosexual implication of turning into a woman been the most pathogenic factor, it is difficult to see how he could have recovered retaining this idea.

Transvestitism

In fact Schreber was now a transvestite: he "moves about his room half naked, stands in front of the mirror in a very low-cut vest, decorated with gay ribbons, gazing at what he believes his female bosom" (S. 400). He "liked to occupy himself by looking at pictures of naked women, even drew them, and had his moustache removed" (S. 384). He believed that his body was covered with female nerves, "the nerves of voluptuousness". He bought sewing material and female toilet articles (S. 429) and took "pleasure . . . in small feminine occupations (S. 388), for instance sewing, dusting, making beds, washing up, and so on" (S. 271). The "cultivation of femaleness" became essential for his well-being: "if only I could *always* be playing the woman's part in sexual embrace with myself, *always* rest my gaze on female beings, *always* look at female pictures, etc." (S. 285, also 417).

Schreber's behaviour cannot be understood in phallic and genital terms, nor in terms of libidinal drives directed towards other persons. It is very different from homosexuality in which a man *qua* man desires sexual relations with another of the same sex. Clearly passive homosexual urges, whether conscious or unconscious, should be sharply distinguished from the confusion about their own sex invariably found in schizophrenics. That in the primary fantasy of change of sex or belonging to the opposite sex, homosexuality is likely sooner or later to play a part secondarily, is undisputed. However great the importance ascribed to homosexual libidinal drives in Schreber's illness, fundamentally they remain a secondary issue. Homosexual behaviour, or homosexual wishes, as also anxiety about them, may be entirely due to primary uncertainty and confusion in sex identity and need never appear in the disease picture. One might say that the more overt homosexual behaviour or transvestitism, the less frankly psychotic the patient, a view supported by the course of Schreber's illness.

The primary delusion of a change of sex may appear in patients in various guises, often as the only symptom: complaint of excessive hairiness in women, lack of hairiness in men, symptoms associated with 'change of life' in women and even men, following hysterectomy, complaints about voice being too high or too low, the breasts being too small or too flat, differences between the right and left halves of the body, etc. Examples could be multiplied *ad infinitum*. Not uncommonly female patients complain of having a male mind in a female body, and male patients that they have a female mind: and request their body be altered accordingly, by surgery and hormones. When supported by physicians, especially endocrinologists, and surgeons, it accounts for the cases of change of sex reported in the newspapers. These two entirely different types of homosexuality have been consistently confused in psychoanalytic theory, in fact have never been distinguished, because of adherence to the doctrine of libidinal wish-fulfilment as the basis of psychiatric symptom formation.

Fairbairn (1943) criticized "the inadequacy of the classic conception that libido is primarily pleasure seeking". According to this, opposition of the ego or superego to unapproved libidinal drives results in 'defence neuroses'. Homosexual urges opposed by the superego and warded off by the mechanism of projection give rise to such libidinal conflict. Psychoneurotic symptoms are therefore postulated to be a compromise formation between the repressing and the repressed. But many features of psychoses can only be understood as a break-through of unconscious fantasies. Sense of reality is lost to the extent that these fantasies become autonomous. Ideler (1848) said "When an idea breaks through the actual life circumstances, insanity ensues".

It seems to us that further study of the psychoses may force this issue, and show that lack of psychotherapeutic success with psychotic patients, as well as the lack of advance in theory, is due to adherence to the libido theory of psychiatric symptom formation.

Procreation Fantasies

Archaic procreation fantasies have no ego or superego disapproval. The wish to produce or create, which can ultimately be traced to the urge to procreate, is intrinsically egosyntonic. It finds no opposition in ego, superego, or personality but can clash with reality. The innate urge to give or prolong life with its connotation of denying or averting death and ensuring immortality, is one of the mainsprings of human activity, and, by sublimation, of creative activity in both sexes. It is a wider, more primitive concept than reproduction, both in the history of the individual and of mankind. Thus ' pregnancy fantasy ' carries limitations avoided by the term ' procreation fantasy '.

Schreber's Memoirs themselves are such a sublimation. He hopes he " will be the middle man, through whose personal fate the knowledge I have gained will spread fruitfully far and wide " (S. 337–338). He believed the " knowledge that a living God exists and the soul lives on after death, could only come as a blessing to mankind " (S. 294); and that his experiences " when generally acknowledged as valid—will act fruitfully to the highest possible degree " (S. viii). He speaks of " a new race of human beings from the spirit of Schreber " (S. 288), and of the draft of his Memoirs being titled " From my Life ": " the content of my revelations was immeasurably richer than . . . in the Memoirs " (S. 195–196). Finally either " my unmanning will be accomplished with the result that by divine fertilization offspring will issue from my lap, or alternatively great fame will be attached to my name, surpassing that of thousands of other people much better mentally endowed " (S. 293, 294).

Schizophrenia

Freud showed the importance of projection of homosexual libido in symptom-formation but did not explain the clinical entities of paranoia, paranoid schizophrenia, or Schreber's illness. His endeavour to describe Schreber's psychosis as a mixture of two illnesses was not an advance; ' double pathology ' thereby introduced, glosses over the clinical fact pointed out by Bleuler (1912) that one is dealing with different aspects of one and the same disease process. Freud, we submit, analysed one part-aspect and the more superficial of Schreber's psychosis. Confirmation of our opinion can be adduced from the fact that projection of unconscious homosexuality has since been claimed to account for many other conditions, such as alcoholism, drug addiction, jealousy, even 'normal' character traits. In any case conflict over unconscious homosexuality with attendant castration fears could not account for schizophrenia in female patients, despite Freud's (1915) *tour de force* on a female patient with 'paranoia'.

The content of Schreber's psychosis is not unique. Schizophrenics regularly are in doubt about the nature of their sex,* commonly speculate on religious matters, particularly the end of the world, speak of sexual transformation, and live through pregnancy and birth fantasies. These last centre around bowel function or the interior of the body; hence the common delusions of poisoning and refusal of food which Schreber also showed, which represent fear of impregnation fantasies.

Hypochondriacal Delusions and Reality Sense

It has been shown that Schreber's delusions of procreating, giving birth, and changing sex formed the deepest layer of his psychosis. These fantasies appeared predominantly as somatic hallucinations; his delusions and hallucinations centring on the outside world may be regarded as elaborations and rationalizations by which he attempted to account for them. The key to the understanding of his psychosis therefore lies primarily in his hypochondriacal delusions, as they also form the connecting link between his two illnesses: the first "a serious attack of hypochondria (S. 379) passed without any occurrences bordering on the supernatural" (S.35).

When hypochondrical symptoms are conceded psychic significance they are almost always diagnosed as hysterical, irrespective of the setting in which they occur. Freud even speaks of Schreber's hallucinations as "hysterical mechanisms" (F. 464, 459). In either case they are classed as neurotic, "mature"; the operation of primitive psychotic mechanisms is disregarded (Macalpine, 1954).

* Such fundamental doubt about their sex, though seldom expressly stated in the literature (Bleuler, 1951; Rosen, 1953), we have found an invariable feature of schizophrenia (Macalpine, 1954; Macalpine and Hunter, 1953, 1954 a, 1954 b, 1955).

The term " hypochondriacal delusion " itself implies a psychotic mechanism. When such delusions are bizarre or grotesque, as for instance when Schreber felt that his abdominal organs had been removed and his body was an empty sack extending into his thighs (S. 152), they are obviously psychotic. When such fantasies appear in milder, more usual and acceptable form (and as isolated symptoms in patients attending medical and surgical out-patient departments), as when Schreber felt that his bowels were " stopped up " (S. 153), the psychotic background may go undetected, and they may be incorrectly attributed to neurotic libidinal or aggressive discharge phenomena, or investigated and treated as organic disease. Because such patients are often not " neurotic " in the loose sense of the term, nor obviously suffering from an " anxiety state ", psychiatric origin of such hypochondriacal symptoms may come as a surprise to the physician (Macalpine, 1952).

In retrospect the ' mild ' hypochondriacal symptoms of Schreber's first illness, such as insomnia, concern over loss of weight, and palpitation, can be regarded as ' psychotic ', because the same symptoms ushered in his second illness.

Psychoanalysts seem to make the diagnosis of psychosis dependent on the presence of frank hallucinations and delusions relating to the outside world, despite the fact that these were classified as only secondary symptoms by Bleuler (1911) and not included among his five primary symptoms. In the absence of hallucinations and delusions " neurosis " is often diagnosed, because preservation of reality sense, " reality testing ", is taken as the criterion. In this way mild, and less mild, psychotics are often misdiagnosed and treated as psychoneurotics. Wertham (1949) remarked, " In private practice schizophrenics are diagnosed and treated as if they were neurotics, whereas in hospital practice neurotics are diagnosed and treated as if they were schizophrenics ". The pitfalls of placing so much importance on reality sense for the purpose of distinguishing neurotics from psychotics—which is really the old distinction between alienated and not alienated—is clearly demonstrated in Schreber's case : according to the expert medical witness his reality sense was so little impaired at the time of his Appeal, that he took an almost decisive part in the proceedings in Court himself, and was praised by the Judges for having conducted himself and his case in so clear and logical a manner. Yet they had no doubt that he was mad, from perusal of the Memoirs and his description of his " oddities of behaviour ". Freud however felt that Schreber's sense of reality was so much restored that his state could be described as "an asymptotic wish-fulfilment". Freud also took the beginning of Schreber's psychosis to be marked by his first obvious delusions and hallucinations, which only occurred several months after his admission into Flechsig's Clinic.

Freud speaks of Schreber's hypochondriacal delusions as onanistic fears, putting them on a level with castration anxieties and masturbatory guilt. But 'hypochondriasis' is only in its early stages accompanied by anxiety and fear. Later, anxiety and fear of disease are replaced by a conviction of disease, no longer amenable to reason: "overt anxiety is no part of a purely hypochondriacal state of mind . . . one of the essentials of the hypochondriacal concept is . . . the absence of anxiety or similar affects . . . The affect in hypochondriacal preoccupation is . . . a type of interest, not of a fearful kind . . . a conviction and not a fear of disease". It is "an affective condition best characterized as interest with conviction and consequent concern" (Gillespie, 1929). Such patients wander from doctor to doctor, from hospital to hospital: "The great desire to be cured induces him frequently to change his physician and his treatment" (Griesinger, 1861). "The sufferings of the patient . . . are most vividly real, and it is impossible that he should forget them till they cease" (Gull, 1868).

"The hypochondriacal states represent the mildest, most moderate form of insanity . . . While they, of course, share with the others the generic character of dejection, sadness, depression of mind, diminution of the activity of the will, and of a delirium which corresponds to this mental disposition, they yet differ from them in this characteristic manner—that in these states the emotional depression proceeds from a strong *feeling* of BODILY *illness* which constantly keeps the attention of the patient concentrated upon itself; that, consequently, the false opinions relate almost exclusively to the *state* of *health* of the subject, and the delirium turns constantly upon apprehensions of some grave malady—upon unfounded and curious ideas regarding the nature, the form, and the danger of this his disease. This feeling of bodily illness is sometimes general and vague, sometimes it resolves itself into particular anomalous and disconnected sensations . . . One cannot help being struck with the remarkable similarity between this process and the production of hallucinations in general . . . The higher degrees of hypochondria . . . gradually pass, partly through increase of the feeling of anxiety, partly through the fixing of certain attempts at explanation, not only into true melancholia, but even complicated with delusions (ideas of being surrounded by an invisible agency, of being the victim of evil machinations, influenced by magnetism, etc.). That considerable degree of self-control also which hypochondriacs still possess, often disappears during each exacerbation. Could the physicians only observe these paroxysms as freely as they can at any time in severe cases in asylums, all doubts concerning the mentally morbid nature of hypochondriasis would very soon disappear" (Griesinger, 1861). All this is clearly demonstrated in Schreber's Memoirs.

Dr. Weber called Schreber's illness paranoia, and says in times gone by it would have been called "partial insanity", because despite severe mental disorder Schreber showed "presence of mind, unimpaired memory, orderliness and logic of thought" (S. 457). Many such patients "live in the world without difficulty, following their profession (S. 470). Whether the delusional ideas refer to the condition of the patient's body (the hypochondriacal form), or to the field of politics, religion, sex, etc., is without great importance for judging the total state" (S. 457).

Clearly the psychoanalytic proposition that by the criterion of "reality testing" a division of mental diseases into "neurosis" and "psychosis" can be effected is illusory. The overwhelming majority of psychotics, namely the mild and early ones, particularly the hypochondriacal form, study of whom would give insight into the frankly alienated in mental hospitals, are thereby artificially forced into a separate category of disease. This has proved a serious obstacle to understanding psychoses, perhaps by giving rise to the mistaken notion of a separate group of mental illnesses, the neuroses.

Psychotherapy

Had Schreber been in psychotherapy and given the accepted interpretation of unconscious passive homosexual wishes towards his father, then Flechsig and eventually God, had his resistance to them been traced to his ego or superego warding off these drives or his being unable to pay the price of such wishes, i.e. to accept castration, it is anybody's guess what might have happened to him. We stated earlier that the question has repeatedly been raised why the paranoid patient should not be able to accept such interpretations, why he should be so sensitive and resistant towards his homosexual wishes. The answer may be simply that it is not unconscious homosexuality which makes him ill. If patients are even made worse by such interpretations, as we quoted from the literature earlier, this in itself should be a hint not only that the theory is wrong, but a pointer to where it may be wrong. A patient already in doubt about his sex identity and fearful of a change of sex—a trend which may appear psychotic to the patient himself, as it did to Schreber when he speaks of "the attacks made on my reason"—is naturally made even more uncertain, more anxious and more deluded by inexact interpretation of passive homosexual wishes. Far from reducing anxiety, such interpretations increase it by lending the weight of reality to budding delusions. On the other hand, to confront a patient with his anxiety and depression in terms of uncertainty in his own identity, to try and understand and trace out such body fantasies with him, often leads to amelioration of symptoms, sometimes surprisingly quickly.

POSTSCRIPT

Feuchtersleben (1845), who introduced the term psychosis in the first textbook of psychiatry ever written, ends his introductory historical survey with the following passage:

"Instead of the notions of the somatic, psychical, and mixed views stated above, and the doubtful foundations upon which they rest, you will now naturally wish to be informed which of them are the views that these lectures adopt, or what others they will propose, in order that you may be guided by something not negative, but positive. A well-grounded answer to this point can only be furnished by the lectures themselves; but from our preliminary basis thus much may be premised. The maladies of the spirit alone, *in abstracto*, that is, error and sin, can be called diseases of the mind only *per analogiam*. They come not within the jurisdiction of of the physician, but that of the teacher and clergyman, who again are called *physicians* of the mind only *per analogiam*. The maladies of the body alone, *in abstracto*, for instance, of the brain or the nerves, without mental alienation, are not diseases of the mind, but of the body. The notion, *mental disease*, must therefore be deduced, neither from the mind nor from the body, but from the relation of each to the other. The question does not turn here on the external cause of psychopathies, which may be either psychical or corporeal, nor upon what is called the proximate cause, which is inscrutable, because the relation between body and mind is inexplicable; the question is respecting the phenomenon itself. Where psychical phenomena appear *abnormal*, there is mental disorder which has its root in the mind, so far as this is manifested through the sensual organ, and has its root in the body, so far as this is the organ of the mind. To search after the phenomena in which these relations are revealed, with the unprejudiced eye of experience—to investigate them scientifically in every point that is of importance to the physician, and to collect them in one whole, is the province of medical psychology, upon which we are now about to enter."

REFERENCES

Abraham, K. (1908). The Psycho-sexual differences between Hysteria and Dementia Praecox. In: *Selected Papers of Karl Abraham.* London, 1948.

—— (1913). Restrictions and Transformations of Scoptophilia in Psychoneurotics. In: *Selected Papers of Karl Abraham.* London, 1948.

Battie, W. (1758). *A Treatise on Madness.* London. Reprinted in "*A Psychiatric Controversy in the Eighteenth Century*". By R. A. Hunter & I. Macalpine. London, 1955.

Baumeyer, F. (1951). New Insights into the Life and Psychosis of Schreber. *Int. J. Psychoanal.*, **33**, 262.

Bayle, A. L. J. (1822). *Recherches sur l'Arachnitis Chronique.* Paris.

Binswanger, L. (1911). Analyse einer hysterischen Phobie. *Jb. psychoanal. Forsch.*, **3**, 239.

Bivin, G. D., & Klinger, M. P. (1937). *Pseudocyesis.* Bloomington.

Bleuler, E. (1911). *Dementia Praecox oder Gruppe der Schizophrenien.* Leipzig. Trans. by J. Zinkin. New York, 1950.

—— (1912). Review of Freud's "Psychoanalytic Notes upon an Autobiographical Account of a case of Paranoia". *Zbl. Psychoanal.*, **2**, 343.

Bleuler, M. (1951). Forschungen und Begriffswandlungen in der Schizophrenielehre 1941–50. *Fortschr. Neurol. Psychiat.*, **19**, 385.

Boehm, F. (1930). The Femininity Complex in Man. *Int. Z. Psychoanal.*, **16**, 185.

Brody, E. B., & Redlich, F. C. (1952). *Psychotherapy with Schizophrenics.* New York.

Browne, J. Crichton (1875). Skae's Classification of Mental Disease. *J. Ment. Sci.*, **21**, 339.

Brunswick, R. M. (1940). The Preoedipal Phase of the Libido Development. *Psychoanal. Quart.*, **9**, 293.

Cameron, N. (1944). The Functional Psychoses. In: *Personality and the Behaviour Disorders.* Edited by J. McV. Hunt. New York.

Clouston, T. S. (1904). *Mental Diseases.* London.

Cramer, A. (1895). Abgrenzung und Differenzial-Diagnose der Paranoia. *Allg. Z. Psychiat.*, **51**, 286.

Critchley, M. (1943). Electro-Convulsive Therapy. Article in *Medical Annual.* Bristol.

Cullen, W. (1777–78). *First Lines of the Practice of Physic.* Edinburgh.

Dawson, W. R. (1929). *The Custom of the Couvade.* Manchester.

Eisler, M. J. (1921). A Man's Unconscious Fantasy of Pregnancy in the Guise of Traumatic Hysteria. *Int. J. Psychoanal.*, **2**, 255.

Evans, W. N. (1951). Simulated Pregnancy in the Male. *Psychoanal. Quart.*, **20**, 165.

Fairbairn, W. R. D. (1943). The Repression and Return of Bad Objects. In: *Psychoanalytic Studies of the Personality.* London, 1952.

Fenichel, O. (1945). *The Psychoanalytic Theory of Neurosis.* New York.

Ferenczi, S. (1911). On the Part Played by Homosexuality in the Pathogenesis of Paranoia. In: *Sex in Psychoanalysis.* New York, 1950.

Feuchtersleben, E. v. (1845). *Medical Psychology.* Trans. by H. E. Lloyd & B. G. Babington. London, 1847.

Freeman, T. (1951). Pregnancy as a Precipitant of Mental Illness in Men. *Brit. J. Med. Psychol.*, **24**, 49.
Freud, S. (1894). The Defence Neuro-Psychoses. In: *Collected Papers*, **1**, 59.
—— (1895). The Justification for Detaching from Neurasthenia a particular Syndrome: The Anxiety-Neurosis. In: *Collected Papers*, **1**, 76.
—— (1895). Psychotherapy of Hysteria. In: *Studies in Hysteria.* By J. Breuer & S. Freud. New York, 1936.
—— (1900). *Interpretation of Dreams.* London, 1948.
—— (1905). Fragment of an Analysis of a Case of Hysteria. In: *Collected Papers*, **3**, 139.
—— (1908). On the Sexual Theories of Children. In: *Collected Papers*, **2**, 59.
—— (1909). Notes upon a Case of Obsessional Neurosis. In: *Collected Papers*, **3**, 356.
—— (1911). Psycho-analytic Notes upon an Autobiographical Account of a Case of Paranoia (Dementia Paranoides). In: *Collected Papers*, **3**, 390.
—— (1914). On the History of the Psychoanalytic Movement. In: *Collected Papers*, **1**, 287.
—— (1915). A Case of Paranoia running counter to the Psycho-analytic Theory of the Disease. In : *Collected Papers*, **2**, 150.
—— (1917). *Introductory Lectures on Psycho-analysis.* London, 1949.
—— (1923). A Neurosis of Demoniacal Possession in the Seventeenth Century. In: *Collected Papers*, **4**, 436.
—— (1924). Neurosis and Psychosis. In: *Collected Papers*, **2**, 250.
Gillespie, R. D. (1929). *Hypochondria.* London.
—— (1938). Psychological aspects of Skin Diseases. *Brit. J. Derm.*, **50**, 1.
Gillies, H. (1950). Schizophrenia. In: *Recent Progress in Psychiatry.* Edited by G. W. T. H. Fleming. London.
Glover, E. (1932). On the Aetiology of Drug Addiction. *Int. J. Psychoanal.*, **13**, 298.
—— (1946). Eder as Psychoanalyst. In: *The Yearbook of Psychoanalysis*, **2**, 269. London.
Gottschalk, L. A. (1947). Systematic Psychotherapy of the Psychoses. *Psychiat. Quart.*, **21**, 554.
Griesinger, W. (1861). *Mental Pathology and Therapeutics.* Trans. by C. L. Robertson & J. Rutherford. London, 1867.
Griffin, F. J. (1939). A facsimile of the Novae Species Insectorum, 1759, of J. C. D. Schreber. *J. Soc. Bibl. nat. Hist.*, **1**, 221.
Gull, W. W. (1868). Hypochondriasis. In: *The Published Writings of W. W. Gull.* New Sydenham Society, London, 1894.
Harley, J. (1869). *The Old Vegetable Neurotics.* London.
Haslam, J. (1810). *Illustrations of Madness.* London. Reprinted in: *Selected Readings in the History of British Psychiatry.* Edited by R. A. Hunter, I. Macalpine, and L. M. Payne. London, 1955.
Haymaker, W. (1953). *Founders of Neurology.* Springfield.
Heinroth, J. C. (1818). *Lehrbuch der Störungen des Seelenlebens.* Leipzig.
Henderson, D. K., & Gillespie, R. D. (1951). *Text-book of Psychiatry.* 7th Edition, London.
Hendrick, I. (1939). Contributions of Psychoanalysis to the Study of Psychosis. *J. Amer. med. Ass.*, **113**, 918.

Hoffmann, J. (1889). Progressive Neurotische Muskelatrophie. *Arch. Psychiat.*, **20**, 660.
Hofmeister, B. (1894). Diabetes Mellitus. In: *Clinical Lectures on Medicine and Surgery, 3rd Series.* New Sydenham Society, London.
Hunter, R. A. (1954). Problems in the diagnosis of early Schizophrenia. Paper read at Annual Conference of the British Psychological Society, Nottingham.
Ideler, K. W. (1848). *Der Wahnsinn.* Bremen.
Jacobson, E. (1950). Development of the Wish for a Child in Boys. In: *The Psychoanalytic Study of the Child*, vol. 5. London.
Jones, E. (1942). Psychology and Childbirth. In: *Papers on Psychoanalysis.* London, 1948.
—— (1951). Personal communication.
Katan, M. (1949). Schreber's Delusion of the End of the World. *Psychoanal. Quart.*, **18**, 60.
—— (1950). Schreber's Hallucinations about the 'Little Men'. *Int. J. Psychoanal.*, **31**, 32.
—— (1952). Further remarks about Schreber's Hallucinations. *Int. J. Psychoanal.*, **33**, 429.
—— (1953). Schreber's Prepsychotic Phase. *Int. J. Psychoanal.*, **34**, 43.
Klein, M. (1946). Notes on some Schizoid Mechanisms. In: *Developments in Psychoanalysis.* London, 1952.
Kline, N. S., Tenney, A. M., Nicolaou, G. T. & Malzberg, B. (1953). The Selection of Psychiatric Patients for Research. *Amer. J. Psychiat.*, **110**, 179.
Knight, R. P. (1940). Relationship of latent homosexuality to the mechanism of paranoid delusions. *Bull. Menninger Clin.*, **4**, 149.
Kraepelin, E. (1913). *Psychiatrie.* 8th Edition, vol. 3. Leipzig.
—— (1918). *Hundert Jahre Psychiatrie.* Berlin.
Lettsom, J. C. (1778). *History of the Origin of Medicine.* London.
Lewis, A. J. (1950). Psychological Medicine. In: *Textbook of Medicine.* Edited by F. W. Price, 8th Edition. London.
Locke, J. (1690). An Essay concerning Humane Understanding. London.
Macalpine, I. (1950). Development of the Transference. *Psychoanal. Quart.*, **19**, 501.
—— (1952). Psychosomatic Symptom Formation. *Lancet, i.*, 278.
—— (1953). Pruritus Ani. *Psychosom. Med.*, **15**, 499.
—— (1954). Critical Evaluation of Psychosomatic Medicine in relation to Dermatology. In: *Modern Trends in Dermatology*, 2nd Series. Edited by R. M. B. MacKenna. London.
—— & Hunter, R. A. (1953). The Schreber Case. *Psychoanal. Quart.*, **22**, 328.
—— & Hunter, R. A. (1954 a). Concept of Transference in present-day theories of Mental Disease. Paper read at the International Congress for Psychotherapy, Zurich.
—— & Hunter, R. A. (1954 b). Psychoanalytic Theory of Psychosis. *Brit. J. Med. Psychol.*, **27**, 175.
—— & Hunter, R. A. (1955). *Schizophrenia* 1677. London.
Mead, M. (1949). *Male and Female.* New York.
Menninger, K. (1942). *Love against Hate.* New York.
Meyer, A. (1904). Trends in Modern Psychiatry. *Psychol. Bull.*, **1**, 217.
—— (1917–18). Psychiatric Diagnosis. *Amer. J. Insanity*, **74**, 163.

Meyer, A. (1928). The Evolution of the Dementia Praecox Concept. In: *Schizophrenia (Dementia Praecox)*. New York.
—— (1933). British Influences in Psychiatry. *J. Ment. Sci.*, **79**, 435.
Morel, B. A. (1860). *Traité des Maladies Mentales*. Paris.
Nasse, F. (1818). Über die Benennung und die vorläufige Eintheilung des psychischen Krankseyns. *Z. Psychische Aerzte*, **1**, 17.
Niederland, W. G. (1951). Three Notes on the Schreber Case. *Psychoanal. Quart.*, **20**, 579.
Nunberg, H. (1920). On the Catatonic Attack. In: *Practice and Theory of Psychoanalysis*. New York, 1948.
—— (1921). The Course of the Libidinal Conflict in a case of Schizophrenia. In: *Practice and Theory of Psychoanalysis*. New York, 1948.
—— (1938). Homosexuality, Magic and Aggression. In: *Practice and Theory of Psychoanalysis*. New York, 1948.
Pelman, C. (1903). Review of "Denkwürdigkeiten eines Nervenkranken" by D. P. Schreber. *Allg. Z. Psychiat.*, **60**, 657.
Perry, W. J. (1918). *Megalithic Culture of Indonesia*. Manchester.
—— (1923). *Children of the Sun*. London.
Pfeiffer, R. (1904). Review of "Denkwürdigkeiten eines Nervenkranken" by D. P. Schreber. *Dtsch. Z. Nervenheilk.*, **27**, 352.
Rank, O. (1909). *Myth of the Birth of the Hero*. New York, 1952.
—— (1912). Völkerpsychologische Parallelen zu den infantilen Sexualtheorien. *Zbl. Psychoanal.*, **2**, 372 and 425.
Redlich, F. C. (1952). The concept of Schizophrenia and its implications for therapy. In: *Psychotherapy with Schizophrenics*. Edited by E. B. Brody & F. C. Redlich. New York.
Reil, J. C. (1803). *Rhapsodieen über die Anwendung der Psychischen Curmethode auf Geistes-zerrüttungen*. Halle.
Romberg, M. H. (1840–46). *Nervous Diseases of Man*. Trans. by E. H. Sieveking. Sydenham Society, London, 1853.
Rosen, J. N. (1953). *Direct Analysis*. New York.
Sanborn, F. B. (1898). *Memoirs of Pliny Earle*. Boston.
Schreber, D. G. M. (1856). *Medical Indoor Gymnastics*. Trans. by H. Skelton. London, 1856.
Smith, G. Elliot (1919). *Evolution of the Dragon*. Manchester.
—— (1929). *Migrations of Early Culture*. Manchester.
Stengel, E. (1948). Application of Psychoanalytic Principles to the Hospital In-Patient. *J. Ment. Sci.*, **94**, 773.
Tausk, V. (1919). On the origin of the 'Influencing Machine' in Schizophrenia. *Psychoanal. Quart.*, 1933, **2**, 519.
Tuke, D. H. (1882). *History of the Insane in the British Isles*. London.
—— (1891). *Prichard and Symonds*. London.
—— (1892). *Dictionary of Psychological Medicine*. London.
Vogel, R. A. (1777). *Academicae praelectiones de cognoscendis et curandis praecipuis corporis humani adfectibus*. Göttingen.
Wertham, F. (1949). Discussion of paper by N. D. C. Lewis: "Criteria for early Differential Diagnosis of Psychoneurosis and Schizophrenia". *Amer. J. Psychotherap.*, **3**, 4.
Ziehen, T. (1894). *Psychiatrie*. Leipzig.
Zilboorg, G. (1941). *History of Medical Psychology*. New York.